Psychotherapy and Counselling in Practice

The many different therapeutic models in use today can lead to blind spots in clinical practice. This important and timely book gives a balanced synthesis, based on actual cases, evidence, practice and experience, to describe the process of psychotherapy and identify the fundamental elements that lead to good outcome across all its schools. In the course of developing a consistently reliable, effective, practical psychotherapy, Digby Tantam pinpoints four essential principles: addressing the person's concerns; taking into account their values and personal morality; recognizing the role of emotions; and binding it all into a narrative treatment for symptom relief, resolution of predicaments, release from addiction or sexual problems, and finding happiness through intimacy. This book is essential reading for psychiatrists or clinical psychologists looking for a straightforward framework for short-term psychotherapy and anyone working long-term with patients using a psychotherapy model.

Digby Tantam is Clinical Professor of Psychotherapy at the Centre for the Study of Conflict and Reconciliation at the University of Sheffield, and a partner in Dilemma Consultancy in Human Relations.

Psychotherapy and Counselling in Practice

A Narrative Framework

Digby Tantam

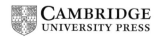
CAMBRIDGE
UNIVERSITY PRESS

PUBLISHED BY THE PRESS SYNDICATE OF THE UNIVERSITY OF CAMBRIDGE
The Pitt Building, Trumpington Street, Cambridge, United Kingdom

CAMBRIDGE UNIVERSITY PRESS
The Edinburgh Building, Cambridge CB2 2RU, UK
40 West 20th Street, New York, NY 10011-4211, USA
477 Williamstown Road, Port Melbourne, VIC 3207, Australia
Ruiz de Alarcón 13, 28014 Madrid, Spain
Dock House, The Waterfront, Cape Town 8001, South Africa

http://www.cambridge.org

First published 2002

Printed in the United Kingdom at the University Press, Cambridge

Typeface Minion 10/12pt   *System* Poltype® [V N]

A catalogue record for this book is available from the British Library

Library of Congress Cataloguing in Publication data

Tantam, Digby
Psychotherapy and counselling in practice : a narrative framework / Digby Tantam.
    p.   cm.
Includes bibliographical references and index.
ISBN 0 521 47963 0 (pb.)
1. Psychotherapy.   I. Title.
RC480.5.T36   2002
616.89'14–dc21   2001035261

ISBN 0 521 47963 0 paperback

Every effort has been made in preparing this book to provide accurate and up-to-date
information which is in accord with accepted standards and practice at the time of publication.
Nevertheless, the author, editors and publisher can make no warranties that the information
contained herein is totally free from error, not least because clinical standards are constantly
changing through research and regulation. The author, editors and publisher therefore
disclaim all liability for direct or consequential damages resulting from the use of material
contained in this book. Readers are strongly advised to pay careful attention to information
provided by the manufacturer of any drugs or equipment that they plan to use.

Although case histories are drawn from actual cases, every effort has been made to disguise the
identities of the individuals involved.

To Emmy, inspiration, lover, and friend

Contents

Preface

This book is principally designed for the psychiatrist or clinical psychologist in training who is searching for a straightforward framework for short-term psychotherapy. It will also be of value to psychotherapists who are trained in longer-term therapy. Mental health professionals whose work involves supportive psychotherapy should also find this book useful in extending and developing their skills.

Practical psychotherapy, the subject of this book, is a brief psychotherapy which is designed to be easily integrated with other mental health practices. No specific therapeutic approach, or modality, is espoused although the reader may find elements of short-term psychodynamic psychotherapy (Beck et al., 1979; Luborsky, 1984; Strupp & Binder, 1984), existential therapy (Deurzen, 1979), strategic and systems approaches (Haley, 1963), client-centered counselling (Egan, 1990), problem-solving methods, and others.

Practical psychotherapy is therefore an eclectic therapy. This does not mean that it permits a free choice of whichever method happens to appeal to the therapist but that treatment 'is empirically based and client-driven (rather than theory-guided)' (Novalis, Rojcewicz & Peele, 1993). Practical psychotherapy is, like other eclectic therapies, rooted in evidence-based practice and thus changes as new evidence comes forward. The practical psychotherapist selects from 'a repertory of proven techniques without theoretical basis' and may 'change techniques as the therapy proceeds, based on observations of what is effective . . .' (ibid.).

Practical psychotherapy may be used supportively. Supportive therapies are more than keeping the client going whilst time does the healing, or the provision of non-specific social support. Rather, they presume that people need therapy because they are temporarily overwhelmed with life-problems and not because they are defective, or in need of correction. Supportive therapies mobilize the client's own cognitive and emotional resources to overcome these life-problems. Clients of supportive therapists are not expected to reform their characters, although they may choose to do so. Nor are they expected to unthinkingly carry out symptom-relieving procedures, although they may choose to make use of any procedures which are offered to them.

Three research findings dominate studies of psychotherapy process and outcome: (1) that the approach used has little effect on outcome (Stiles, Shapiro & Elliott, 1986); (2) that different practitioners get different outcomes, even though they are using the same approach; and (3) that experienced practitioners are more similar in their behaviour during therapy than inexperienced practitioners, irrespective of the approach in which they originally trained.

A parsimonious interpretation of these findings is that effective, experienced practitioners have discovered what works in practice, in which situations, and with which people. This may mean that all effective practitioners are eclectic, but it may mean more than that. Jerome Frank (1993) supposed that there is an orderliness to effective therapy which reflects basic psychological and social healing processes, processes which he termed 'remoralization'.

In the course of developing a practical psychotherapy, and in my preparation of this book, I have come to consider that the following are essential dimensions of remoralization in psychotherapy, at least in westernized cultures: addressing the *concerns* that a person has about their situation; respecting the *values* of a person; recognizing that people are guided by *emotions* and the *emotional meaning* that every aspect of therapy conjures up; and finally, binding all of these elements into a jointly constructed treatment *narrative*.

Using these four elements to produce an effective treatment is what practical psychotherapy – and this book – are about.

A note on terminology

Anyone writing a book on psychotherapy has to choose his or her words carefully. This is most acute when deciding what to call the people who are not the therapists. Some are students, trainees, supervisees or analysands. But what about the others? Are they also students? Well, yes, in a sense. They are also collaborators, enquirers after truth, users, consumers, visitors and, sometimes, customers. Many of these latter terms are used for the people whom doctors would call 'patients'. It does seem to me that suffering is what impels people to seek out a psychotherapist. This word seems appropriate etymologically, but it has inextricable medical connotations. It is therefore anathema to many counsellors or psychotherapists who eschew the medical model. I have racked my brains to find an English word which is the inverse of 'therapist'. 'Therapee' seems artificial. 'Therapand' is an unfortunate hybrid of a Latin and a Greek root.

I can think of no better word solution than to use the word that is in currency among counsellors – the word 'client'. The origin of this word in the Latin word for 'leaning' is awkward. It is also a word that has connotations of a business relationship, and this is unpalatable to many mental health professionals. However, that is also a strength. The fact that advertising agencies, bank managers and solicitors also have clients does put the clients of therapists in good company.

I have sometimes used an even more provocative term – 'treatment' – from time to time. This has been when I have wanted to stress the directedness of some therapies. Spurning this word because it has connotations of physical treatment widens the unnecessary gap between the different professions involved in mental health care, in my view. However, I do recognize that not all therapy is about treatment. Some is about discovery or releasing a person's talents and creativity. No single word is precisely synonymous with therapy. Helping implies that the therapist knows where the therapy is going, which may not be true. Nor is therapy always educative, one of the other commonly used synonyms. Sometimes I have used the word 'therapy' when there has been no doubt that it is psychotherapy that is under consideration, but when this might be in doubt or when I wished to be a little bit more formal, I have spelt this out by using the word 'psychotherapy'.

Words are the tools of the psychotherapist, and also the weapons. Connotations matter, hence the explanation.

Acknowledgements

The original plans of this book were formulated whilst I was on a study tour in the United States, and I am grateful to the University of Warwick for financial support, to Professor William Sledge, Professor Tim Beck, and, especially, Dr Jon Borus for their assistance and support, and to many therapists who gave up their time to discuss psychotherapy issues, including Dr Simon Budman, Dr Bruce Rounsaville, Dr Fred Wright, and Dr Judy Beck. At that time I was committed to a procedural approach to psychotherapy, believing that there were active ingredients which needed to be purified. Since then, I have experienced a crisis in my personal and intellectual life which has changed much, including my understanding of psychotherapy. It is therefore more than usually true to say that without Professor Emmy van Deurzen this book would not have been written, and I am indebted to her for that and for much else. Emmy has also made many valuable comments on the book in its first draft and has unerringly indicated passages where a loss of readability indicated a need for more thought. My knowledge of existential psychotherapy is largely gained from her, as was the potential usefulness of the concept of self-deception on which she has written extensively. Nick Huband has also read Chapter 8 and parts of Chapter 2, for which I am grateful. Finally I would like to thank my publishers, Jocelyn Foster and, subsequently, Richard Barling, who have been very patient whilst these changes took place, and then took root.

Introduction

Psychotherapy has been shown to be effective in relieving depressed mood (Elkin et al., 1985) and is more effective than other treatments in panic disorder (Clum, Clum & Surls, 1993). It enables a person to change habitual ways of behaving (Szapocznik et al., 1990) and thinking (Hollon & Beck, 1994), and to improve social relationships (Winston et al., 1994). It may also be pursued as a form of self-knowledge, to improve job or marital prospects, or in the course of training. It may be provided on a one-to-one basis, to couples, in groups of strangers, or in families. People may seek out psychotherapy for themselves, or they may be pressured to have it. Similarities with counselling, with being a friend, with team-building and other motivational activities, with being a good parent and with good medical care have been claimed by many. Psychotherapy also has techniques in common with self-help, and with self-treatment guided by a book, computer or personal organizer (Newman, Consoli & Taylor, 1999). Some would claim that is just common sense, others that it is nonsense, yet others that it is the religion of our age. None of these is a position that I hold. About the only thing that everyone does agree on is that it is different from physical treatment.

This book will not address all these extensions of psychotherapy. The concentration will be on psychological therapy provided by a therapist to a person voluntarily seeking treatment for a psychological problem.

Often this problem will be diagnosable as a mental disorder, such as depression, anxiety, substance abuse or a personality disorder. However, concentrating solely on the symptoms that the client is experiencing may prevent the therapist from appreciating that the client may also be overwhelmed by an upheaval in personal relationships and a re-appraisal of deeply held spiritual beliefs. Jerome Frank, recognizing this wider context, wrote of states of demoralization rather than states of distress, and emphasized the remoralizing effects of psychotherapy.

Demoralization may be the prelude to clients losing their hold on their place in the world, and to suicide. But a demoralized person may also be in the process of *reculer pour mieux sauter* – falling back to take a better run up to a big jump. Existential psychotherapists emphasize that a crisis of personal values is both a danger and an opportunity (Deurzen, 1998). The psychotherapist needs to be sensitive to these dimensions, and to adopt a psychotherapeutic method which not only treats dis-ease, but promotes healing.

Docherty et al. (1977) contrast 'relating to the client as a diseased organ or object of study and as a disturbed person'. They conclude that both perspectives need to be maintained in a collaboration between client and mental health worker. These authors were writing in the context of their involvement in schizophrenia research, and in schizophrenia it is appropriate to consider that the client has a 'diseased organ'. The same may be said to be true of people with some other psychological disorders, for example developmental disorders or affective psychoses.

However, I strongly believe that the metaphor of a diseased organ is wrongly applied to personality. Indeed I am doubtful about the value of the term at all, except as an actuarial predictor of common variance in large groups of people. People do think of themselves as suffering from a brain disease called schizophrenia or of sometimes being, more simply, 'out of their heads'. They do not usually think of themselves as the victims of their personality, but as active agents seeking to overcome obstacles and to achieve goals.

There will be little mention in this book of personality, or personality disorder therefore. This is not to say that there will be no recognition that some problems – or concerns, as I termed them in the Preface – are more deeply seated than others. Mental depth is an everyday metaphor which makes no presumption that the mind is an organ. Glover (1988) suggests that deeper beliefs are more central ones, and that the more central a belief is, the greater the number of other beliefs that would be affected by a change in it. A longer period of persuasion and reflection is required to change deeper beliefs, and longer therapy is required to change deeper problems (Kopta et al., 1994).

However, it is not always easy to know how deep a problem is for another person. Kopta and Howard (Kopta et al., 1994) found that chronic distress was not a deep problem very often. But there is often a temptation to assume in assessing clients for psychotherapy that the longer a problem has continued, the more therapy will be required to treat it.

In fact, the reader will find little in this book about the assessment of the suitability of clients for brief psychotherapy. This is partly because the current state of the literature does not provide an evidence basis for the assessment methods currently in use (Tantam, 1995b). It is also because I think that the function of assessment is not to select which clients are suitable for the psychotherapy on offer, but which treatment is suitable for the client. Sometimes this will be treatment that the therapist is competent to give, and sometimes not. Sometimes the therapist may be competent to give the treatment, but it will be perceived – by the client, or by a third party who is paying for the treatment – to be too expensive, in time or money, for the benefit received. Rarely, the therapist may advise the client that the risks of treatment making them worse outweigh the possible benefits.

The task in the first interview is therefore to establish what are the client's preoccupying concerns, and what might be done about them. This will be the subject of Chapter 1.

Being depressed, becoming disabled by obsessive–compulsive disorder, or indeed having any other psychological problem, is not like having bad headaches or a wonky knee. The experience of depression includes hopelessness and a sense of personal failure. Values that have previously gone unchallenged become problematic. A person might ask him- or her-self, 'Is depression a kind of weakness?' or 'Why can't I just pull my socks up?'. Developing a psychological disorder is often experienced as a crisis, like a long-term relationship breaking up or losing one's job, which requires a reassessment of personal values. Even if the preoccupying concern of the client is, 'Help me to get better', this will be in the context of a crisis of personal values. Psychotherapists cannot ignore either request. They must be able to provide technical help in relieving symptoms where that is required, but also be able to acknowledge the spiritual crisis.

The values of the therapist, and the values inherent in the treatment, must be values which enhance the value of the client. When this occurs, when there is congruence between a therapist's and a client's values, outcome is enhanced (Kelly & Strupp, 1992). Another task in the first interview is to identify the client's own values, and in what way they have been called into question by the client's crisis. How to do this, and how to plan a treatment which will address the client's need to re-establish a stable set of values, is considered in Chapter 2.

Assessment is often taken to be a means of ensuring that clients do not drop out of treatment. It is true that non-compliance is a major reason for treatment failure. It is easy to neglect it by assuming that people drop out because they are improved, or because they were not suitable for the treatment. In fact, there are many institutional practices which make people lose confidence in the treatment that they are being given, and consequently drop out (Tantam & Klerman, 1979).

Dropping out should be taken seriously, but not by excluding clients who might drop out. Rather, treatment should be designed to give the client the hope and satisfaction in the treatment that will make drop-out unlikely. The characteristics of treatment that might influence client compliance with psychotherapy have received little attention. Klerman and I (Tantam & Klerman, 1979) found, in a study of a community mental health centre, that the client's first impressions of the centre were one of the strongest influences on whether they would drop out later. The analogy with food is obvious. If I don't like the flavour of something, I may swallow what I have in my mouth, but eat no more. If I'm really offended, I spit it out. Usually this is a judgement that is made as soon as a new food is tasted, but it can also happen if the flavour becomes unpalatable, for example if I chew a food for too long. The analogy holds true for this, too. In the mental health centre study, most people who were going to drop out did so shortly after their first contact. Others dropped out later, but usually after a first contact with a new clinician.

Since that study, I have been more and more persuaded that these immediate emotional reactions are important in affecting compliance with many aspects of treatment and that they consequently affect outcome. I have also come to think that the immediate emotional reaction aroused by a new experience has the same origins as the emotional reaction to a new food. I therefore think that it is legitimate to apply the same term – flavour – to both.

Choosing which treatment to recommend to the client is partly a matter of choosing which flavour of treatment is most palatable, and is discussed in Chapter 3 when the range of different treatments is considered.

The reader might by now be aware that practical psychotherapy is not a new school of psychotherapy but a framework of good clinical practice, into which different psychotherapeutic techniques can be incorporated. Indeed it may have wider generality, as a framework for mental health interventions generally.

What makes me think that there is a framework? The best evidence is that relationships, stories and musical compositions all seem to share some developmental sequences in common. The ur sequence is pre-verbal: taking in (eating, listening, data gathering), playing (digestion, thinking, transformation) and giving out (excreting, acting out, responding). Managing a long-term relationship requires that these sequences are respected. In the case of therapy, they must be applied to the exchange, to the session and to the whole of the long, punctuated conversation between the therapist and the client. The topic of the conversation must be of concern to both client and therapist. The metaphors and imagery used must have a flavour which is palatable to the client. And the values which the two speakers hold must be congruent. This is also true of the values about the conversation itself. There will need to be a mutual acceptance of the values of openness and honesty, for example. Another value which is important to brief therapy is empowerment. The client needs to know the ground rules of the conversation and to feel confident that they know what is expected of them. He or she needs to know what kind of conversation it is.

It is an excessive burden, for both client and therapist, to think that the therapist is there to help the client. People are far more inclined to work to improve themselves and their situation than many mental health workers believe. Conversely, specific interventions of the psychotherapist are less helpful than the moments of self-discovery or empowerment that occur in successful psychotherapy. The conversation is not, therefore, one in which advice or guidance is given. Rather the therapist works to talk ever more honestly with the client, touching, with greater and greater emotional intensity, on the client's concerns.

The conversation that is most similar to this is not the helping or advice-giving one, but the negotiation. Both sides want to reach the same goal. Both are unclear at the beginning what they can concede. For it to succeed, both sides need to respect each other, and particularly to respect the real difficulties with which each has to contend. Both sides need to expect that they will sometimes get exasperated with each other, but to be committed to work through that.

It is useful in a negotiation to keep regular minutes, particularly of decisions that have been reached, and to open each session of the negotiation with a statement of these decisions. I think that this also applies to therapy – at least to therapy that is being conducted along these lines. Good note-keeping is therefore necessary. Records should always be made of new findings, of commitments by the therapist or the client, and of summaries of what has been said and what has been achieved. The summaries constitute the narrative of the therapy for both therapist and client. The more they contain what the therapist and the client 'really' think, the better the outcome of therapy will have been.

The process of narrating the therapy is discussed in Chapter 4. It is considered in relation to the first assessment interview and the subsequent formulation, in relation to period reviews during the course of treatment, and to the final summary. These reviews may also correspond to the need to write letters to referrers, after the first assessment and after discharge.

The first four chapters of the book cover what is needed for the first assessment interview. They should therefore be read before this assessment takes place. It might be thought that this is a disproportionate amount of emphasis on a one or one-and-a-half hour session. There are good reasons for this. I believe that once psychotherapist and client have agreed what it is important to talk about and how to talk about it, it may require little expertise from the psychotherapist to make sure that the subsequent conversation is therapeutic. Or, in other words, the client will ensure that he or she uses the time effectively once he or she identifies what his or her preoccupying concerns are, and what approach might be taken to them. The concerns and the approach are usually identified in the assessment interview.

Psychotherapy is rarely quite as simple as this. A person's concerns may change or become more radical. The approach that seemed right at the assessment may no longer seem right later on.

Therapies are like conversations. With the possible exception of the very briefest, they often consist of repeated cycles. Each of these is initiated by a new, perhaps deeper, preoccupying concern being negotiated. Each may result in the exploration of different, sometimes more fundamental, values.

Each has a different flavour. The story of what happens in each is also different. These four elements – concern, value, flavour and narrative – therefore continue to need careful attention and re-discussion throughout the treatment.

Chapter 5 introduces the narrative approach to psychotherapy. Narratives become of particular importance in psychotherapy when they fail. It is then that psycho-dynamic or psycho-analytic approaches, which emphasize the relationship between the client and the therapist, become particularly relevant. Relationship-orientated approaches are dealt with in later chapters of this book, and readers may find that they are more understandable after reading Chapter 5.

Chapters 6 to 10 are each devoted to a different preoccupying concern. The sequence in which the concerns are presented is the most common sequence in which they emerge in psychotherapy. The final chapter addresses some of the problems that might arise when matters do not follow this orderly structure. What might be preventing the therapy from progressing and how the therapist can monitor their own work to ensure that they are not contributing to this non-progression are both discussed in Chapter 11. Some general principles of dealing with crises are then applied to some of the other challenges that may arise during therapy, such as a client expressing strong personal feelings for the therapist, or the emergence of a serious health problem. Chapter 11 is about saying goodbye . . .

Emphasizing the importance of discovering the client's real concern and de-emphasizing the conduct of the therapy sessions is not to belittle the skill of the psychotherapist. Combining emotional intuition and intellectual judgement to sift out what is 'real', and to know when the therapeutic conversation is going towards or away from it, is very skilful indeed. This is particularly true when the client is not participating fully or wholeheartedly in the conversation.

What might prevent someone from participating fully? Answering this question adequately means suspending a natural tendency among health professionals to blame clients for treatment failure. It might be easier to do this by considering therapy as a negotiation. Why do negotiators fail? Why do people sometimes negotiate dishonestly? One reason is that the negotiations are a sham, to satisfy some third party who wants an agreed solution or to make it possible to claim at a later stage that negotiations have been tried, but failed. Another reason is that what one of the parties really wants is too shameful or embarrassing to disclose, and so it is concealed behind another demand. Negotiators may realize that the process of the negotiation will draw in other elements that they would rather not have examined. Finally, the negotiator may doubt the trustworthiness of the other side, and fear exploitation. This may be a realistic, or an unrealistic, fear.

What, then, about resistance? What about the refractory client?

It is clear to any experienced practitioner that a significant proportion of clients do not do well in their therapy. Many of these clients drop out of treatment prematurely. The emphasis of the analytic therapies on the client's negative feelings for the treatment or for the therapist does not seem misplaced. And conversely, the forced optimism of therapies which deny these negative feelings seems naïve. The analytic approach seems to me to be in error in attributing these negative factors to the client's psychology. This has been a prolific source of theorizing, but at the expense of moving theory into the subjectivity of the inner world, and away from objective realities like the power, income or status differentials which separate therapist and client. Even more importantly, attributing negative factors to the client prevents a consideration of whether they are due to a failure of the therapist's understanding or formulation of the problem.

Throughout this book, I shall assume that our clients are putting as much energy as they can into overcoming the difficulties about which they consult us. This value seems to me to be an essential one to practical psychotherapy, and gives a flavour to this approach that, I hope, fosters a collaboration between client and therapist which is to the benefit of both.

1

Establishing the concerns

Why start with the consideration of concerns?

Starting a book about psychotherapy with a discussion of concerns is appropriate because it is a concern about something that takes people to a therapist in the first place. People seeking psychotherapy may be concerned about the symptoms of a psychological disorder. More usually, even if they have a psychological disorder, their concern is about a crisis in relationships or in everyday life – an existential crisis (Coursey, Keller & Farrell, 1995).

What is a concern?

Concerns are '. . . the more or less enduring disposition to prefer particular states of the world. A concern is what gives a particular event its emotional meaning' and emotions 'arise from the interaction of situational meanings and concerns' (Frijda, 1988). Concern is therefore 'a motivation construct. It refers to the dispositions that motivate a subject, that prompt him to go in search of a given satisfaction or to avoid given confrontations' (Frijda, 1986, p. 334).

An example of a concern

Alan suffered brain damage at birth. Despite this and the developmental problems consequent on it, he had been able to get to university, but found that he was unable to make friends or be taken seriously by his peers. His awareness of that diminished when he was with his family, with whom he had a close relationship, and, unless he thought or talked about the university, he had no particular distress about his social isolation when he was at home. When he returned to university, many incidents during the day reminded him of his social difficulties and made him angry and resentful. His resentment was associated with the feeling that other people should treat him better, and he often sat alone in the university bar watching other people together, and nursing his own distress.

Alan's resentment is a kind of concern. He was on the look-out for people who dismissed him because of his disability, and who did not respect his ideas or his personality. He believed that he was as good as the next person, but that other people did not recognize this. These beliefs were such that when Alan was put in mind of them, he would feel angry rejection or, if he was also lacking in self-confidence, miserable self-pity. Other people sympathetic to him would also feel anger or sadness on his behalf. However, less friendly people would feel more hostile and rejecting because they would find the flavour of Alan's concern unpalatable. He had a chip on his shoulder, they would say.

Concerns reflect what is important to a person and, as Frijda points out, may give rise to many different emotions. Frijda (1988) writes, 'One suffers when a cherished person is gravely ill; one feels joy at his or her fortune or recovery . . .' Disability is a very important issue for Alan, and is therefore one of his major concerns. Overwhelming concerns may lead a person to seek relief from a doctor, a priest, a counsellor or a psychotherapist.

Mrs Wright was on her way to London for one of the regular monthly meetings of the charity for which she worked. As usual on these trips, she had brought some work with her but, as usual, she was lost in not unpleasant reverie. The journey seemed no different from many others until the train braked so hard that she was nearly thrown from her seat, and an elderly lady across from her did actually fall to the floor. Mrs Wright felt her heart take a sudden bound, and her mouth went dry. It was some moments before the thought formed in her mind that: 'We are going to crash'. Almost immediately there was a bang followed by repeated sounds of metal tearing. Mrs Wright hardly noticed. She had been thrown forwards almost over the seat in front of her and shortly after thrown sideways as the carriage in which she was travelling twisted onto its side. She fell onto the window, which had shattered. She was lucky not to have been cut by the glass. A man that she had noticed before was not so lucky. He was thrown with great force from one side of the train to the other, and glass penetrated his face, causing copious bleeding. Mrs Wright felt overwhelmed with horror as his blood splattered her. She was shocked to find herself thinking not of this man's injuries, but of the possibility that he might be infected with HIV and that the virus might be transmitted to her.

This is an extreme example of an overwhelming concern about personal safety. Mrs Wright wanted relief from the flood of unpleasant emotion that the situation, and her concern about it, had released. One component of psychotherapy, and of medical or psychological practice, is to provide the sort of relief that Mrs Wright was seeking. Some of the techniques that can be used are discussed in Chapter 6.

Concerns and psychotherapy

Concerns orientate us in our environment. They enable us to prioritize occurrences and to ensure that happenings that activate our deepest concerns get, *ceteris paribus*, most of our attention (Oatley, Jenkins & Stein, 1998). This process most often occurs outside awareness. In fact, when the concern leads imperceptibly to an action that takes care of the concern, we may have no awareness of there being a concern at all. Others, such as psychotherapists, might be able to infer the concern from observing a pattern in our actions, however. If no immediate action suggests itself, we may become aware of the concern because we become aware of feelings and thoughts associated with it. We might experience ourselves concentrating on a problem, or finding ways round a difficulty. We might experience ourselves on the defensive, or using our winning ways. We might, in other words, have to self-consciously recruit learnt means of resolving the concern. Very often this will be successful. But sometimes, it will not. It is these situations, of unassuaged concern, with which psychotherapists are concerned.

Concerns are normal. They engage us with the world. A lack of concern, perhaps associated with indifference, apathy or boredom, may also lead a person to consult a psychotherapist or, more often, to lead someone else to recommend psychotherapy. I do not think that psychotherapy is going to be practical for someone who has no concerns. But it may be enough for a person to feel concerned about their lack of concern. In fact, as we shall see in Chapter 10, concerns that are hidden are often the ones that most destroy happiness.

The three elements of a concern

Frijda's use of the word concern is subtle and ambiguous, befitting a term that is to be useful in psychotherapy where both subtlety and ambiguity are highly prized. Concern can be used as a feeling, as in, 'Jane's back late. I'm feeling quite concerned'. It can be used as an indication of thought, as in, 'Our first concern should be to find out whether she has already left the party'. Or, it can be applied as Frijda probably intended it, to values, as in, 'You're always so concerned when Jane's away. I think that you care more about her than you do about me'.

Of the very many ways in which human action can be classified, a three-fold classification has emerged as the most influential in psycho-therapy. It has been argued that a preference of three-fold models reflects familiarity with three spatial dimensions. Harre has also suggested that models of the mind do not reflect reality, but create – and therefore restrict – it (Harre, 1979). We should, therefore, treat any model of the mind with some scepticism. However, this does not apply solely to the models used by psychotherapists, but also to our own commonsense psychology which blinkers us as much as any other model, if we let it.

Case example

Howard was admitted to an observation ward, having arrived at work, bought a cup of coffee as he always did, and then repeatedly gone up to people in the lobby saying, 'I don't know what to do next'. He had a bruise on his forehead, and was obviously confused. He had cycled to work, and it was assumed that he had either had an accident, leading to a head injury, or that it was a confusional state. Over the next 3 days, Howard's state improved. On the second day, he began ringing his colleagues, apologizing that he had missed appointments with them, but was unable to make alternative appointments as he had no sense of his future plans. He later said, 'It was as if my mind had gone silent'. Normally, there would be constant chatter of plans, thoughts, ideas, hopes, and so on. That had all disappeared. There was only the now. On the third day, he was no longer clinically confused and he was allowed to go home. His condition returned to normal over the next week, but there was a nagging problem about what had caused it.

Howard reasoned that even if he had no conscious memory of what had happened to him, he would have an autonomic memory. He therefore set out on his bicycle to undertake the same journey to work. This time, though, he stopped regularly to take his pulse. It increased at the beginning of the journey as he began to exercise, but then remained at the same rate until he approached a section where there were large trees. The rate went up progressively as he approached a particularly large oak, which had a limb over the path along which he was cycling. Stopping under this limb, Howard realized that if he was at full stretch he would have struck it with his forehead. Standing under it, straddling his bike, he felt uncomfortably anxious and he concluded that it was here that he had had his accident. He would probably have fallen off, and then remounted to continue his journey, but with a frontal lobe deficit. He could complete the journey and buy his coffee as he always did, because these plans were already 'laid in' and did not require conscious deliberation. When they had been completed though, and he had to think about what he had to do that day anew, his deficit had become apparent.

Howard was concerned, following his head injury, that there was some hidden danger in his environment. It was hidden from his thought by amnesia, but it was detectable using his emotions, and the different memory system subserving them (Ikeda et al., 1998). Since Howard had no conscious memory of what had caused the injury, his anxiety was the only manifestation of his concern that he should not be injured in a similar way in the future.

Had he not conducted his experiment, Howard would be in the same situation as any other animal which has been injured in a particular place. The animal learns, or as the jargon goes, is conditioned to experience fear in association with stimuli associated with that situation. This fear might extend to other stimuli of a 'similar' kind (see Chapter 5 for a consideration of what 'similar' means in this context).

Animals, including people, live in an environment which contains many conditioned stimuli. The anxiety that these stimuli evoke is the means by which the animal demonstrates its concern for its physical safety. The Howard case indicates that the concerns of people, too, may be furthered by emotions elicited by the environment without the mediation of thought although, as I shall argue in Chapter 5, the emotions may be complex and are by no means restricted to anxiety.

Howard was not content to rely on instinct to preserve him from further harm. He wanted to know what had caused it. Having conducted his experiment, he would not only have his feelings to alert him to possible danger, he would be able to use his conscious appraisal of his environment to look out for trees with overhanging branches. Howard, as it turns out, was not a devil-may-care person. Had he been, he might have taken a different attitude to danger than he did. Rather than avoiding tree-lined paths, he might have sought them out, to show his lack of fear, even to free himself from any such mundane concern as a fear of injury. It is likely, although there is no evidence to prove it, that this devil-may-care attitude would not have been present during Howard's convalescence. It would most likely have returned when he started again to be aware of plans, wishes and long-term goals, as he began to be, just before discharge. Howard's concern to preserve himself may have been subordinated to a more important concern for him to see himself, or to be seen, as 'macho'.

The reader will note that there is a ternary model implicit in this description of Howard. The three elements are emotions, attentive appraisal, and values. It is interesting to note that, in Howard's case, it appears that these elements are differentially affected by the head injury, recovering at different rates. It may therefore be, although further study of people recovering from head injury would be needed, that when a person is concerned about something, three distinct neural substrates are involved. What matters more for the purpose of this chapter is that when a person expresses a concern, or when we speak of a person's concerns, we are referring to 'emotions', 'attentive appraisal' 'and values'. These three terms are not meant to be exhaustive. There are many other independent aspects of mental function. Each of these aspects of concern also draws on previous experience and thinking. Emotional responses are affected by the emotional meanings, which are discussed in Chapter 3. Attentive appraisal takes place in relation to beliefs. For example, Howard's appraisal of the threat of the tree was determined by his belief that tree trunks are harder than heads. Values are also informed by beliefs, and particularly the strongest beliefs – convictions – which seem to be beyond question.

The ternary model of psycho-analysis

In many psychotherapeutic approaches, a particular mental agency, often called 'the unconscious', is held to be responsible for emotional responses and for impulsive actions following on from emotions. The concept of the unconscious was particularly developed by Freud (Freud, 1940), but he had a number of influential forerunners (Ellenberger, 1970). A great deal of twentieth century thought has been shaped by the awareness of man's animal nature, as Nietzsche termed 'the unconscious' (Nietzsche, 1977).

As is well known, Freud developed his ideas about the unconscious more as his thinking developed. He presumed that there were two unconscious agencies – the 'It', which was man's animal, 'primitive', nature, and the 'over I', which was a crystallization of social prohibitions, created by the child's experience of paternal repression. These two, the It and the over I, or, as Strachey renamed them, the id and the superego, battled it out for the ear of the third agency of the mind, the 'I' or ego. The ego is not quite the self, but comes closest to what philosophers call 'the agent'.

Freud, too, therefore had a ternary model of mental function. It was based on conflict rather than partnership, and it placed considerable emphasis on men and their struggle to master themselves.

Freud's immense success in popularizing the idea of the unconscious has meant that his contribution has over-shadowed not just psychotherapy, but popular culture. It is difficult to escape this grandparental influence. Freud was an extremely fertile and wide-ranging thinker who made new contributions in very many areas. Even defending and criticizing Freudian psychology has become a major literary industry. It is almost certain to turn out to be as pointless as arguing about Paracelsian medicine was in the seventeenth century. I do not intend to contribute to it.

Freud's preoccupations have been passed on to younger psychotherapists, and continue to influence, sometimes adversely, the development of the profession. Freud was preoccupied by seductive women and repressive men, by childhood, by sexuality, by mental struggle, by the psycho-analyst's power to know what others did not, by the rightness of civilization, and by the dangers of man's 'animal nature' (Midgeley, 1979).

A psychotherapist in training today cannot remain neutral to Freud. His name, like the concept of the unconscious, has become a sort of rallying call. Joining another camp is not an answer: cognitive-behavioural psychotherapists, existential psychotherapists and interpersonal psychotherapists all have their characteristic concerns too.

What I try to do in this book is to set aside these concerns as much as I can without necessarily setting aside the ideas with which they have been linked.

What is a concern?

I have already noted that a concern has three elements: emotion, appraisal and value.

Richard was a young man with autism, preoccupied by the world news. He was convinced that some disaster was at hand, and would often wake his mother in the night to ask her for reassurance. She had a recurrence of a breast cancer, and was already very stressed. She could not deal with her son's difficulties, which she attributed to his autism. He was referred to a psychotherapist, who quickly discovered that his mother had never told him about her state of health, although he had guessed it. She did then tell him, on the advice of the psychotherapist, and the psychotherapist suggested to the young man that his concern about his mother may be at least as important as his concern about the whole world. His behaviour improved. Some months later, his mother died and, within the next 12 months, so did the young man's father and grandfather. He was completely unprepared, became depressed, and began to drink heavily.

The three components of Richard's concern are obvious. He valued security above all things, and was therefore preoccupied by the possibility of disaster. His world was suffused with anxiety about death, which gave particular emphasis to the threat of war. And he was trying to work out what he could do to avert the catastrophe that he felt was looming.

Richard's concern was 'real'. His history dates from a time of cold-war tension when many people were starting to commission nuclear bunkers in their back gardens. But this was not the concern which was really bothering him. The really bothersome concern was no more nor less real, but it was a bigger concern or, as Stock Whitaker puts it, a more preoccupying concern (Whitaker, 1985).

The therapist was aware of the three components of Richard's concern, but made the mistake of thinking that Richard's real concern was that his mother might be concealing a relapse of her illness. But, as events showed, Richard had legitimate concerns about independent living which were, arguably, the real concerns that he was experiencing all along.

How does the discussion of concerns differ between medical or psychiatric practice, and the practice of psychotherapy?

Very little one might say, if ordinary everyday medical practice is considered, since people going to doctors are just as concerned about the emotional and spiritual significance of their problems as people going to psychotherapists. But the goal of the physician or psychiatrist is different. She or he must behave as a positivist, and find out whether the concern is real in the sense of being material.

Doing this involves many activities which are similar to those of the psychotherapist in an assessment. There has to be a recognition that clients may withhold information to protect themselves, others or the doctor. They may misinterpret experiences, and they may be unaware of important information which has to be elicited directly or even inferred.

Assessment

Activities are often collectively called 'clarification', and I will use that term too. However, it is important to note that clarification is not merely a process of exposing what is there. The person doing the clarifying is concerned, too, to achieve a particular end, and this influences what becomes clear.

A few years ago, it was a common practice for trainee psychiatrists to include, in their mental state descriptions, expressions like: 'Depression. Present subjectively, absent objectively'. What this purported to mean was that the person who complained of depression did not look depressed. But such statements were often the consequence of a hard-pressed junior psychiatrist meeting an unhappy person threatening to take an overdose in casualty in the middle of the night. The junior psychiatrist is concerned not to 'block a bed' or to be made to look a fool in the morning when the client is discovered to be a regular user of mental health services and, as the consultant may disparagingly term him, a 'known personality disorder'. But the psychiatrist is also concerned not to appear in the coroner's court and have to explain why a person who says that they are going to kill themselves was not taken seriously. So the psychiatrist starts out his or her clarification of the client's symptoms with the intention of making clear whether or not the client is 'objectively depressed'.

The medical paradigm is that clarification of the concern leads to a pattern which the doctor can recognize as being caused by an abnormality of bodily functioning. In ordinary practice in many medical specialities, and especially in psychiatry, this paradigm is an ideal. The normal process is that the doctor recognizes a pattern which can be changed by some intervention, and the bodily malfunction is either inferred or unknown. However, either way, clarification leads to an intervention which deals with whatever is causing the things which are concerning the client. And this is backed up by the supposition that, sooner or later, the bodily malfunction will be discovered.

Many psychotherapists consider that this paradigm can be made serviceable for psychotherapy by widening the range of possible causes to include memories and learnt responses. Traumas, maladaptive learning, insecure attachment and negative automatic thoughts have all been proposed as causes of psychological disorder. This adoption of a causal model of psychotherapy has many advantages. It enables easier dialogue with other mental health professionals. It is a tried and tested paradigm, which lends itself to research. It avoids blaming clients with mental disorder.

However, it has two disadvantages. Being considered to be mentally ill is, according to the causal model, to be considered to have emotional difficulties caused by external factors. Most people believe that they are responsible for the character or abilities that protect them from reacting badly to adversity (Rogers & Pilgrim, 1997), even if they do not consider that they are responsible for their immune system's capacity to fight infection. For many people, becoming mentally ill is therefore to have given up responsibility. The more the doctor tells someone that they cannot help themselves because their illness is, like pneumonia, caused by something that is out of their control, the more problematic it is for the client. If the client values self-control highly, he or she may pretend to agree with the doctor, but think that the doctor does not really understand mental problems. If the client goes along with the doctor, it may be difficult for him or her to know what they are responsible for. Perhaps getting angry that the lunch is late is also caused?

A second disadvantage is professional. In the ordinary world of medicine, a client who coughs up blood may be successively visited by an infectious diseases specialist, a chest physician and a surgeon. Each may clarify the problem in such a way as to make it out to be particularly susceptible to their style of intervention. The infectious diseases doctor may get a history of night sweats and a lack of BCG immunization, and the surgeon might emphasize the long history of smoking and the irregularity of the enlarged regional lymph nodes. However, their disagreement can normally be resolved by further physical findings. There is a constraint set on their rivalry by this appeal to a shared material world. If the proponents of tuberculosis as a cause of haemoptysis begin to outnumber the proponents of carcinoma, it is likely to be because they predict these physical manifestations more accurately and not because they are better politicians.

When a cognitive-behavioural therapist uncovers negative automatic thoughts and a psycho-analytic psychotherapist uncovers transference problems, both seeing the same client, how can their different points of view be resolved? The evidence seems strong that different psychotherapy modalities are more similar in their effects than they are different (Stiles, Shapiro & Elliott, 1986). Even if this were not so, it is clear that there is a substantial non-specific effect in psychotherapy (Frank, 1984) and that almost any intervention can be effective some of the time and in some people. There can therefore be no definitive test of outcome which shows one account to be true, and another not.

Causes and reasons

Another way of contrasting medical and psychotherapeutic practice is to say that the former is about finding a cause for the client's concern, and the latter is about finding a reason for the concern. Clarifying the cause for concern leads to a diagnosis which, it is assumed, would be reached by any competent practitioner discussing that concern. Clarifying the reason for a person's concern leads to a consensus between the client and the psychotherapist about why the concern has arisen, and it is recognized that a different consensus might be reached by another practitioner. This is not just because there are many reasons for a person acting as they do, for there are also many causes. It is because the concern may exist long before the reason for it has been formulated (Tantam, 1999b). This is not to say that reasons are merely epiphenomena of causal chains. Once brought into being, they are causally effective.

A woman notices that her husband is abstracted. 'You're hallucinating again', she says to her husband, 'because you didn't take your tablets.'

A . . . 'You forgot to take your tablets.'

B . . . 'You don't like those tablets.'

The cause of the husband's hallucinations is the fall in his medication levels. His wife thinks that there is a reason for this, but neither of the reasons could have been causally effective. There was no act which corresponded to forgetting, nor to not liking, and so no act on the husband's part corresponding to either reason could have caused him not to take the tablets. But both of the reasons given by the wife are likely to have future causal consequences. She may institute a medicine diary if she considers her husband to be forgetful. Or she might get angry with him and try to change his motivation to take the tablets by indicating that his dislike of them will certainly be outweighed in the future by her dislike of him hallucinating.

Medical psychotherapists may need to consider the causes of their client's concerns, but are principally concerned with the reasons for them. The evidential criteria that they bring to bear on reasons are very different to those that apply to causes (Tantam, 1999b). That means that the process of clarification of the concerns is different too.

It is different partly because, like psycho-analysis, it is interminable. Since reasons for an action or an event may be brought into being after the action or event, fresh reasons can always be advanced. Indeed, in writing up many of the illustrations in this book, I have seen possible new reasons for the actions of the people that I describe.

Being a bit more practical about concerns

It would be a much simpler world if everyone knew what they were concerned about, and were able to express their concerns clearly and in a way that readily led to resolution. In fact, in this simple world, psychotherapists and counsellors would probably not be needed. For it is to psychotherapists and counsellors that people turn when they do not know the causes of their mental dis-ease. As the client said to the doctor, 'What's my problem? If I knew that, I would not need to come to see you'.

Lotty B. wakes in the small hours, wet with sweat and with her heart pounding. She is due to be admitted to see a surgeon in the morning for assessment of a lump in her breast.

(1) She has been dreaming of being at the dentist, but something had gone wrong and it was not as it should have been. More horrific. She feels somewhat calmer when she wakes because she hears her husband calmly breathing next to her. She snuggles up to him, and he mutters in his sleep. She thinks of how good he is, and drops off to sleep again.

(2) She has been dreaming of being at the dentist, but he is pulling out her nipple, not her teeth. As she wakes, she remembers the lump, and she is sure it is cancer. Her husband feels her rapid breathing and restlessness and wakes. They talk about the possibility. What he would do, and what she would do, if she does have cancer. She feels less alone with her fears, and realizes that even if it is cancerous, life will not stop immediately. There will still be much to live for. Her heart slows down, and her anxiety returns to manageable levels.

(3) She wakes out of a dreamless sleep, straight into the feeling that she is dying. She can't breathe. She struggles upright, and manages to slow her breathing down but there is nothing she can do about her heart. She knows that she will not get back to sleep that night. 'Surely there must be something very wrong with me', she says to herself. 'It must be cancer.'

Lotty B.'s anxiety dream in 1. is obvious and, as we would say, understandable. Her anxiety is resolved by a direct influence over her feelings through the relationship with her husband. She identifies with him, and with his quiet breathing, and that quietens her. Then she re-experiences the closeness of their relationship – as attachment theorists would say, how securely they are attached – and that further calms her.

In 2., Lotty remembers the dream. It has a propositional content, distorted but recognizable in the dream, accessible to her on waking, and understood by her husband. The concern leads directly to reflection and planning. 'Even if it is cancer, life does not stop.' The concern that presents intrusively and overwhelmingly is that there can be no future after the diagnosis, but her husband allays this concern when he indicates that he will continue to feel for her even if she does have cancer: '. . . life does not stop'. It seems to be this concern – that life will change after the diagnosis – that is the reason for Lotty's anxiety, and not her concern that she may die of cancer at some time in the future. Once it is allayed, she feels calmer.

Lotty B's panic in 3. is without propositional content. A sleep EEG would have shown that she awoke not from REM sleep, but from stage 4 sleep. This is often interpreted to mean that this type of panic attack is physiologically triggered and is without propositional content. The fact that Lotty is unable, even after waking, to put any meaning to her feelings, and that she concludes herself that the panic is merely the effect of a bodily disturbance, seems to bear this out. Panic attacks like this recur night after night, and are one of the commoner reasons for a mental health consultation.

What do these illustrations show about reasons and concerns?

We surmise that Lotty has some different concerns in each of these situations, and one concern that is the same. The different concerns relate to the quality of her relationship with her husband, and the kind of contact that she wants from him.

The concern which is common to all the situations is the emotional meaning. All of the dreams involve anxiety. In the first dream this meaning is not linked to the operation, but to the dentist, and it is merged into the emotional meaning of her husband sleeping beside her, suggesting that her concern is about separation.

The concern is much more explicit in the second situation. It is briefly about the dentist, but shifts quickly to the surgeon. This new concern seems much more overwhelming, because it is so much more threatening. Indeed, it is so threatening that the dream seems to be a sort of escape from the real danger, whilst preserving some of the feared elements, for example the interference with her breast. However, locating the anxiety in the forthcoming surgical appointment, and away from a story about the dentist, moves it on further. Lotty realizes that she is most concerned not, as a therapist might expect, that she will die or that she will suffer, but that she will become alienated from her husband. This is a concern which translates directly into a social action: a request to her husband which he convincingly answers – he will not abandon her, their life will go on.

In the third situation, there is no mention of a husband and Lotty's concern remains tacit. However, it seems possible that her anxiety attack is not merely coincidental with the appointment on the following day, but is linked to it, and that she does have the same concern as her avatars.

Preoccupying concerns

In her excellent book on group psychotherapy (Whitaker, 1985), Dorothy Stock Whitaker introduces the notion of a preoccupying concern. These are concerns which are fundamental to many other concerns, and which have a strong emotional flavour. This type of concern may colour an individual's reactions to many situations, and may occasionally manifest itself in a strong emotional reaction. Preoccupying concerns, like Lotty's, may be overwhelming, and yet not seem resolvable. They may intrude on a person's everyday actions, and create an emotional backwash that engulfs everything else. It is this kind of concern that usually takes a person to a friend or a healer. And it is this concern which the successful friend or healer locates and addresses.

Short-term dynamic, analytic or existential therapy is based on the assumption that it is a preoccupying concern or concerns which bring a person to the therapist. Clarifying the concern, or sometimes clarifying a sequence of linked concerns, is the main therapeutic activity of all these approaches, and is discussed in Chapter 9.

Another example of a preoccupying concern

Edward was coming to the end of his Master's degree. He had made a number of friends at university, and had enough money to enjoy himself. But he was dissatisfied. His life had not been as straightforward as he had hoped. He asked to see a psychotherapist because he had decided that he suffered from 'dysthymia', and wanted to discuss treatment options. The therapist reviewed Edward's history of broken relationships and of projects enthusiastically embarked upon, only to be dropped, his early separations from his parents, and his tendency to become anxious especially on leaving people he loved, and his depression when he felt rejected. The therapist suggested that Edward might have a deeper concern – to find someone or something on which he could rely and which would give him security and care.

Edward partly accepted this way of looking at his problem, but remained convinced that he did meet DSM-IV criteria for dysthymia and that he should receive drug treatment. He also pointed out that he was not so concerned about being close to people. He was, after all, a pretty successful guy.

The therapist was concerned not to reinforce Edward's view of the matter, and arranged a further meeting to discuss psycho-dynamic therapy. Edward did not attend.

Edward's concern was not the salient concern that brought him to see the psychotherapist. It was his concern that he had attention deficit disorder. The Lotty of the third situation – the one who just had an anxiety attack – would probably have expressed her salient concern as gaining relief.

Clients who come to see psychotherapists are not always as concerned as the dynamically orientated psychotherapist to understand why they feel as they do. They may want relief (see also Chapter 6), to be happy again (see Chapter 10) or, rarely, to understand why they keep getting into the predicaments that they do (see Chapter 9). They are, in other words, concerned about the kind of help that they will get.

Concerns about treatment

Many dynamically orientated psychotherapists believe, rightly in my opinion, that the emotional determinants of problems are considered far too rarely. They believe, therefore, that the clarification of a person's preoccupying concern, with its substantial emotional component, should be a more frequent response to problems. Organizational consultancy based on psychodynamic principles is successful, precisely because it provides explanations of the behaviour of people in organizations in terms of their emotional needs.

However, there are some circumstances when meeting an emotional need, or providing an emotional explanation, causes affront, not benefit. Consider the following:

Sugar-cane workers who were receiving benzodiazepines for treatment of palpitations and 'ataquos dos nervos' were found to have low blood sugars, due to overwork on a poor diet.

A disgruntled wife threatened to leave her husband because every time that she asked him why he was home late from work, and whether he had been seeing another woman, he told her that she was pathologically jealous.

The starvation faced by the sugar-cane cutters and the husband's conceal-ment of his activities from his wife were ignored by others dealing with the problem. Maybe the others felt that they were helping, but it was practical help that was wanted and not emotional intervention. Denying this practical help increased the supplicant's sense of inadequacy and impotence. The importance of intervening only when a person is ready for it is stressed in motivational interviewing, a technique developed for the treatment of alcohol problems (Miller, 1983) but also applied more widely (Fowles, 1992).

One way to identify a person's concerns about treatment is to ask what they were hoping to get from the consultation (Lazare, Eisenthal & Wasserman, 1975).

Mr Hill had been diagnosed as having paranoid schizophrenia. He believed that he was the Saviour, and spent many hours, often until the early hours of the morning, reading the Gospels. Every so often he became more distressed and thought-disordered. Admission to hospital would be required, his medication would be increased and he would eventually settle down. It was thought that his wife was quite intolerant of his delusions, and that from time to time their relationship became acrimonious. On one occasion, he rang the doctor request-ing an urgent appointment, and the doctor assumed that he wanted to be admitted to hospital because of rows with his wife.

Mr Hill was apparently more psychotic, but he seemed also to be expectant. The doctor asked him if there was anything that he hoped that the doctor would be able to do for him. With great hesitation, Mr Hill raised the question of Easter, which was just a few days away. Was it necessary, he asked, for someone who was the Saviour of the world to be crucified at Easter? Because, he said, he did not want to die. The doctor reassured him that the fact that one Saviour had died at Easter did not rule out the possibility of other sorts of Saviours, who might never be crucified. Mr Hill seemed much reassured by this, and went home a calmer man. On subsequent meetings with the doctor, he said he thought that he might have been mistaken that he actually was Jesus Christ. Perhaps he was another sort of Saviour.

I do not think that Mr Hill would have brought up his concern unless he trusted the doctor to take it seriously, and not to ridicule him. Like many people with schizophrenia, he knew that no-one else would recognize that he was Jesus Christ, even though he was convinced that he was, himself. He could predict the humiliating rejoinder that doctors may sometimes make to clients who step out of the client role.

Fortunately, Mr Hill and the doctor had already established a mutually respectful therapeutic relationship. Had this been their first meeting, matters might have been different. The concerns that clients have about consulting a psychotherapist may determine the extent to which other concerns can be expressed.

Concerns about the therapeutic relationship

Going to see a psychotherapist is frightening. There may be enquiry into intimate matters, and perhaps judgement made or implied about one's personal behaviour. It is also disempowering. Psychotherapy remains an arcane undertaking, about which the therapist appears to know a lot, and the client little. The client's request for treatment may be rejected, if they are found 'unsuitable'.

The client may have high hopes, and delight in the opportunity of finally finding someone who will listen to their view of the world and their problems in it. But there will always be some negative expectations. They will be associated with a concern not be rejected, humiliated or shamed by the therapist.

Empirical research about shame indicates the dangers. In a diary study of women attending psychotherapists who had been sexually abused in childhood, Macdonald and Morley (2001) showed that some of the women decided during the course of their therapy to disclose the abuse to their partners for the first time. In a proportion of cases, the partner allowed the woman to express her feelings about the abuse, and accepted them. In these cases, the disclosure lessened the shame that the woman felt about the abuse. In other cases, the partner tried to get rid of the problem, rather than accept the reality of the woman's feelings. Very often, the partner's reaction was to get angry with the abuser, and sometimes to threaten to harm him or damage his reputation. In these cases, the woman very often felt more ashamed as a result of the disclosure.

An example of a concern about the trustworthiness of the therapist

Mr Slovoboda, a 40-year-old academic, came to his second selection interview in a hostile frame of mind. He was Czech, but brought up in Africa, most of the time by different uncles and aunts, or friends of the family. His parents had split up, and neither had wanted to raise him. He had been, as he said, searching for psychotherapy for 18 years. Since the first interview he had been ruminating on a remark that the assessor made, to the effect that not everyone benefits from therapy. He had concluded that this remark had been made to lay the groundwork for further treatment to be refused.

Mr Slovoboda was convinced even before he came to the first interview that he would be refused what he sought. This was, in fact, the most important theme of his life. He had been refused the care of his parents, and had concluded that others had kept them from him. He had begun a restless and intrinsically hopeless search for substitute care, but was always ready to identify those who would impede him and to fight to overcome them.

Mr Slovoboda's treatment never began. He had a series of mutually frustrating meetings with a psychotherapist who tried as hard as she could to be helpful to him. Mr Slovoboda was preoccupied with defending himself against her. He assumed that any help that would be offered to him would only be second-rate and that he should therefore refuse it.

The therapist's concerns

Psychotherapists are not without their concerns about therapy. The beginning therapist's preoccupying concern is likely to be 'not getting it wrong'. Mr Slovoboda's therapist who was working with a new consultant wanted particularly to show that she could be helpful. These concerns may sometimes be difficult to be put to one side, and may prevent the therapist from being fully aware of the client's concerns.

It is sometimes useful for beginning therapists to remember that psychotherapy shares many commonalities with other mental health practice. The skills that have been learnt there – or indeed in work as a teacher, parish priest or other professional concerned with the personal development of others – are the basis of psychotherapy skills. Even more importantly, the lessons about the limits of the professional's influence that are learnt in these other pastoral actitivies also apply to psychotherapy.

One of the greatest challenges for the beginning therapist is to determine the limits of their responsibility to their client. What if a client is suicidal? What if they report having committed a crime? More mundanely, but more commonly, what should the therapist answer if the client says, 'I came to you to get help with my problem and here it is, 4 weeks later, and I do not feel any better'?

The therapist needs to be clear about the limits of his or her own agency.

He or she is responsible – morally, professionally and sometimes legally – for what he or she does. But the therapist is not responsible for the client's actions. The therapist is not responsible, therefore, for taking away the client's concerns. This is an important difference from other types of practice.

Example of agency

Mr Y. goes to see his family doctor, complaining that he can't hear very well. Examination of the ear indicates that it is normal, but the doctor promises to arrange an audiogram. The client is relieved of having to do anything further, except wait. He may continue to worry, but he does not have to think what to do. If people ask him what is wrong with his hearing, he says that he does not know but is waiting for the results of tests, and this satisfies the enquirers. The doctor has become the agent dealing with Mr Y.'s hearing problem.

In fact the audiogram is normal, and the doctor tells Mr Y. that he need not be concerned about his hearing, because it is normal. Mr Y., who has come to the surgery confident that his hearing will be sorted out, finds all his old concerns returning, and protests that he still can't hear. He is so perturbed that the harassed doctor refers him to the practice psychologist.

She asks Mr Y. if he accepts that the tests are normal. He says that he does: he can hear sounds well enough, but he cannot hear what people say to him. She asks him if the problem is that he cannot take in what people say, and Mr Y. says, 'Yes. That's it exactly'. So far, the psychologist has not accepted responsibility for Mr Y.'s concern. She has only clarified what it is. It would now be possible for the psychologist to take responsibility for this new concern, and vie with the doctor in curing the problem. Mr Y. could be given some attentional exercises, for example, or the psychologist might investigate Mr Y.'s language processing.

Neither of these approaches would be wrong in principle, although both might be wrong for Mr Y. But neither would be psychotherapeutic. The psychotherapeutic approach is not for the psychologist to take responsibility for Mr Y.'s concerns, but to assist Mr Y. to find a way to follow these concerns to their conclusion. She might, for example, say to Mr Y: 'Do you have difficulty in taking in what everyone says, or is it just particular people?'. Mr Y. might say that he has particular difficulty in taking in what his daughter says. Further clarification might lead Mr Y. to the realization that he has his biggest problems when his daughter talks to him about her feelings about her upbringing.

What the psychologist has done is to help Mr Y. to clarify his concerns. She has not taken responsibility for them. Mr Y. remains responsible for what he hears, and does not hear. However, his concern has changed. He is now concerned that he can't hear what his daughter says about her feelings about her upbringing. And this new concern seems to be one that Mr Y. is more likely to be able to do something about than his previous blanket concern that his hearing was failing.

The psychotherapist's stance on agency and responsibility is not an easy option. It has to be balanced by a greater commitment to the autonomy of the client, and to the right of the client to confidentiality. Changing attitudes to the responsibility of mental health professionals to third parties have undermined their duty of confidentiality to their clients. Some agencies may require professionals to report to an investigative body a client's disclosure of actual or suspected abuse of a child. If a client tells a doctor of their intention to kill or injure another person, that doctor is ethically required to warn the potential victim or to take other steps to protect the third party. But even today, many psychotherapists take the view that, while they might do everything in their power to persuade their clients against a course of action that might harm others or themselves, they should be very reluctant to act independently to prevent it. This caution continues despite a ruling by the Californian supreme court in re Tarasoff that a psychologist has a duty to warn a possible victim.

As a house physician, I admitted a late middle-aged man who had just had a heart attack. His heart was failing and a chest X ray showed that there was substantial pulmonary oedema. There was no question about the diagnosis, or the possibility that he might die. He refused admission and insisted that he wanted to go home. He was slightly confused but understood that he had had a heart attack and that he might have another, or he might get more severe pulmonary oedema. He could give no good reason for wanting to go home other than that he would feel better there. My reality was that he was seriously ill and needed to be in hospital. My concern, in his place, would have been to do everything to save myself. His reality was also that he was seriously ill, but in those circumstances he believed that it was better to be at home (and I have to say that more recent research supports his position to some degree). His concern was to be psychologically safe, and that meant to be in a familiar environment.

I was so concerned that I asked a psychiatrist to see him who concluded that the client was not compulsorily detainable and no obstacle was put in the client's way of leaving hospital.

It is not possible to discuss deeply personal aspects of someone's life without it touching on concerns that one has oneself. In this instance, I was afraid that I would be seen by others to have done less than I should have for a client of mine. I have found over the years that I often need to consult colleagues in cases where I am afraid that I have not done enough. My instincts continue to be somewhat over-protective. I would, for example, warn a victim. But I recognize that there are times when this limits my ability to have a completely trusting relationship with those clients who want complete trust.

Sometimes these preoccupying concerns of the therapist stand in the way of dealing with the preoccupying concerns of the client. It is for this reason that many psychotherapists undertake a personal therapy as part of their training. This is not a complete solution to the problem of what may sometimes be termed counter-transference. The psychotherapists' concerns are not always due to their personalities or their past experiences, but may reflect their present circumstances, including their working practices. All psychotherapists need to be aware of their own concerns, and how these concerns might impinge on their work. Some clues about how one can monitor this, and what to do about it, are discussed in Chapter 11.

Identifying concerns

Some time ago, it used to be said that computers were changing our lives, and were taking over many of the tasks presently carried out by people, such as traffic control, record-keeping . . . and psychotherapy. This over-hasty conclusion followed on from work such as that of Marks and Carr (Carr, Ghosh & Marks, 1988), showing that phobias can be treated by a suitably programmed computer.

For clients who know that they have, say, agoraphobia, and are willing to consider this to be a learned behaviour which can be unlearned, computer-based treatment may be excellent. People are rarely so clear about their problem and its solution when they first see a psychotherapist, just as it is not usual for people to attend their doctors complaining of idiopathic hypertension, and asking for beta-blockers.

Doctors are used to having to clarify a person's concern. More transactionally minded doctors are aware that this may involve negotiation, as Balint (1957) noted, but there is reassurance in the knowledge that there is a 'real problem' to be found which can be demonstrated by tests or the response to treatment.

In psychotherapy, a person may have many concerns. Some of them will be causal ones, which can be addressed by appeal to an objective standard, such as the diagnostic criteria of depression. Others, and these are the ones that are of most interest to psychotherapists, cannot be. Enquiry into these concerns will often generate others, and enquiry into those will generate yet more . . .

Sometimes, as in the second Lotty illustration (see p. 19), the client themselves will indicate which is the preoccupying concern. But this may not always be the case.

Roger was a man with a history of angry, sometimes violent, confrontations with other men. He was referred for psychotherapy because of his increasing anxiety and depression. He spent the whole of the first session talking bitterly about having wasted his life. He related this to pursuing a career which was one that his father wanted for him, but which he did not want for himself. The next

session he talked only about his interest in his work, his wife's lack of understanding of it, and her lack of support for him. The therapist addressed both of Roger's concerns with understanding and empathy. He concluded that Roger had been emotionally deprived and hoped that he could make up for this in the therapy. As if to refute this, Roger rang to cancel the next session, saying that he did not think that anything could be gained by discussing his problems with the therapist, who did not seem to be able to understand his problems, which were just too deep.

The therapist wrote to Roger with a new appointment, and Roger came regularly for some weeks. After a while he started to describe his travel problem. He could never travel any distance from home unless he could be sure that he could contact either his wife or his father on his mobile phone. Very often he did ring them. When his father was away, he would have great difficulty in getting to work.

Camilla had an anxiety disorder. Over the 3 months during which she intermittently attended a general psychiatry out-client clinic, she spoke about her mother's abandonment of her, the threatening behaviour of one of her children, and her very poor home circumstances. This led to a home visit by the psychiatrist, after which Camilla failed to keep her out-client appointments and was counted as having dropped out of treatment. She was re-referred 6 months later, still with anxiety. After the first assessment, she had to be admitted to hospital with a head injury, and whilst on the ward, she developed some alcohol withdrawal symptoms. A great light dawned for the psychiatrist who asked Camilla at their next meeting why she had always denied heavy drinking. She said that it was always her intention to admit to it. Indeed, she knew that it was the reason that she was so anxious. But she just hated to think of herself as an alcoholic.

Both Camilla and Roger entered spiritedly into talk about concerns – in Roger's case about his emotional deprivation and in Camilla's about her anxiety. However, despite the apparent liveliness of these discussions, these were concerns that the therapist had formulated. They were not the preoccupations of the clients. Roger was preoccupied by his dependency on his father to be safe from anxiety, and Camilla about her alcoholism. However, they were both ashamed of these problems and so were also concerned to conceal them.

Useful therapy only began when the therapist found a way to focus on these preoccupations. These were the things that 'really' mattered to them.

But what does it mean to say that they 'really' mattered? There is no objective reality involved. How can the therapist recognize that a concern is the preoccupying one, the one that really matters?

When doctors think of reality, they often think of illness or death. Such things are givens that we all have to accept, irrespective of culture, religious belief or intelligence. Because of their regular contact with these realities it is easy for doctors to believe that they have a better grasp of reality than most. It is also easy for them to be contemptuous of those who try to challenge their position, either by pointing to the cultural determinants of illness or, more fancifully, by adhering to non-rational beliefs in life after death. However, the reality of biology is no more privileged than social or psychological realities. And each of these realities may be as pressing as the other.

Hilda was filled with shame. She had been admitted with a depressive illness which had partly responded to antidepressant treatment, but she continued to avoid every social situation and to take the blame for anything that went wrong. She was being seen in psychotherapy by a psychiatric registrar to whom she confessed after many weeks of wide-eyed fear that she was a bastard. Hilda rarely used words as bald as this and the registrar noted that she would need considerable encouragement to explain. The explanation came in fragments over the next 2 weeks. The story, when put together, related to when she was 15 years old. For some reason she had to get a copy of her birth certificate, and she discovered that her father's name was missing from it. She asked him why this was, and he said, 'You're a bastard, that's why. You're illegitimate'. She felt, as soon as he said it, that she had known this all along – that, in fact, she did not deserve to be legitimate. It turned out that the man that she had known as her father was in fact her father, and that he and her mother had only married in a secret ceremony when she was 11. It did not matter that, biologically, she was the daughter of her parents. What mattered was the social reality that she had been born out of wedlock.

One way of resolving conflicts about concerns is for the therapist to decide which concern is realistic. This was the method used by Freud who posited 'reality-testing' as a criterion of psychosis. This assumes that there is one reality, and that the doctor knows it. Neither of these assumptions is sustainable. The reality of Hilda's situation, as far as the doctor perceived it, is that she was the daughter of her parents, and therefore not a bastard. This was not Hilda's reality. The doctor never knew that that was. Perhaps Hilda suspected that she was not, in fact, her father's daughter. Perhaps she had knowledge about her paternity which she would not admit even to herself. What matters is that there was no unique reality. The doctor's insistence that the reality was that Hilda was the daughter of a married couple and therefore had no cause to be ashamed of her birth was an assertion of how the doctor viewed illegitimacy.

If the doctor focusses the treatment on his or her 'reality', the treatment will become unduly influenced by the concerns which are most real to the doctor. These will, in turn, reflect the doctor's own beliefs and culture. As in the cases of Roger and Camilla previously mentioned, there is a danger that an insistence on reality as the doctor sees it will obfuscate, and not bring out, the preoccupying concerns of the client.

Evidence-based approach to concerns

The current emphasis on the randomized controlled trial and evidence-based treatment reflects the powerful reach of the cause-and-effect model of medicine. It recognizes the fact that people may complain to their doctors of many different physical or mental symptoms, but that these can be translated into recognizable diseases whose life history can be predictably altered by medical interventions. The evidence of the disease and the evidence of the impact of the intervention can both be measured.

An evidence-based approach presumes that certain symptoms or signs are consistent indicators of particular states, and that certain interventions have particular impacts on those states. These presumptions are most readily accepted if the state is a state of the brain or the body which can be independently demonstrated. As Szasz (1960) has pointed out and has subsequently repeatedly reasserted over the last 40 years, there are no differences in the bodies and brains of people with psychological problems that might not also be found in people without any disorder.

It seems unlikely to me that psychotherapy will ever become reduced to a procedure which can be applied according to defined rules. The need for creativity and intuition on the part of the therapist will always limit the scope of an evidence-based approach in psychotherapy. However, this is not to say that evidence can be ignored, or that it has no place at all.

William was in his 40s. He had been married to Enid for 15 years, and their sexual lives had been fulfilling until Enid had a brief affair at a conference that she was attending. She regretted it deeply, and gave a full account to William. After several weeks of soul-searching, he decided that he could forgive Enid and he wanted the marriage to survive. But he was a changed man. He became anxious and hesitant where he had been decided before. He found it increasingly difficult to get a full erection, and after a few months, could rarely get enough of an erection to penetrate Enid. During the second consultation about his anxiety, William hesitantly brought up his fear that 'he could no longer satisfy his wife'.

Evidence-based intervention 1
William was prescribed sildenafil by his doctor. This did not restore his erection to normal, but did restore it enough that he could penetrate Enid. William felt reassured that he could satisfy her again, and that the marriage was saved. But he did not enjoy sex as he had before, and found that he was accepting more invitations to activities that he would do on his own, without Enid.

Evidence-based intervention 2
William and Enid were referred to a sexual therapist. They were treated by a modified Masters and Johnson method at first, which reduced William's anxiety

and improved his erection, although the effects were gradual. As the therapy progressed, Enid's lack of desire for William came to the fore. Her affair was discussed in the light of this. William recognized that he, too, had been attracted by a work colleague and had imagined asking her out. When this came out, Enid spoke about a previous relationship with a man she was to have married, but who went off with a colleague of hers. She had always half expected that William might treat her similarly. They both expressed angry disappointment with each other, and then sadness that they had neglected each other. William's erectile dysfunction improved but his ability to sustain an erection was dependent on Enid's arousal, and that was variable. Both realized that they had to make a fresh start to restore their marriage, and began by planning a long holiday abroad.

Both of these therapies were effective, and even though the brain state corresponding to William's impotence is not known, and is anyway not pathological, both interventions are evidence-based. Both sildenafil (Goldstein et al., 1998) and sexual therapy (Hawton, Catalan & Fagg, 1992) have been shown to be effective in treating male erectile incompetence. However, the two interventions are targeted at different concerns, and also reflect the different concerns of the person treating William.

The physical intervention was more effective for the physical symptom, but there is some suggestion that there remained marital problems which might, yet, have undermined William and Enid's relationship. The psychological intervention was probably less effective for the physical symptom, and was certainly more time-consuming. But it did uncover the problems in the marital domain and may have given William and Enid a better chance of resolving these (Hartman, 1983).

A busy genito-urinary surgeon seeing many people like William might feel that there really is no alternative to physical treatment and, of the possible options, sildenafil is clearly the least invasive. Why complicate matters looking for deep explanations? And why withhold a perfectly effective treatment? Marital satisfaction is a personal, not a professional, concern. Physical symptoms are what should concern doctors.

A psychotherapist might be concerned that focussing on the symptom will distract both William and Enid from getting to grips with what may be more important concerns. Taking tablets for erectile dysfunction anyway turns sex into a performance, and distracts from the fact that it is intercourse – an enacted dialogue between two people which conveys relationship. Problems need to be worked out, not suppressed.

The professional concerns of the psychotherapist and of the surgeon are clearly different. It is not appropriate, as sometimes happens, for the surgeon and the psychotherapist (or the general psychiatrist and the psychotherapist, or the general practitioner and the counsellor) to discount the concerns of the other. Moreover, it is important for each of them to recognize that applying the evidence-based approach to William's concern may reflect the therapist's concern to be effective and not William's own concerns.

William's first concern will be to feel at ease with the therapist. Unless he is, he is very likely to drop out of, or otherwise not comply with, treatment. The therapist and the setting will have an emotional flavour which William and his wife must find palatable, and so too will the therapy. Evidence for this readily observed effect has proven more difficult to obtain in practice (Messer & Meinster, 1980).

Some support comes from an unusual quarter. In a clinical trial of lumpectomy versus mastectomy for breast cancer, Fallowfield et al. (Fallowfield et al., 1990) found that about a third of women who had surgery were depressed or anxious. Conservative treatment in which only the tumour was removed (lumpectomy) was followed by just as much anxiety and depression as more radical mastectomy in which the whole breast was removed. The anxiety and depression are therefore a response to the fact of having cancer, and not to the surgery. Women who were given a choice of treatment did not get less anxious or depressed than women who were not given a choice (often they were not given a choice because they agreed to participate in a randomized trial). However, women who had consultants who normally offered their clients a choice between lumpectomy and mastectomy were less depressed at follow-up than women who had consultants who did not give their clients the choice.

This study suggests that lumpectomy and mastectomy do not have a distinctly different emotional meaning, but that different styles of doctoring do have a distinctively different meaning or at least result in different emotional outcomes. Doctors who give their clients the freedom to choose convey that flavour of openness to their clients even if, because the client has consented to be in a clinical trial, she does not end up having the choice.

Evidence-based approaches are limited in their application because there is often not enough evidence. But they are also limited because evidence about the interpersonal factors in health care, such as the evidence about doctors' styles mentioned in the previous paragraph, is hard to come by. Randomized controlled trials can provide evidence about erectile dysfunction, but not about Enid and her fears of abandonment, or William and his emotional detachment.

The evidence-based approach depends on finding a dysfunction, and on defined and repeatable measures which will reduce that dysfunction. But categorizing a problem as a dysfunction may offend the values which are inherent in the concern. William and Enid may be preoccupied about William's erectile dysfunction precisely because they do not consider it to be a physiological malfunction, but as a reflection of their waning love for each other. Whilst they may be concerned to overcome the problem, they will be concerned to overcome it by restoring this love rather than by just fixing William up.

The fact that the referral was to a surgeon ensured that the concern that would be dealt with was the physical one of failed erection. Referring William and Enid to a sex therapist made it more likely that the concern that would be recognized was a relationship one. Does this indicate that clients should choose the practitioner whose concerns are the nearest to his or her own?

Whose concern is it anyway?

Perhaps it is not necessary to find out much about the client's preoccupying concern. Indeed, perhaps this is a mirage. Maybe it is more important as a therapist to be clear about one's own professional concerns and to expect that clients who do not share these concerns either do not get referred, or do not enter treatment.

This is, in practice, how much of psychotherapy assessment and planning works. Particular therapists have their own take on the world – attachment theory, object-relations, faulty cognitions, or whatever – and they construe the difficulties of the people that they assess in terms of whichever of these they espouse. A good fit, and the client is taken on for treatment. A poor fit, and the client is refused treatment, or drops out an early stage. Drop-out rates are difficult to establish in psychotherapy, and probably depend on the setting. In one study of a community mental health centre in the US (Smoller et al., 1998) – a situation which approximates to the National Health Service – clients missed 60% of appointments with a mental health professional, including those offering psychotherapy. Clinical experience suggests that more clients may leave treatment by unilateral termination than by agreement.

Some might argue that non-compliance is really an expression of self-selection, and that the clients who drop out are the ones who would not benefit anyway. However, in one study, it was found that clients who were not considered to be good prospects for psychotherapy were more likely to drop out. But if poor-prospect clients persisted in treatment, their outcome was as good as good-prospect clients (McCallum & Piper, 1990). It therefore appears that clients who drop out do so not because they will not benefit from the treatment, but because they find the treatment unpalatable.

There are two other considerable disadvantages to this self-selection method. The first is that if clients are not able to make a clear choice – if psychotherapists form misleading impressions of their clients, or if there is a limited range of psychotherapists available – decisions may not be made freely and with full information.

The second disadvantage is even greater. Making explicit a person's preoccupying concern is often the first stage, and sometimes an essential stage, to it being resolved. Psychotherapists who dodge the possibility of clarifying the preoccupying concern are therefore denying their clients an important therapeutic possibility.

Many psychotherapists, while conceding this, believe that their treatment approach, i.e. their concerns about what matters psychologically, is so bound up with their values and the emotional flavour of the treatment that it cannot be compromised. This view presumes that the psychotherapist cannot adapt his or her values, and suit his or her emotional flavour, to the client. I do not believe this to be so. In fact, as will be shown in the later section on the practical steps to defining concerns, I think that therapists should adapt themselves in just this way, and that this can be done without sacrificing integrity.

Is the client always right?

The client-centered or person-centered approach has been an influential one in counselling and psychotherapy. According to this approach, it is essential that the therapist adopts an attitude of positive and unconditional regard for the client. This means that the therapist respects the values of the client, and responds to the client's concerns. Lotty's husband, in the second illustration given previously (see p. 19), adopted a person-centered approach.

Client-centered therapists respond to the client's concerns, and avoid intruding their own. If clients were always able to articulate their preoccupying concerns, assuming that no barriers are put in their way by the therapist or the treatment situation, it might be expected that the client-centered approach would be the optimal one for psychotherapy – if, that is, client-centered therapy is as inoffensive in its emotional flavour as it might seem to be. But, of course, blandness may be quite as disgusting to some people as strong flavours are to others. For one thing, person-centered treatment may just not seem powerful enough to be effective (Shapiro, 1981).

However, putting the flavour of the treatment to one side, is it true that client-centered approaches are generally the most effective at identifying preoccupying concerns? So far as I know, there is little research evidence on this point. However, many psychotherapists, particularly those influenced by psycho-analysis, are of the opinion that no amount of facilitation will overcome an innate resistance to the declaration of what most concerns a person.

My experience is that the power of this resistance varies from person to person, and from situation to situation. Some people in almost all situations, and many people most of the time, are reasonably transparent. They are willing to express their concerns as soon as they feel that they are in a relationship where it is safe to do so. Other people may have a profound reluctance to betray deeply felt beliefs or emotions to anyone. People with emotional disorders, or people whom psychiatrists might consider to have personality disorders, are more likely to conceal their preoccupying concerns.

Most people seeking psychotherapy are preoccupied with a concern about a recent life event. They will have no deeper concerns to conceal. A short-term counselling or psychotherapy approach, which accepts their expressed concerns without trying to uncover 'deeper' interpersonal problems, will therefore be right for them. One such approach, sometimes termed 'problem-solving therapy' is a successful intervention for many emotional disorders in primary care (Catalan et al., 1991). It assumes that if a person can be helped to think about a problem in a new way, for example by considering a wider range of options, they can find a solution. It is not a criticism of the approach to point out that it also assumes that an emotional disorder is always something to be removed, that persistent and intrusive emotions are never guides to right action, but are only obstacles. Nor is it a criticism to point out that it assumes that everything a person apprehends about a situation, and their concerns within it, can be expressed in words.

It would be a criticism if problem-solving therapists did not recognize that there are clients who need something more. These are the clients who say, 'Yes, but . . .', or do not have any particular concerns, or who want to know what to do, or who just want to be happy or fulfilled. They are people who cannot put their concerns fully into words. A different operational policy will be needed for a service that deals with them, one that takes account of the salience of struggle or conflict in their lives.

Jill was in her 30s and was referred because of anorgasmia. She had been married for 9 years, and both she and her husband had busy jobs which often took him away from home. She has always loved horses, and most of her spare time was spent looking after and riding two ponies. Their sexual life had never been fulfilling to her, and she described herself as having a low sex drive. At the time of referral they had not had sex for 6 months. Jill was agreeable to her husband being involved in a modified Masters and Johnson approach (Bancroft, 1989), but although the therapist wrote to him asking him to accompany Jill, he rarely did. Sensate focus exercises were suggested, but the couple rarely found time to carry them out. More and more strains between Jill and her husband emerged as the therapy continued, but Jill refused to consider them as anything other than due to her lack of sexual interest. Eventually the therapist proposed to make appointments only when Jill could attend with her husband, and Jill agreed to ring to make the next one once she knew her husband's schedule. Nothing more was heard.

Jill's concern was with her lack of sexual drive, but the therapist became increasingly concerned with the quality of the relationship between Jill and her husband. Jill was, in the therapist's view, wilfully blinding herself to the obvious: that on her husband's trips away, he was finding sexual satisfaction with someone else. Or rather, Jill had concluded that if ever this possibility was explicitly addressed, the conflict between herself and her husband would be uncontainable.

Concerns as we tell them to others

Jill may have been frightened of the irresoluble nature of the conflict that openly expressing her concern about her husband's fidelity would engender. Her exploration of the concerns about her sexual life therefore reached an impasse when they raised a more wide-ranging concern about the quality of her marriage. (I consider in later chapters that there may have been other reasons for her rejection of the therapy, for example that it began to challenge some of her values, or that its flavour was becoming repugnant, or that the picture of herself that she was developing was not one which she wanted to accept.)

However, in presenting our concerns to ourselves, we undertake what Goffman called 'face-work' (Goffman, 1969). We edit and change our concerns so that they seem more acceptable, or more soluble. A simple example of this is the common observation that we explain other people's conduct by reference to their personality, but explain our own behaviour by describing the situations to which we react.

What applies to what we say to ourselves about our behaviour applies a fortiori to what we say to others about it. This is especially so in cultures where there are strong social norms.

Case example
Jaya's parents were from Pakistan, but she had been born in the UK. She had a serious weight problem which worsened every time her father tried to arrange a marriage for her. On one occasion, some years before she was referred to the psychotherapy service, she had returned to Pakistan for a betrothal service but had tried to hang herself before it had taken place. Or so she said, in one unguarded moment. She denied it later. As she did any criticism of her father, or the existence of a boyfriend whom she secretly hoped to marry but who her family thought was too poor. She has shown her psychotherapist a photograph of the boyfriend once, but denied even that later.

Jaya's social mores required her to obey her family in her choice of marriage partner. Hers was not a wilful personality and she genuinely wished to do so. But, so far as the psychotherapist could make out, she was in love with a man whom her parents had spurned and she was unwilling to give him up. She could not express this concern to her therapist, perhaps not even to herself. Her account of her life, as she presented it, was that she had a physical problem with her weight which made her unattractive to potential suitors, and her father wanted it fixed.

It must be expected in psychotherapy that a person is unable or unwilling to present their most troubling concerns immediately. It behoves the therapist to create a facilitative environment in which the client can gradually discover them. How to do this is the subject of the next chapters. However, it has already been noted that there may be reluctance for the client to consider what antecedent concerns might lie behind the presenting one. The therapist might come to think that a person is failing to be concerned about something to which she or he should really be alert.

I have already noted that there is no objective standard by which the therapist can say, 'This is a real concern'. Nor can the therapist often say, 'Evidence shows that . . .'. But it will often be the case that the therapist might think that they know what their client may really be concerned about, even though the client does not admit it. In the case of such a conflict arising, can therapists assume that they know when they are right?

Consensus or conflict between therapist and client?

A client once defined for me the difference between counselling and psychotherapy. 'Counsellors', she said, 'listen. Psychotherapists interfere'. I took it that by interference she meant the kind of conflict that was referred to in the last paragraph.

Counselling, particularly of the person-centered kind, proceeds on the assumption that, given a sufficiently facilitating environment, a person can reveal their preoccupying concerns to a skilled listener. Psychotherapy begins with the assumption that there will be conflict between the client and the therapist over what is revealed. Psycho-analytic psychotherapists formulate this conflict as occurring because clients resist giving expression to 'deep' or 'unconscious' concerns. Existential psychotherapists consider that some degree of self-deception is endemic in all of us as we compromise between the different poles of paradoxes inherent in the life-situations into which we have fallen. Other psychotherapists consider that there are ingrained misperceptions or habits which blinker the client.

Conflict about 'real' concerns, or 'real' motives, is almost always present in negotiations, and one or other party may articulate what they believe the other is concealing as a means to move the negotiation along. This may not always have the desired effect (see Chapter 10) in 'ordinary' situations although it is a standard tactic in psychotherapy.

Case example
Sylvia had a history of chaotic eating with episodes of weight loss, of deliberate

self-harm, and currently, of anxiety. She described her work as a primary school teacher, where she was known for her impeccable appearance and perform- ance. I asked if one of her concerns was that people never found out about her more chaotic, emotional side. She said that was true. I asked what happened when something in the lives of one of her pupils touched her greatly. She said that, although there were tragic family circumstances sometimes, she never allowed herself to become emotionally involved. I said that I was surprised that she was able to do that, and yet remain open to the children. She said that it had never been a difficulty. She loved her work. Later in the interview, she described her relationship with her fiancée. He was very kind to her, and she felt com- pletely accepted by his family. But there were times when she felt that he did not know her at all.

Sylvia herself was concerned about the two very different sides of her person- ality. She described how she never showed her 'out of control' side at work, and my saying that she was concerned that people never found out about this side of her was simply summarizing and reflecting back to her what she had said to me, although re-framing it as a concern. Later, I hinted at another concern – emotional isolation, and distance from others – which Sylvia did not accept but which, from previous knowledge of the consequences of splitting emotional life in this way, I thought would come back later in the therapy.

I believed, having spoken to Sylvia, that she was a passionate person who had, perhaps for family reasons, chosen to try to suppress her emotional side because she thought that it was bad or selfish. I presumed that one of her preoccupying concerns was to be taken by others as unselfish and rational, but that a deeper, concealed concern was to be accepted as the passionate person that she was.

What does my conversation with Sylvia, and my inferences from it, say about clarification? Firstly, there is a process of linking disparate concerns together. This is common to all expert enquiry. Secondly, there is a process of interpretation, that is uncovering a new meaning. Both of these processes occur in all therapeutic methods, even those that purport only to reflect back what the client says. However, they are strongest in psycho-analytically derived therapies, where the process of interpretation has acquired a status far beyond its everyday origins in dream interpretation. It sometimes seems that, to a psycho-analyst, interpretation is like reading a book written in a code that no-one else knows.

A misleading example
Sherlock Holmes's first case turned on a message so damning that it gave James Trevor a fatal stroke (Conan Doyle, 1981). The message was: 'The supply of game for London is going steadily up. Head-keeper Hudson, we believe, has been now told to receive all orders for fly-paper and for preservation of your hen-pheasant's life'.

Holmes gave two interpretations of this message. The first was obtained by breaking the code, and writing down the first word, and every subsequent third word. The encoded message was: 'The . . game . . is . . up . . . Hudson . . has . . told . . all . . fly . . for . . your . . life'. However, Holmes recognized that there was also a message in the words omitted from the coded instruction. These filler words were disproportionately drawn from field sports, and Holmes deduced that the sender of the message was therefore a landed gentleman, to whom words like 'head-keeper' and 'hen-pheasant' would readily come to mind. Were Conan Doyle to have commented on this passage, he might also have said that the message had an additional emotional meaning which arises from the connotations of many of the words used in it. 'Fly-paper' conjures up getting caught like a fly. 'Game', 'keeper', and 'pheasant' conjure up hunting, and being fattened up only to be shot in the end. 'Preservation' has the same connotation, but in addition means 'being preserved after death'. The use of all of these words gives the passage a scary feeling which adds to the eeriness of the story as Conan Doyle tells it.

This simple message therefore has three possible interpretations. There is the intended message which relates to the sender's understanding of the world, to his intentions. There is another message which says a lot about what interests him, what he values. And there is a further meaning which conveys the emotions of the sender to the reader.

Every communication has at least these three kinds of meanings. I deal with emotional meaning in Chapter 2, and with values in Chapter 3. However, even if we restrict our interpretation to what a person 'really' intends, we shall normally find that there is no deep intention encoded in a person's concern that could be revealed in the way that Holmes revealed the message to Trevor.

There is a good reason for this. People often do not have reasons for what they do, only causes. They perceive themselves as reacting to situations, rather than imposing their own goals on others. Within a situation, a person may have a goal. Sylvia was always smart and well-groomed at work because she thought that was what the situation demanded. She had goals related to this, for example to buy suits which were right for work. But she did not have an overall goal to split her life into two parts – one emotional and chaotic, and one coping. That just happened.

Although situations may cause a person to act as they do, they can find reasons for their actions in retrospect. And these reasons, once enunciated, influence future causal dispositions to act. However, there are many possible reasons that will fit one cause. Interpretation is about hitting on the right reason, but if there are many possible reasons, what can this mean?

Holmes knew that he had found the right interpretation because, as he remarked elsewhere to Watson, 'Watson, if you received a message which said, "Fly, everything is known", what would you do?' Holmes knew that

Trevor was a man with an uneasy conscience. If even Watson would be moved to uneasiness by the message, 'Fly, all is revealed', Holmes knew that Trevor would be crushed by it. Holmes therefore knew that his interpretation was right because the message it revealed clearly had the power to bring about what Holmes had observed to happen – that Trevor shot himself.

Even though interpretation is not like decoding a message, and the Holmes example is therefore misleading, the example does correctly indicate that rightness of interpretation is about supplying reasons for people's actions which increase the effectiveness of those actions. This is not without its ethical problems, neither for Holmes nor for the psychotherapist. Had Trevor been unable to interpret the message sent to him, and asked Holmes to do so, it is not clear to me what Holmes's most ethical course would have been. We know the consequences of the decoded message, but had Holmes refused to decode it, Trevor may have passed the next few days in false security until he was arrested, tried and hanged.

An example from industrial relations

In October 1999, Jaswir Tega had an argument with a foreman at the Ford car plant in Dagenham, in Greater London. He was shouted at and shoved by the foreman, who was white, and Mr Tega complained to higher management who decided not to suspend the foreman. Subsequently, some 1200 workers from the paint, trim and assembly sections at the Dagenham plant refused to return to work after the morning tea break. The action was continued by the night shift. It was the first mass walk-out at the plant in 10 years. Action continued until the CEO of Ford, Jacques Nasser, flew to London, and investigated the situation personally. He concluded that there was an unacceptable level of racism at Dagenham, and instituted corrective measures saying that he, too, had been a victim of racism. Mr Nasser also met one of the workers who had striven most against the racist culture in Dagenham, congratulating him on his stand and promising him the company's backing.

The workers at Dagenham probably had many concerns, as usually happens in a walk-out. What the CEO did was firstly to accept that their preoccupying concern was racism, and then to interpret the walk-out as a legitimate protest against it. This could not have been an easy interpretation to make, since the UK managers had indicated the myriad ways that Ford was already tackling racism and, by implication, the inefficacy and inadvisability of this particular protest. However, it helped that Mr Nasser identified with the racially harassed workers, and that he was independent of, and superior to, the local management team. As it turned out, there had been instances of racism that subsequently indicated the wisdom of his action. Dagenham had a very racist culture.

Clarifying the focus

Clarification first leads to the preoccupying concern, and then to the heart of the concern, its 'focus' (Balint, Ornstein & Balint, 1972). Other psychotherapy authors have used other terms, but with similar meaning. Balint stressed the circumscribed nature of the concern, originally introducing the term 'focus' as the main issue to be addressed in short-term analytic therapy (Balint et al., 1972). This term is now used by many brief psychotherapists. Malan (1979) defines the focus to be the conjunction of a hidden feeling or impulse with anxiety and with a particular defence and a particular person who elicits the feeling or the impulse. Hinshelwood has written of the 'point of maximum pain', to mean the apparent origin of a psychological disturbance. Luborsky has described the core conflictual relationship theme (Fried, Chrits-Christoph & Luborsky, 1992), and Beck the negative automatic thought. All are proposed as the points to which the client often recurs during therapy because of their importance to him or to her as stumbling blocks for the client, and as leverage points for change. In the next two chapters, we shall see that the focus might be an emotional meaning, or a value, but in this chapter, the concentration will be on focussing on actions which have failed.

Case example

Donald had lost his mother in his teens, and had then fallen out with his new stepmother. He had gone to live with his girlfriend and they were soon married. His early working and married life were interrupted by his developing tuberculosis. However, he was a hardworking man and he spent years of dutiful service as a gas fitter. Some 5 years before referral, his wife developed multiple sclerosis, and he developed a hiatus hernia. He was operated on and whilst he was in hospital, he was made redundant. He felt that he could not protest, but he developed further gastro-intestinal symptoms which were diagnosed as irritable bowel syndrome. At the time of referral, he could hardly leave the house because of his various gastro-intestinal complaints. His surgeon had, he thought, washed his hands of him and the psychotherapist was his last resort. There was an exaggerated and dramatic quality to Donald's symptoms, and it was easy to see why the surgeon had concluded that they were 'functional'.

Donald's preoccupying concern was with his pain and his borborygmi. Despite the various other difficulties that he had faced, and was facing, his symptoms preoccupied him completely. There was no question then about the preoccupying concern, but what should be the focus? Should it be his anger about the various losses that he had suffered through his life? Should it be his anxiety about his financial problems and his wife's health? Each of these foci has very different entailments. The former implies that Donald is right in concluding that the surgeon no longer thinks his symptoms have an organic basis, because they do not. The symptoms are somatized – 'depressive equivalents'. Focussing on the depression should relieve them completely. Focussing on anxiety does not rule out a physical problem, because anxiety and autonomic arousal might worsen gut dynamics. Moreover, it is a contemporary here-and-now focus, rather than a focus on the past. A focus on depression takes Donald's symptoms as a communication, and therefore an action. A focus on anxiety brings to the fore the way in which Donald has woven his symptoms into his actions.

These implications were not lost on Donald. In fact, he was exquisitely sensitive to the humiliating idea that he might be 'doing it himself'. Any suggestion of this had such an unpalatable emotional flavour that Donald would not only have rejected it, but rejected the whole treatment. The assessor was in a quandary. Having outlined some of the different ways of looking at the problem, he suggested that Donald keep a diary (see Chapter 7) and that a decision about the focus be put off until the next session.

At that session, the psychotherapist noticed in the diary that Donald had very unusual eating patterns. He would never eat when he was out, for example, and this meant that he would often go hungry for a whole day. On other occasions, when he was at home, he would eat a normal amount but would avoid any food that was bulky. The psychotherapist was, by this session, also more knowledgeable of the after-effects of the operation that Donald had had. It had many more side-effects than he had realized, and they were similar to those experienced by Donald. The psychotherapist began to think that Donald's exaggerated behaviour was due to his embarrassment about his symptoms, and that he had misled his previous medical advisors about their true severity. It was decided to make the symptoms the focus of treatment, and to discuss dietary and other measures which Donald could adopt to minimize them.

What is psychotherapy after all?

Many readers might protest at this conclusion of Donald's treatment. Surely it would have been much better carried out by a specialist nurse attached to the gastro-intestinal unit? The psychotherapist would have agreed with this too. Fortunately, he was medically qualified and had some experience as a general practitioner. Otherwise it would have been quite inappropriate for him to have made dietary recommendations. The fact that there was no-one else to undertake the treatment is a pragmatic justification, but it does not answer the question, 'Was this psychotherapy?'.

The quick answer is, 'No'. All the information that the psychotherapist had gained about Donald's personal experience – everything that he knew about the lousy deal that Donald had received – was all put to one side. The treatment intervention was diet and practical suggestion. However, the psychotherapist did use his skills in specific ways. Firstly, he was not taken in by Donald's exaggerated illness behaviour, like others had been. He did not assume that there was no illness. Secondly, his understanding of Donald's life enabled him to see why Donald would be so concerned to conceal his physical problems, and yet be so blind to the exaggeration of his symptoms that these attempts at concealment had caused. Donald hated confrontation. He did not stand up to his stepmother or his father, but left home instead. He did not protest the redundancy notice from his employers. He was not angry with the surgery which had left him so disabled. He did not want to talk about his symptoms or to have emotional discussions with others about them. He preferred to deny them. However, denying them led to him not just failing to manage them, but to their exaggeration in his attempts to conceal them. Coughing when his borborygmi were loud, for example. The mannered nature of the cough just drew attention to him even more – the very opposite of what he wanted.

It needs a psychotherapist to understand how a person might find themselves locked in a predicament, and then choose a course of action which appears to make matters worse for themselves. It needs an understanding of a person in the context of their personal world. Non-psychotherapists can easily assume that a person 'wants' to be the way they are. That it suited Donald to be 'ill'. Such formulations are born of the avoidance of anxiety in ourselves. It is hard to contemplate a series of contingencies that leads to the life that Donald led without fearing that something similar could happen to oneself. Each of us is insulated from such existential anxieties by the limits of our empathy. If that fails, there is always refuge to be taken in the thought that 'he must have brought it on himself'. But the obverse of the insulation of his friends and carers from Donald's situation was his isolation in it. It needed a psychotherapist's skill to be able to experience the world as Donald saw it without insulation, and to deal with the anxiety that was engendered in some other way.

Psychotherapy involves the application of the clarifying skills outlined in this chapter. But it also requires the ability to respect and work with the values of other people, and to enter into the other person's emotional world, however bleak or frightening. These skills are considered in the next two chapters.

2

Values

Psychotherapists sometimes seem unable to accept the simplest things without questioning them, or looking for hidden meanings. This is not because of an aversion to doing, although it may become linked to this, or because psychotherapists are odd or different. Psychotherapists are, however, committed to understanding other people in a more rigorous way than is usually the case. Psychotherapists all share this fundamental value, but they may be very different in some of the other values that they hold. These differences are considered in this chapter.

Values are important in psychotherapy because:
- Values determine identity
- They are the basis of ethical practice
- Good outcome depends on a compatibility of values between the therapist and the client

My values are me

Values are beliefs, often convictions, about what is right or good. Along with concerns and wishes, they constitute the 'me' that a person describes when someone says, 'Tell me about yourself' and they reply, 'Well, this is me: I hate racism, I love ice-cream, I want five children . . .' or 'I love Beethoven, fast cars, dogs and Rugby football. I hate sitting around, chatting and East Enders'.

People do not wear their values on their sleeves. In fact, it may be very difficult for some people to describe their values at all. Values have usually to be inferred from the client's discourse, which is more likely to be about plans, wishes or feelings.

One way that psychotherapists try to infer a person's values is to consider not only what someone has said, but why they have said it, and why at that moment. Doing this means putting the client's utterance 'in brackets' as phenomenologists would say. The process is comparable to the Biblical scholar who tries to set aside a twenty-first century understanding in order to reconstruct what the writer of St Matthew's Gospel meant when he wrote of Christ's 'resurrection'. Indeed, the term for this kind of biblical exegesis – hermeneutics – has also been applied to psychotherapy (Chessick, 1990).

Biblical scholars are concerned to know more about human reactions to the divine. Other proponents of exegesis, of looking 'behind' what is being said, have different concerns. Feminist or Marxist literary critics, for example, look 'behind' texts and other cultural manifestations to disclose the operation of power relationships between men and women, and capitalist and worker.

Psychotherapists, too, may be concerned about power relations, particularly when inadvertent psychotherapy practices perpetuate the domination of the client by the therapist, a state of affairs that is in neither's interests in the long term. However, when psychotherapists look behind what their clients say, they are often particularly concerned to find out the values that their clients have about therapy and, even more importantly, the values which determine the direction of their clients' lives.

Some of these values are so important that, if they are taken away, it leaves a person feeling as if they no longer know who they are, or what their identity is. Indeed, the brainwashing of American airmen captured in the Korean war consisted of systematically challenging and overthrowing the airmen's belief in America, in capitalism and in the love of their families (Lifton, 1989). Similar processes may operate in cults and in abusive families, and have the same destructive effect on identity.

'Helping'

Psychotherapy is sometimes counted as one of the helping professions. I have no hesitation in going along with this, if it means that psychotherapists seek to benefit their clients. Some psychotherapists would not accept this, arguing that even this modest statement implies that the psychotherapist exerts some sort of control over the therapeutic outcome. Their suspicion of the word 'help' derives from the values which it connotes, of doing or fixing or making good. When someone asks someone else for help, he or she implies a willingness to put him- or herself in the other person's hands, and that he or she values the hoped-for benefit more highly than the autonomy that he or she is sacrificing.

Levi-Strauss (1983) describes a traditional healing practice in Central America. This involved confining the ill person alone in a house until he or she was in a high state of arousal. The house would be surrounded by neighbours shouting encouragement. At a propitious moment, the healer would enter the house, bite the part of the victim's body which the healer thought was the location of the illness, leave the house again with 'the disease' in his mouth, and then spit it out on the ground outside in view of the neighbours. The healer would then announce that he had cured the illness.

Levi-Strauss particularly describes a healer, whom we might call Paco, who learnt his trade in one particular district where the healers bite a piece off a raw chicken before they enter the sick house. When these healers spat out the disease, they spat out the piece of chicken flesh, feathers and blood which they had carried in their mouths. Paco moved to a new area of Central America where the healers did not spit out bits of chicken, but he carried on doing this. It had a profound effect. He was hailed as a supreme healer who could actually demonstrate the real disease, whilst his colleagues only spat out saliva and blood, a very insubstantial disease altogether.

Paco became famous. Not only that, he cured more people than his colleagues. When Levi-Strauss heard about him, his successes were in the past, however. Paco had become disgusted by the deceit on which his healing was based, and refused to practise it any more.

Paco helped people more than his colleagues, but he duped them more comprehensively too. Paco did not quit because he discovered that his clients were worse as a result of his treatment than they would have been otherwise. He quit because he valued honesty over beneficence. His clients may not have shared these values. Neki has argued that in the Indian sub-continent, autonomy – the fundamental right which is abrogated by deceit – is less important than it is in the West (Neki, 1976). Perhaps this is also true in Central America, in which case the advantages of Paco's beneficence might have been considered, by those of his peers who adhered to a utilitarian ethical system, to have outweighed the disadvantages of his dishonesty.

Beneficence and respect for autonomy are two of the four values that many medical ethicists cite as fundamental, following their formulation by Beauchamp and Childress (1979). The other two are non-maleficence and justice. Applying these principles in practice may not be so easy. Particular difficulty is created by the potential conflict between respect for autonomy and beneficence which confronted Paco.

Roger had been married to Jean for over 16 years. After being in therapy for a year, he came to see that his marriage had never been fulfilling, and he parted from Jean.

Jo had been having blackouts for years. She would not lose consciousness but would suddenly 'come to' in some strange place. She had sudden mood changes, too, and on several occasions had contemplated suicide. She went into therapy when she was 19 years old, and her therapist asked her a good deal about her childhood. After the third session, Jo dreamt that she was lying on a bed and that a shadow drifted over her. She was paralysed and although she wanted to scream, no sound would come out. She had a stabbing pain in her genitals and then woke up. For a long while she could not work out where she was, thinking that she was back in her childhood. Following discussion with her therapist, Jo concluded that she had been sexually abused by her father when she was a child. She went home and confronted him, and in the ensuing quarrel, during which her mother took Jo's side, Jo's father, who was asthmatic, developed status asthmaticus.

Winifred had been in therapy for 3 years. She believed that her life had been improved out of all recognition by the therapy. She believed her therapist to be one of the great men of his generation. When she discovered that he had founded a trust to promulgate his teaching, she made a donation of £10 000 to it, with the request that her therapist should spend it in any way that he wanted.

It is conceivable that the therapist was helpful in all of these examples. Perhaps Roger and Jean thrived once they had separated. Maybe Jo's father, once his asthma was back in control, would admit that he had abused Jo and she could be freed of the shadow over her life. And maybe Winifred's therapist was a highly ethical practitioner who created a training fellowship for new students in her name, giving her an enduring sense of fulfilment. But it is equally possible that the outcome would have been much less obviously helpful. Roger might have discovered later that he had really loved Jean, but now there was no going back. Jo's family might have broken up without Jo ever really knowing whether she had been abused or not. Winifred, far from having a fellowship endowed in her name, might have had the mortification of seeing her therapist in a new car which she could not help but think was bought with her money.

It is clear that the beneficence of psychotherapists and counsellors is much harder to assess than that of other members of the helping professions. Indeed, as we have already noted, some psychotherapists are reluctant to consider themselves to be in the helping professions at all. In the absence of beneficence as a guide, respect for autonomy becomes the regnant moral principle. Most of us would be inclined to question the ethics of a therapist who had encouraged Roger to leave Jean, had suggested to Jo that her dream indicated that she had been sexually abused, or had told Winifred that, if she was grateful for her treatment, a cash donation would not be amiss.

One of the cornerstones of respect for autonomy is informed consent. It is tempting to think that applying this procedure makes a deeper consideration of values unnecessary. However, the very fact that clients are required to sign forms, or are given lists of side-effects and are asked to make decisions in relation to them, places a priority on some values over others. It is consistent with the values of conscientiousness, but not with humanity, with education but not with openness, with defensiveness but not with trust.

Truthfulness, honesty and effectiveness

Family therapists have recently embraced post-modernism. This strongly conveys the value that there can be no objective criterion of 'the truth'. This value, which readers might think has already found some echoes in this and earlier chapters, might seem to underlie and substantiate the value that parents, or society, may be held responsible for the difficulties of their children, or of individuals. For, if the post-modern approach is right, this is just one 'reading' of reality and is not at all inconsistent with parents believing that they have struggled hard to make something of their children, as most parents believe.

If there is no absolute truth, is it a problem for family therapists – and researchers – if parents think that they are being victimized by theories which seem to hold them responsible? After all, it is the parents who have misunderstood the situation. They have assumed that the truth of their way of looking at things is put in jeopardy by the truth of the experts' way of looking at matters.

There is something unsatisfactory about relativism of this kind. People generally come into therapy precisely because they wish to understand what they can do to make things better, not just for themselves, but for close others whose welfare is tied up with theirs. Establishing a consensus about a situation may be the first step for many people in resolving a predicament. For most people, the process of arriving at a consensus is not an arbitrary one. It is a process of establishing the truth for all to see.

Actually, the matter has been stated a little more starkly than it is. Everyone recognizes that there are many truthful statements that can be made about any particular situation. People say, when faced with this knowledge, not just, 'Tell me the truth', but 'Tell me the honest truth'. Honesty and truthfulness are not the same.

Mrs Evans had spent many years trying to discover what was wrong with her daughter. Eventually she found an expert who diagnosed the daughter as having an autistic spectrum disorder. This seemed to explain many things about her, and her mother was relieved. However, she then began to think of her husband. He, too, seemed a very egocentric man. The marriage had become increasingly dissatisfying to Mrs Evans over the years, and she now reflected on her husband's lack of success at work, and his lack of friends. Did he, too, have Asperger syndrome?

Mrs Evans persuaded her husband to see the same expert who had seen her daughter. The expert wanted to know why Mr Evans had come. What difference would it make if Mr Evans was diagnosed as having an autistic spectrum disorder himself? Mrs Evans said, truly, that knowing about her husband's difficulties in communication would help her to understand him better, and perhaps to get less angry with him if she realized that he could not help reacting as he did.

However, the expert wondered if Mrs Evans was being honest about her reasons. Although she was speaking the truth, the expert wondered if discovering that Mr Evans had an autistic disorder would not provide a reason for Mrs Evans to leave him, on the grounds that her husband had a disorder which placed such strain on his partner that it had become impossible to live with him.

Family therapists may, if they feel that the end justifies the means, also be 'economical with the truth'. A paradoxical injunction may be used in this way, with a client being advised to continue with a symptom that the therapist knows to be destructive in the hope that the client will rebel against the advice, and do the opposite. The shmaglotz, a healer in the community of Ethiopian Jews living in Israel, has a similar value when dealing with couples in conflict. Lies and dishonesty are justified if they enable the couples to reconcile (Sharon & Schwartzman, 1998).

It would be wrong to decide which value – truth, honesty or reconciliation – is the fundamental one. However, one of these values does need to be taken as absolute. In a western situation, as we have seen, truth is not an absolute value any more. Westerners no longer regard any relationship as indissoluble. It has too often been recognized that parties in conflict might be better off separating rather than staying together. Therapists in most cultures in the UK will be out of step with their clients and with society if they base their approach to dealing with conflictual predicaments on the assumed value that reconciliation will be the best solution.

Authority and pathology

Paco's colleagues, in the vignette above, seemed to value effectiveness over honesty. Mrs Evans valued the truth over honesty. However, both assumed that the therapist had a special authority which gave him the right to impose his scheme of understanding on his clients and their nearest and dearest.

Authority of this kind might be welcomed by the client who values fixed relationships between people based on their social position. For a client who feels oppressed by society's arrangement of power, the therapist's authority may be unwelcome or unacceptable.

One particularly important perquisite of authority in the mental health field is the right to pathologize.

Telling someone that they have a personality disorder, even more sending this verdict to a family practitioner, may have devastating consequences. The client may not just feel it is a false verdict, or that it is unfair to make such a judgement without offering a remedy. The client may reject the system of values which attributes their struggle with life to a disorder.

This discrepancy in values is clearly seen in the different ways that people view anxiety. Existentialism emphasizes the impossibility of living in the world without experiencing concern (Sorge) about it (Heidegger, 1927). These concerns lead to constant anxiety (Kierkegaard, 1960). Existentialists emphasize that having concerns, and experiencing anxiety, are not pathological states, but consequences of having opened one's eyes to life as it is. Other psychotherapeutic approaches suggest that concern is an indication of friction between different aspirations or emotions, and that clients should be encouraged to free themselves of concerns and their attendant anxieties. Psycho-analytic theory, for example, suggests that concern only arises from a discrepancy between the world that a person wishes for and the world that he or she experiences.

Commonsense psychology is equally divided. This is obvious if we contrast being careless with being care-free (Sorge is also commonly translated as care). Most of us want to be free of care without being careless. The contrast is perhaps more apparent than real. Heidegger had in mind the inevitable concerns of living, dying, loving and facing pain: what Jaspers called 'limit situations'. However, it is usually at moments of exceptional challenge that these concerns surface. Life is mostly frittered away in concerns about competing or overcoming particular people in particular situations. These are not 'limit' situations. It is easy to see that another person's concern to further their own projects at the expense of others is petty. It diminishes, rather than enhances, the stature of that person in our eyes. Concerns, and cares, of this kind we can clearly do without.

Mrs Williams had been known as a 'perennial neurotic'. She was repeatedly admitted to hospital for treatment of agitated depressive episodes, which were often triggered by relatively minor life events. On the admission when I looked after her, as a newly appointed psychiatry trainee, she unexpectedly developed bacterial meningitis, and nearly died. Following her transfer back from the general hospital, I found her strangely changed. She seemed much calmer. I asked her what had happened and she said, 'Well, you know that I nearly died. But I didn't. Compared with that, all the little things I worried about are so unimportant. I really don't know why I did used to worry so much about them'.

The everyday concerns that engage most of us are linked to our desires and our conflicts, as Freud, Lacan and others have argued. We interpret concerns as indicating where our life seems to pinch or pull at us, and we think that this indicates that something is wrong with our lives or with ourselves. We think of life as being full of cares and dream of a life without care. And this seems right. People who have not a single care in the world may seem admirable. But they are less admirable if one lives with them, because then it is apparent that not caring also means not caring for others, or what others hold dear.

If I lie awake being concerned about a client, I may imagine my next meeting with the client and think about what I will say if the client says, 'I don't seem to be any better, doctor'. Or, I might imagine standing in a coroner's court or meeting a family member, and thinking what I would say to the question, 'Why didn't you admit her when she said that she would kill herself'. My feelings during the course of these imaginings may be anxious or hopeless, but I am likely to judge them as appropriate to the situation. I may recognize that they have a purpose in drawing my attention to something which needs reflecting upon.

Ethics

Paco's story could be taken as one example of the many ethical dilemmas which face psychotherapists. Many better examples exist, however, and interested readers might, for example, consult Holmes and Lindley (1995), or look at the web-page for the course on ethical and legal issues in the behavioural sciences at Antioch University (http://college.antioch.edu/~dfriedman/ssc300a.html).

This chapter is not about ethics. It is about the interaction between values and concerns. Values are easy to overlook in one's own culture, hence the use of a Central American example. In fact, one of the principal challenges of cross-cultural psychotherapy is to accommodate the different values of client and therapist. Further consideration will be given to this later in the chapter. For now, the main issue is that the people of Levi-Strauss's story valued a healer who could remove the disease, and valued a healer even more highly if what caused the disease was made manifest. We can infer that these people did not value autonomy so highly. Their explanations of disease contained no references to their own previous actions. Nor did they consider that slighting some dangerous adversary, such as a witch or an ancestor, could cause disease. Nor did they value knowledge. They did not want to know much about the illness, or about different kinds of illnesses. However, they were willing to give the same value that our culture accords to entertainers or sports people to a healer who could bite out their diseases.

One might suppose that healing techniques used in other parts of the world would not be so highly valued in Central America. Pilgrimage, for example, would give the individual too much autonomy. Drinking decoctions of scriptures – a popular remedy in all parts of the Islamic world – would have little value in a pre-literate culture. Exorcism might be more successful, although the lack of privacy involved in the removal of the disease and the fact that the disease agent was spiritual rather than physical might make this a less highly valued option.

It will be clear to the reader that every healing method incorporates values. One of the points of this chapter is that these values have to be congruent with the values of the client if the client is to participate wholeheartedly. The Levi-Strauss story also makes a second important point: that the values of the healer, too, need to be congruent with the healing method. In the story, the migrant healer valued honesty more highly than the relief of suffering, and was willing to deprive future clients of the latter in order to feel secure in the former. In the language of medical ethics, the healer placed a higher value on autonomy (which is diminished by deceit) than on beneficence (Gillon, 1994). In doing so, he was at variance with his clients who, as their attitude to illness suggests, valued beneficence highly, but placed little value on autonomy. This discrepancy between the values of the healer and of his clients exemplifies a third major point to be considered in this chapter. What should the psychotherapist do if her or his values are discrepant with those of the client? Should one or other change their values and, if so, who, and how far?

Congruence of values

Empirical research indicates that therapists whose values are moderately similar to their clients are more effective than therapists who have different values. However, this statement conceals a complex picture. Some values are not relevant to outcome: sexual morality, for example, and probably political convictions. Other values are of particular importance to a few people. Most important amongst these is religious persuasion. Clients with strong religious principles expect that the values of the psychotherapy should be consistent with them, and will reject a psychotherapeutic approach that is not.

Clients' values do change during treatment too. Clients may become more open or more tolerant, for example. But there are certain values which are sticking points, on which there needs to be a consensus without which treatment cannot continue successfully. These are values that cannot be changed without a person feeling that they themselves are being so fundamentally changed that their social existence is in question. These are the values that constitute 'me', which have been discussed in an earlier section.

The client's treatment values

Clients will have values which determine the kind of help that they want. Some clients will value being fixed up much more highly, for example, than exploring deeper issues. Other clients will have quite different values. These are values which are linked to particular preoccupying concerns. The order of the chapters in the later part of this book has been arranged to reflect some of these values, which are:
- Gaining relief
- Finding out what's doing this to me

- Changing something about me
- Finding happiness

Implicit in these concerns are other values, which are considered in each chapter. They include how highly the past is valued over the present, whether sharing something with a group diminishes people or enhances them, and whether a problem arises because of a situation or because of something that the person has done. This last value is linked to how people perceive themselves in many situations. In the psychological literature, it is referred to as the 'locus of control'. Clients are said to have an external locus of control if they consider that someone or something else holds the control over their life difficulties. Therapy that alters a person's ability to deal with, or cope with, external difficulties is said to be directed towards an external locus of control. Having an internal locus of control means that a person believes that their difficulties are due to failings in their own efforts or understanding. Therapy that seeks to change a person's beliefs or some other characteristic is directed towards an internal locus of control. Clients have higher expectations of a therapy approach which is congruent with their perceived locus of control, whether or not this is internal or external (Foon, 1986).

Very little of what happens in therapy is value-free. A therapist who is flexible in his or her therapeutic arrangements, for example seeing clients in the evenings or at weekends, or conducting therapy over the phone or using the internet, may have values which are congruent with clients who value modernity or efficiency. But other clients may consider that this flexibility implies that the therapist does not value their private life, or undervalues human contact, and will be put off.

3

What life means. Emotional flavour

Just as we swallow food because we like it not because of its nutritional content, so do we swallow ideas because we like them and not because of their rational content (Asher, 1972)

This chapter sets out in more detail the third of the four ruling ideas in this book. Concerns and value have already been considered. The next two chapters deal with narrative. This chapter deals with what might be less familiar concepts, emotions and emotional flavours, and emotional meanings.

An emotional flavour is the capacity for something, a familiar object or a close other person for example, to induce a particular emotion in us. I shall call the something an emotor to avoid having to spell out all the different things that can induce an emotion. Emotors induce emotions without going through the appraisal stage. They plug straight into the emotion brain. They acquire their emotive capacity by associative learning, and I shall give examples of this below, but we experience them as having this capacity inherent in them. If I see a body, covered in blood, lying on the road, I might think, 'a road traffic accident', and I may start to work out how I feel about stopping to help, but long before that, I will have felt horror, fear, compassion and other more idiosyncratic emotions. If I am with a trained paramedic who has seen this sight many times before, he might say, 'It happens every day. What are you getting so upset about? You know the statistics for accidents along this road'. But I would be inclined to reply, 'Just look at all the blood', as if nothing else was needed for the emotions to be aroused in me but looking, for the emotions were inherent in the body lying there.

Flavours are apprehended without words, as moods or feelings. But, like other moods or feelings, they demand an explanation. This explanation will usually be an account of why the emotor has the flavour that it does, that is an account of the emotional meaning of the emotor. My account of why I feel such strong feelings about seeing the victim of a road accident might be, 'I often cycle along this road. I'm imagining that it's me lying there, not him'. The emotional meaning of the accident would therefore be, 'It could have been me'.

Why give emotions such importance? What about relationships?

The reader may have noticed that relationships, including the therapeutic relationship, have often been referred to, but relationship is not included as a ruling concept. Relationship theory is a substantial area in psychology, and it has been proposed as a theoretical basis for psychotherapy (Derlega, et al., 1992). Unfortunately from the point of view of the psychotherapist, the dominance of social-exchange theory and its derivatives has tended only to consider how the parties in a relationship are maximizing their rewards, and minimizing their costs. It does not account for the 'emotional' or 'irrational' behaviour which seems so important in ordinary human interaction and in psychotherapy. Relationship theory has diversified much more in recent years to take in naturalistic studies, conflict theory (Gottman, 1999) and attachment theory (Bartholomew, 1997). The latter are touched on briefly elsewhere in this book.

Scheff has argued persuasively for a richer sociology (Scheff, 1997) which takes account of social integration. He (Scheff, 1990) considers that every social interaction involves communication, often mediated non-verbally, about what he calls the 'social bond'. He suggests that '. . . human behaviour is determined in large part by activities relevant to the bond . . .' (ibid., p. 179). In particular, the social bond is the prerequisite of any relations within the primary group. Two families of emotions are particularly important in ensuring that social bonds remain strong: the shame family (shame, humili- ation, ridicule and embarrassment) and the pride family (in which I will include its inverse, disgust). It is interesting to note that psychotherapists, too, make frequent use of this adhesive metaphor. Psychotherapists suppose that people have an innate stickiness which 'bonds' or 'attaches' them to other people and which results in aggregations of people becoming 'cohesive'.

Shame or disgust constrain relationships in ways that are of particular importance in psychotherapy. I think that they provide a better window on the therapeutic relationship than to study it directly, at least using the current theories of social relationship. This is the reason that I have made social emotions, and not relationships, one of the fundamental concepts in this book.

Shame and disgust

Shame has been relatively neglected by psychotherapists before Lewis's work, although Fairbairn's (1946) formulation of the schizoid personality seems to be based on shame, even though it is not specifically mentioned by him. At first sight, pride has been far from neglected. Esteem, and particularly self-esteem, is one of the most commonly cited concepts in explaining clients' problems. However, what therapists usually mean by self-esteem is what people think about themselves. What Scheff is proposing is a formulation about feelings in relation to other people: feelings which are engendered by the extent to which another person is approved or rejected by others.

In a paper on one of the founders of object-relations theory, the Scottish psycho-analyst Fairbairn, which I wrote before I became familiar with Scheff's work, I supposed that Fairbairn's complex theory about internal relationships could be replaced by an interpersonal theory of shame and disgust (Tantam, 1996a). There is an obvious parallel with Scheff's formulation.

Shame and disgust are contagious emotions. If one person feels them, they cannot help displaying them, and this display induces shame, embarrassment or disgust in others. Ricks describes the effect that this had on John Keats, the poet. Keats, like other people with social phobia, was exquisitely sensitive to embarrassment. If he was in a party and someone else in the room became rowdy or drunk, causing embarrassment to those around him, Keats would perceive it even if his own companions did not. He would blush, become unable to carry on a conversation, and sometimes would have to leave (Ricks, 1976).

Something of this sensitivity is captured in Keats's poem, 'Endymion', in which the eponymous hero goes on a journey led by various nymphs and spirits, in search of love.

> At last, with sudden step, he came upon
> A chamber, myrtle wall'd, embowered high,
> Full of light, incense, tender minstrelsy,
> And more of beautiful and strange beside:
> For on a silken couch of rosy pride,
> In midst of all, there lay a sleeping youth
> Of fondest beauty; fonder, in fair sooth,
> Than sighs could fathom, or contentment reach:

There follow many lines of voluptuous praise of this sleeping youth, who is the inamorato of Venus. Endymion's reaction to this gorgeous boy is to become 'breathless' and 'impatient with embarrassment'. Fortunately, the Cupids who are stationed around the youth's bed are able to reassure Endymion, something one supposes that Keats's medical student friends did not do in real life.

The delicacy of manners which Keats typifies was an important contributor to the 'refinement' of society and ultimately to the kind of inhibitedness that Freud discovered in *fin-de-siècle* Vienna. But, as Scheff indicates, these emotions play a part in every society and in every relationship.

Psychotherapy relationships are no exception. Scheff quotes extensively from the work of Lewis (1975), who analysed 100 therapy sessions, and concluded that shame is rarely overt in these sessions but is one of the most important factors in determining the bond between the therapist and the client. Shame may also adversely affect the supervisory relationship (Talbot, 1995). This is a perspective on the therapeutic relationship that is only just beginning to be discussed by clinicians (Kaufman, 1996) and social psychologists (Tangney, Burggraf & Wagner, 1995).

One of my PhD students conducted a study of patients in long-term psychotherapy in an NHS service (Macdonald 1999) and found that being preoccupied with shame was often associated with lack of progress in therapy. In an extension of this study in another service, he showed that revealing shameful experiences to a partner or parent was not necessarily helpful. Sometimes the partner would respond with further shaming (see p. 33). This finding is consistent with other studies which show that it may be other people's reaction to something bad happening to oneself that causes the most long-term damage. For example, women who have been raped may be held responsible by their friends or family, and this may make the trauma worse. This is more likely to happen if the woman is already numbed by the shock of what has happened (Winkel & Koppelaar, 1991).

This has implications for us as therapists. To do our job well we have to be able to work with shame without adding to it, and without rejecting someone more.

Emotions as a guide

It may have been the enlightenment that introduced into western culture the notion that emotions are dangerous because they disrupt rational decisions (Oatley, 1992). Whatever its origins, it seems to be a prevalent concept which has coloured attitudes to emotions in mental health. Psychiatrists and psychologists, and psychotherapists perhaps to a lesser extent, are inclined to judge strong emotions as excessive and to consider them as disorders. However, another way to look at strong emotions – a way that values subjective experience more highly than social conformity – stresses the importance of emotions as way markers. Anxiety for an existential psychotherapist, for example, is not an obstacle to be overcome but may instead be an indication of a preoccupying concern which directs attention to a life problem.

Psycho-analytic approaches to emotions have tended to be suspicious of unbridled emotion, too. Psycho-analytically orientated psychotherapists consider anxiety to be the mental equivalent of pain, and redefine other emotions as wishes, drives or impulses which have been banished to the unconscious and where repression should continue to confine them. Some psychotherapists have reacted against this and developed therapies like primal scream therapy, which placed a strong emphasis on emotional expression. The more intense the emotion a person expressed, the more valuable the therapy was thought to be. However, these approaches shared with psychoanalytic approaches the prejudice that emotion was something to be eliminated.

Sartre (1971) wrote a short but powerful book on emotions. He was critical of psycho-analysis and, particularly, of the notion that there was an unconscious mind with its own motives and intentions. He saw emotions as a kind of appraisal, an approach that now dominates emotion theory. 'I am frightened', he wrote, 'because I feel the dark, sinister passage around me, not because I am conscious of myself having a state of fear. I am not therefore mindful of being frightened until something directs my consciousness to my state of mind – but I am certainly aware of what is making me frightened, and this consciousness enters into my purposes as I try to get out of the passage as quickly as possible. I may not be conscious of myself when I am very frightened, but I am certainly conscious of the object of my fear'.

Sartre therefore supposed that we are often not conscious of our feelings, not because they are repressed, but because emotions are part of a background of mental processing (Searle, 1983). What emerges from this background are the objects of the emotion. Getting home safely if we are anxious. Gaining the upper hand if we are angry. It is only if these objects are blocked that we become aware of our feelings or our bodily sensations and in that way become conscious of our emotion. So to return to the example of the scary passage, I may be aware of a certain tautness, a certain focus on getting through it as soon as possible. I may look fearful, but I might not feel frightened until I find the end of the passageway blocked, so that I cannot get out.

A consciously felt emotion is therefore an indication that an object is out of reach, that a plan has been frustrated. This may explain why the failure of plans and emotionality are often associated. Not because emotionality causes plans to fail, but that the failure of plans is associated with emotionality.

This is not to say that emotionality cannot become an end in itself. Sartre also described the situation when a person feels blocked because his or her world does not seem to offer a way forward. People may, according to Sartre, use emotion as a way of magically re-making the world in this situation.

All the authors mentioned in this section shared one idea about emotions: that we rarely become aware of them. This is not necessarily because they are deliberately hidden. The fact is that emotions are apparent to us by their effects, and not by their emergence as feelings in the sensations of which we are aware. Emotions have the effect of orientating attention, prioritizing our concerns, maintaining our social bonds with other people, and, in general, serving as a guidance system.

Oatley defined emotion as 'mental state of readiness for action . . .

normally based on an evaluation of something happening that affects important concerns' (1992, p. 20).

Different people have different dispositions to different emotions, depending on their emotional history. Frijda et al. (1991) have subdivided dispositions into categories like sentiments, passions (used more narrowly than Hume used the word), moods, emotions, and so on, depending partly on their duration. Frijda et al. stress that a person's profile of emotional responses will include slowly changing tendencies to prefer one long-term goal over another as well as the short-lived emotional reactions which are the most obvious manifestations of emotion.

Rationalists' suspicions of emotion become particularly sharp when it comes to people following their heart rather than their head. Notwithstanding this, experience in psychotherapy suggests that, in practice, people do use their emotions as guides at least in relation to the following:
• How to act when plans fail
• Maintaining the social bond
• Making decisions, particularly ethical decisions
• Answering the question, 'Who am I?'

How to act when plans fail

There are moments in life when normality suddenly seems to be disrupted. Sudden bereavement is one example. Scruton quotes Emily Dickinson's description of unexpected bereavement as 'awful leisure' as an example. Emotion scripts guide people when they confront such a caesura (Averill, 1980).

Anya had lost her grandfather. He was 90, and she was 35. She told herself that it was only to be expected. Her mother dealt with the funeral arrangements, and Anya shed a few tears but thought no more about it. She continued working as an oncology registrar, with no break. Her job was a busy one, and she seemed even busier as time went on. At first she put down the fact that she seemed to be at a loose end when she did get home to tiredness. But it got worse and worse. She would come in, make herself a meal, switch on the television and just vegetate. She had no interest in going out or meeting new people. Her boyfriend told her that she was no fun any more, and their relationship gradually attenuated. The crisis came when Anya took 2 weeks' leave, intending to go abroad. But she could not work out where to go or what to do and she ended up just sitting about at home.

Anya went to see her family doctor, who told her that she was not depressed, but did refer her to the practice counsellor. The counsellor asked Anya if she was grieving for her grandfather. Anya found tears welling up and began to talk about what he had meant to her. The counsellor suggested that Anna may need to mourn her grandfather. Had she visited the grave? Did Anya have any photographs of her grandfather?

Anya thought a lot about her grandfather after she got home. He had been a distinguished oncologist himself, in the days before there was much treatment available other than radical surgery and faith in the specialist. She decided to write his obituary and find out whether a journal would print it. Research on the obituary comprised about a month of interviews, and looking through her grandfather's papers. At the end of that time, she really felt that she deserved a holiday, and booked herself one for as soon as she could next take leave.

Oye's family went to a healer saying that Oye was possessed. Ever since his father had died, he had stopped working and just wandered around with no apparent direction. He did not answer immediately when people spoke to him, and sometimes did not recognize people. The healer said that he must have offended his father, and that now his father's ghost was haunting him. He had probably not performed the funeral rights properly, and the healer recommended a visit to all the shrines in the region, making a sacrifice at each one. Oye took the advice and visited three shrines. At the third, he told the priest that his father's spirit had left him. So he returned home and went back to work.

Oye and Anya had both found themselves at a loss as a result of a bereavement. Both of them were pointed towards the need for mourning and both recovered their emotional investment in their own lives once their grieving had been completed.

Maintaining the social bond

Thinking what to do in a situation often involves anticipating how others will react to it, and how it will affect our social bond with them. If they would be ashamed of us or disgusted by our action, we are very likely to think twice before doing it. To the extent that our judgement about other people's reactions are sound, we need never fear being shunned by others if we modify our behaviour according to these anticipations.

A person might sometimes explicitly imagine what someone else – their mother or father, say – would say or do if they knew how their son or daughter had acted. More often than not, though, it is another emotion – anxiety – that acts as the guide. Anxiety, often termed 'guilt' in this context, is a reaction to the risk of discovery.

Jean-Jacques Rousseau stole a ribbon when he was a child, and blamed the maidservant. He writes in his Confessions that: 'When she appeared I was agonized, but the presence of so many people was more powerful than my compunction. I did not fear punishment, but I dreaded shame: I dreaded it more than death, more than the crime, more than all the world . . .'.

It is a fortunate person whose shame and guilt responses are tuned to the norm. Many clients seeing psychotherapists are too shame-prone, and a few too shameless. Sometimes they can be a mixture of both.

David was a good driver in many ways. If he had faults, they were mainly of over-conscientiousness. He would never drive above the speed-limit, even one mile an hour above it. He obeyed every road sign. If he missed one, he was immediately ashamed. He was sure that he would be arrested. However, if he saw a crane, he would turn his head and stare at it, even if it meant that he continued driving with his eyes off the road. Cranes fascinated David. He thought of them as strong and good. He could not imagine that anything connected with cranes could be bad, and was quite unaware how odd his fascination seemed to other people and how embarrassing it could be.

David was unusually sensitive to criticism and to being shamed. He obeyed the law rigidly, almost slavishly, as a result. But when he saw a crane, he lost all his inhibitions, and seemed to be lacking any sense of embarrassment or shame.

Shame, and pride, are experienced fully when a person is self-aware and when they can evaluate their success or failure at a socially defined task. However, their roots probably begin very early on in family life, before the child has language at all (Barrett, 1998).

From about the age of 2 years to the age of 5, children are acquiring a 'theory of mind'. Before this age, children assume that everyone knows what they know (Kagan, 1982). Children without a theory of mind cannot feel fear that they will be discovered and shamed, because they will assume that everyone else will know what they have done. (The reader should note here that the review cited in the previous paragraph by Barrett (1998) leads her to the opposite conclusion. She thinks that pride and shame are mainly about self-as-object, and guilt about self-as-agent. This may partly reflect the fluid boundaries between conceptions of guilt and conceptions of shame.) Guilt – the fear of discovery – therefore develops some time after the child starts to react to shame and guilt. Deception and pretence, too, require a theory of mind (Leslie, 1987). So at the same time as the child is developing guilty anxiety about being discovered in some wrong-doing, and shame, the child is developing the distinction between what they tell other people – their 'me' – and what they know themselves – their 'I'.

The distinction between shame reactions and guilty anxiety corresponds broadly to the differences between psycho-analysts who belong to the object-relations school and those who follow Freud. Klein, Fairbairn and also Margaret Mahler concentrated on identity problems which they thought developed from the child's earliest experiences: the period during which shame and disgust are developing. Freud concentrated on the Oedipal period, and the child's fear of retaliation: this corresponds to the period during which the consequences of a theory of mind are being worked out.

The differentiation between shame and guilt anxiety also corresponds to a distinction made by psychologists with a very different persuasion, for example Kagan. He suggests that there are two dimensions of anxiety-proneness: behavioural inhibition, which is partly temperamental and emerges in the second year of life, and self-blame (Kagan, 1994). Internalizers – those who elsewhere in this book are described as having an internal locus of control – blame themselves for things that go wrong. Externalizers blame others.

Richard was, and always had been, deeply Christian. He was very happily married with six children. When asked how he came to have so many, he got embarrassed. He said that neither he nor his wife believed in birth control. His problem was that he had become afraid that his sperm might leak out and contaminate the surroundings. He imagined that his oldest daughter might get pregnant because she used a towel that he had used. At his worst, he was afraid to post letters in case his sperm was transmitted through the post and fertilized a female correspondent.

Richard was rapidly and effectively treated with cognitive therapy. The approach taken was to tackle his assessment of the risk that someone could be passively fertilized, and Richard quickly saw that he need have no fear that this would happen. He was not ashamed of his sexuality fundamentally, and once his guilt had dissipated he had no further problems. Richard was an internalizer, but he was not inhibited in Kagan's terms.

Roger was a young man of average intelligence who had some difficulties in expressing himself verbally. His speaking had been delayed and he had required speech therapy. There were considerable class and other social differences between his parents. His father was Italian, for example, and had been a dry-cleaner, although for most of Roger's childhood he had successfully pursued a new career as a golfing coach. During his early adolescence, Roger had adopted a lifestyle which was completely at variance to his father. He had got into some trouble with the police, hung around with people that his parents felt were undesirable, and gave up golf, which he had played since an early age. Then his father had become ill. Roger became constantly anxious, tried on one occasion to kill himself, and became preoccupied that he had the same illness as his father. He became increasingly monosyllabic, and his mother began to think that he had a psychotic illness. Roger told her nothing about his anxiety, and nothing about his regret that he did not realize how much he loved his father until after his death.

At interview, Roger's voice and face were inexpressive except that his forehead would briefly, but regularly, corrugate with a tense frown, and his nose would wrinkle with an evanescent expression of disgust. He spoke of not wanting women to see him undressed in case they commented on his lack of development. Recently his friends had called him a 'poof', and he told the psychiatrist that talking about his feelings would only reinforce them in that opinion. He blamed his mother for not understanding him.

Roger had been unable to communicate to his mother that he had felt ashamed of his origins, and that he now felt ashamed of himself. In fact, he had stopped communicating to his mother at all. She had worried that he was becoming psychotic and, unwittingly, had shamed him further. All of this had led to an increasing spiral of behavioural inhibition, but Roger did not hold himself to blame for this. He blamed his mother.

The differences in the case of Roger and Richard show how important it is to differentiate shame and guilt. It is not necessarily the age of onset of the emotional difficulty that matters. Roger became ashamed as he got older. Nor are there hard and fast criteria, although Klein was right, I think, in differentiating suspicious, hostile or over-sensitive reactions to the world (consequences of shame or disgust, I would say) from the depression that is a consequence of self-blame.

Shame may be particularly manifest as shyness about one's body or disgust with one's body (Andrews, 1995). I do not think that Andrews is right in supposing that this type of shame is always linked with childhood abuse. Roger was categorical that he had not been abused, for example. But it may be more common in those who have some infirmity which they find digusting as well as in those who have been disgusted at their bodies being abused sexually.

Shame or disgust may be apparent in behavioural inhibition, or in microexpressions like the nose-wrinkling of Roger, the nose-touching of embarrassment, or easy blushing. Gaze avoidance may indicate shame or guilt too. However, there is no easy means of detecting either of these emotions in many people. We do, after all, try to conceal them as much as we can.

Shame scales (Tangney et al., 1996) and questionnaires do exist but they are rarely appropriate in a clinical setting. What it is important to remember is that shame, or self-disgust, always has three elements:
- Negative appraisal by important others
- An acceptance of this negative appraisal by the self
- Resulting in an impulse to hide

Making decisions, particularly ethical decisions

The philosopher David Hume scandalized his contemporaries by asserting that 'all morality depends on our sentiments; and when any action, or quality of the mind, pleases us *after a certain manner* we say it is virtuous; and when the neglect, or non-performance of it, displeases us *after a like manner*, we say that we lie under an obligation to perform it' (1748, p. 517). Hume was not arguing for hedonism or for the relativism of morality, although it may seem like that. He presumed that there are 'natural sentiments of humanity' such as the love of a father for his children. He presumed that there are many relations between people which are of mutual benefit, and that these are motivated by self-interest. 'But tho' this self-interested commerce of men begins to take place, and to predominate in society, it does not entirely abolish the more generous and noble intercourse of friendship and good offices. I may still do services to such persons as I love, and am more particularly acquainted with, without any prospect of advantage . . .' (ibid., p. 522).

The linking concept for Hume is sympathy. 'My sympathy with another may give me the sentiment of pain and disapprobation, when any object is presented, that has a tendency to give him uneasiness . . .' (ibid., p. 586). There have been many critiques of Hume over the last 200 years, notably that of Kant, but his views continue in currency. Williams (1972), for example, considers that Hume's system contains 'many interesting and valuable things', sympathy being one of the most interesting.

Even if Hume's system is not complete, as Williams concedes, it demonstrates the importance of the contribution of emotions to moral judgement. Once again, it is the social judgements of shame and disgust that are particularly important. The correct application of these judgements is so important that it is regularly practised. People gather at the site of a tragic accident, or become gripped by a crime that achieves notoriety, and in doing so rehearse their own disgust or condemnation. This may have the effect of strengthening the feeling or, sometimes, tempering it with pity or compassion.

One other faculty that is rehearsed at these times is sympathy. It may be increased, as people vicariously share in the loss of a national figure or the death of a child, and it may be diminished. Requests to withhold sympathy may be part of the official reaction to tragedy, as when a Home Office minister indicates that a bombing is the work of an animal. Animals have diminished rights to sympathy. Redefining a human being among them is one way of managing otherwise disgusting or shameful behaviour (Midgeley, 1979).

This is specifically important in working with people who lack empathy, especially those whose sympathy has become abnormally restricted as a result of deviant socialization (Tantam, 1995a).

Darren had what he euphemistically termed an 'old-fashioned' father. Whenever Darren cried or was upset, his father would get angry, calling him a 'wimp' or a 'nancy boy'. If Darren didn't stop, his father would say, 'I'll give you something to cry about' and would punch him as hard as he could. Gradually

Darren learnt to harden his feelings, but by this time his younger brother, Elliot, had been born. Elliot also got the old-fashioned treatment but with the modification that he was told, 'Why can't you be a bit more like Darren instead of the snivelling little runt that you are'. Darren got quite a kick out of this, and felt that he was a hard case unlike other softies like his brother. Darren began to bully Elliot too, and later to bully other boys at school. He discovered that he positively enjoyed the feeling of fear on the faces of softies, although he was careful to treat his small group of hard-case friends rather differently.

Darren's normal sympathetic reaction to the distress of other boys had been suppressed by his father. Darren learnt to treat hard boys as human beings, deserving of consideration, and other boys as softies, whose pleas for mercy elicited no sympathy from him.

Darren would have run the risk in the early part of the eighteenth century of being diagnosed as a moral imbecile but it's not necessary to have an anti-social personality to have subtle abnormalities of sympathy. These abnormalities contribute to the difficulties that many people have in making close relationships, including people with a highly developed sense of morals.

Norma had a neighbour of her own age to whom she had taken quite a dislike. She seemed so 'down in the mouth' the whole time. She never wanted to talk. The few times that Norma had tried to be nice to her, and invite her around, the neighbour, whose name was Mae, had refused.

Mae's name came up in the group during a discussion of neighbourliness. William, who was a bit down in the mouth himself, asked Norma about Mae's family. Norma said, 'It's funny you should ask that. I knew that she has two boys. They seem almost as miserable as her. But I just found out the other day that she lost her daughter a year or so ago from meningitis and her husband left her afterwards. I'm not surprised either. I couldn't imagine living with her'. There was a gasp in the group. Bernadette said, 'How could you say that? The woman has had two terrible tragedies in her life. Wouldn't you be miserable if that happened to you?'. Norma, who was infertile, began to cry. Other members of the group chipped in, and Norma began to talk about Mae in a very different way.

It seemed to the conductor that Norma had no sympathy with Mae because she envied her the children (later in the group, Norma talked about her depressed mother and the conductor revised her judgement about the reasons for Norma's intolerance of Mae). She had cut herself off from Mae's feelings, and was only aware of the direct effect that Mae had on people around her. As the group aroused her sympathy, she was able to experience how Mae herself felt, and instead of being contemptuous of Mae she became sad for her.

Who am I?

Put a spot on the nose of a child and then place them in front of a mirror. Most children who are at least 15 months old touch their noses. Most children younger than 15 months do not (Amsterdam, 1968). This is commonly taken to be the first definite indication that children recognize themselves, a defining moment not just for cognitive psychologists but for psychotherapists like Lacan who considered the specular image to be the foundation of the self. But the self to which Lacan refers is, as we shall discuss in more detail in Chapter 5, the self that is presented to other people, the 'me', the 'self-as-object', as it was termed earlier in this chapter.

Children before the age of 15 months have an identity that is not merely a bodily or a social identity. Fond parents might say, 'she's very quick' or 'he's a bit sensitive' long before the child can recognize her- or himself. These are attributions to the self-as-agent, to the narrator of the self-narrative, not to what is narrated, the 'I'.

Glover has summarized some of the shortcomings of the commonsense notions about 'I'. One of his conclusions is that 'people are more fragmented, or at least more of a federation, than we usually think' (Glover, 1988, p. 107). This view would be shared by many psychotherapists who have come to believe that their clients have plural selves. Glover argues that no test of what 'I' is stands close scrutiny. It is an indexical, like 'here' or 'now', and like 'here' and 'now', does not stand for a particular thing.

Glover attributes the tenacity of the concept of 'I' to the wish to experience oneself as an integrated whole. This experience is tied up with experiencing oneself as an agent.

Hamid had been in a therapy group for about a year. He was referred because of his sudden rages, which were often directed at his wife. His father had been a teacher, and his mother had come from a military background. She had left his father when he was a young teenager. Hamid had initially gone into the Army himself, but had bought himself out, disenchanted. Since then, he had no belief in himself and, despite qualifying as a teacher, he was only just managing to motivate himself to go to work each day. It was a major achievement, or so the group saw it, that he accepted an invitation to accompany a school party to France. The trip was not uneventful. One boy was arrested for threatening behaviour, and Hamid had to persuade the French police not to prosecute. Hamid told the group that it seemed like a year and not a week, and he was more relieved than he could ever remember feeling when the ferry docked in Dover and he realized that his responsibilities were nearly at an end. However, quite suddenly, he stopped feeling himself. It was as if he, Hamid, no longer existed. He could see himself doing things – having conversations, giving instructions, saying goodbye – and when he got home, he could feel himself kissing his wife. But he could feel no direction in any of this, no reason in it. It was all unreal. This state lasted for several weeks.

Hamid was experiencing a common psychiatric syndrome, that of depersonalization, although in his case it lasted much longer than is usual. Its main characteristic is the loss of the feeling of integration that Glover suggests is central to the experience of 'I'. Hamid had perceptions, undertook actions and had emotions, but they all seemed unconnected and therefore remote and lacking in personal meaning.

In psychotherapy practice, as for Hamid, not knowing 'who I am', living life as an automaton, and not knowing what life means, are all linked. A rich emotional life is one of the pre-conditions for having a strong sense of 'I', and for experiencing life as full of meaning. That is because emotions reach out, as Kierkegaard and other existentialists have argued, to the world. They are the vehicle for what Heidegger called '*Sorge*' – care or concern for the world. Losing one's feelings, perhaps because they have been exercised too intensely for too long, as in Hamid's case, means that both identity and meaning are attenuated.

'I am like no other.' My sense of having an 'I' is also linked to my experience of uniqueness and to the differences between myself and other people. As Kant said, to have a conception of myself, I have to have a conception of a frontier between myself and the rest of the world. This frontier does not exist in fact, or even in thought. It is an emotional frontier which, as we shall see in Chapter 5, is maintained by the social emotions that have dominated this chapter – shame and disgust.

Seeking to be an integral self is not the same as seeking to be a unitary self. It is conceivable, as some people with multiple personalities currently argue, that being a community of selves is a desirable state. However, a community *is* integrated. It is harmonious, not simply a collection of individuals or groups of people at odds with each other.

Experiencing life as meaningful and having an inner integrity would, I think, be considered prerequisites for well-being and psychological health for psychotherapists from many schools. Freud hoped that the 'I' would expand at the expense of the 'it': if 'I' means what is integrated, and 'it' means what is separate, then his dictum would seem to be consistent. The humanistic movement's goal to achieve authenticity is also consistent with these aims. Bugental reviews his deepest beliefs about therapy and about himself and concludes that: 'As we discover our own sense of possibility, we uncover more and more of our deeper natures, and thus we lay bare more of our own aliveness' (1976, p. 296). As van Deurzen (1979) writes, 'authentic living brings with it motivation and enthusiasm to do well what is worth doing. This experience of increasing vitality . . . is the hallmark of authentic life'.

I in the interpersonal domain

Emotions have been given a central place in psychotherapy in this chapter. They inform our actions even when we are not aware of them. But it has been assumed that emotions belong to a body. When a person experiences an emotion, we assume that there is a stimulus which is appraised, and assimilated to a remembered stimulus, and that the emotion linked to that memory is evoked. The emotion is experienced as being in ourselves, a reaction to the stimulus. However, it can happen that a stimulus evokes an emotion directly, without a process of recognition, appraisal or recall (Panksepp, 1999). Under these circumstances, the object seems to have a power to make a person experience a particular emotion. This power – emotional meaning or emotional flavour – will be considered in the remainder of this chapter.

Emotional meaning

The capacity to touch important concerns, and therefore to elicit emotions, inheres in almost any aspect of experience, including inner experience. Objects, memories, people, events, places, books, ideas, words . . . all of these may trigger off emotions in the right person.

Case study
Sadie and Tom had been trying to have children for over 3 years. They had gone through an increasingly intrusive series of infertility interventions. None of these had been successful. They had just been told that they were not candidates for in-vitro fertilization, and both of them knew that it was now unlikely that they would ever be able to have children. On the evening of the fertility clinic appointment, they went to a film. They did not choose the film very carefully, and it turned out to have a sub-plot about a woman who abandons her newborn baby. Sadie could not watch the pictures of the baby, and finally had to leave the cinema as she was so upset.

Sadie's overriding concern had been to have children, and the film seemed to speak directly to her. She felt acutely the unfairness of life that one woman can casually abandon a baby whilst she so desperately yearned for one. She knew that she could have seen the film 10 years before and felt untouched by it. It was not a very good film. But in the context of her and her husband's constant attention to the subject, the film hit her emotionally more forcefully than she could bear.

Mediocre films do not arouse much emotion unless they are on subjects about which a person is especially and unusually concerned, as Sadie was. However, some events arouse emotion in everyone. A new baby in the family is one of these.

Roberta was Anna's second daughter. She was a bit worried that the first, Rosie, now aged 2 years, would feel upstaged, and would not take to Roberta. However, when Rosie came into the hospital with her grandmother a few hours after the birth, she immediately smiled at Roberta and wanted to hold her. Her grandmother said, 'Rosie's very pleased to have a new sister', and she was.

Rosie smiled and was pleased by her sister, because very little babies afford that reaction. (This is not to say that a particular baby does not soon develop other emotional meanings. One of these might be, for Rosie, 'rival' and her emotional reactions to her sister may soon change.) Some stimuli are emotive to most people in a culture because children are socialized to experience emotions in relation to them. Most adults have an emotional reaction to genitalia, which would be absent in a one-year-old child for example. There may be some characteristic of the stimulus that triggers an innate emotional response. A newborn baby is one example. Another is the ruined buildings, steep wooded cliffs and rushing torrents which fire the romantic imagination. These afford a sense of awe or wonder. Wordsworth's comment in his poem, 'Tintern Abbey', of 'a sense sublime / Of something far more deeply inter-fused' refers to this reaction in him to this half-ruined building.

There are other stimuli to emotion, which I shall call emotors, which become impregnated with emotion because of their juxtaposition to, or association with, other emotional stimuli. Examples include: pictures of a person's family, letters or underwear of a loved one, a building where a horrific crime took place, a national flag, the word 'spider' to an arach-nophobe, and many more. Some emotors, like the national flag, will be common to many people, while others – like the picture of one's partner – will be common to just a few or even only one person. However, whether they are unique or common to many, each person has to create their own emotors. This might happen because the emotor is present during an upsurge of feeling. Women's underwear is an example. The sight of underwear alone, for example, in a catalogue or on display, may arouse sexual excitement in some post-pubertal men. It could be that the sight simply gave men the idea of sex, or that they imagined the underwear being worn in a sexual context. But a simpler explanation, which accords with many men's experience, is that the underwear is itself impregnated with desirability – with the capacity to arouse desire. Indeed there are some men for whom capturing underwear from a washing line is almost as exciting as a seduction.

Semiologists would argue that female underwear is an indexical represen-tation of a partly clothed woman. Freud, who wrote about this subject from a slightly different perspective in *The Interpretation of Dreams* (Freud, 1965), termed it 'condensation', or pars pro toto. Behaviourists will note that classical conditioning is an example of the creation of an emotor, but I am arguing that there need be no association of ideas. This seems to be in line with current studies of learning in animals (Rodgers & Cole, 1993) and in clinical situations (Carr, Yarbrough & Langdon, 1997). The emotor becomes imbued with the same emotion that was present when the emotor was created. However, Freud and others were right to suggest that an emotor may often be particularly likely to become imbued with emotion because it is part of an emotive whole.

Emotors might also become invested with emotion because of similarity, a relation that Freud called 'displacement' and that semiologists have termed 'iconic representation'. Pictures, corpses, statues, effigies – all of these resemble a person and tend to be able to evoke some of the same emotion as the person depicted.

I have referred to 'emotional flavours' or 'emotional meanings' being invested in things. Clearly, an emotor is not physically changed because it becomes able to trigger off an emotion in someone. Similarly the letters 'a-a-r-d-a-p-p-e-l' do not change when we know that they take on the meaning of 'potato' to a Dutch speaker. What presumably happens is that the word 'aardappel' becomes linked to the word 'potato', which has itself been previously linked with other associations, some of which will be emotions. Hearing 'aardappel' evokes 'potato' and that evokes all the other associations. Similarly, I would suppose, an emotor becomes linked with an emotional experience so that when I perceive it, the links to the emotion are activated, and I experience the emotion. However, our experience is that the *word* itself has a meaning which inheres in it. This seems to be true of emotors, too. When a person goes through the attic, some objects get saved because they have too much meaning. And, if they are thrown away by mistake, the person feels diminished. It feels to us that emotional meaning inheres in emotors.

Molly was bereft. She had been burgled about 3 months before. It had been bad enough feeling that her home had been invaded, but they had stolen an antique clock. It had not been terribly valuable in itself, but Molly had been bequeathed it by her mother. For years, she had become accustomed to think of her mother when she glimpsed the clock, or when it struck the hours. Now there was a sort of void in her. She often felt that she was waiting for something, or missing someone. And then she realized. There was no clock. It hadn't been just any clock. The clock reminded her so much of her mother. Like her mother, it was always busy, always on time, always there. Now the clock, and some part of her mother's continuing presence in her life, had gone.

Projection and emotional meaning

Emotional meanings are experienced with such immediacy that we do not think of them as our reaction to an emotor: we think of the emotor having the capacity to produce feeling in us. Although Molly told people that losing the clock was important because of its sentimental value, not because of its monetary value, this conventional phrase did not capture her experience. Molly felt that she had lost something of herself when her clock was stolen. It reminded her of the time that she had lost her sexual feelings when she had been on antidepressants.

This experience of objects or people having something of ourselves in them has been known to psychotherapists from the earliest days of psycho-analysis. Freud described the purpose of paranoia in a patient as being 'to fend off an idea that was intolerable to her ego by projecting its subject-matter into the external world' (in draft H of his 'Project' written in 1895) (Freud, 1954). Later, Freud wrote that 'internal perceptions of emotional and thought processes can be projected outwards . . . they are thus employed for building up the external world' (1955, p. 64). The term has been used increasingly ever since by psycho-analysts, especially since Klein introduced the term 'projective identification'.

This special case of projection fits situations when so much is projected into another person that it is as if a part of the self is being projected. Klein described this as follows: 'Much of the hatred against parts of the self is now directed towards the mother. This leads to a particular form of identification which establishes the prototype of aggressive object-relations. I suggest for these processes the term 'projective identification'. When projection is mainly derived from the infant's impulse to harm or to control the mother, he feels her to be a persecutor. In psychotic disorders this identification of an object with the hated parts of the self contributes to the intensity of the hatred directed against other people' (1955, p. 102).

The reader will note that, as so often in the writings of psycho-analysts, Klein's knowledge of psychosis seems to be mainly theoretical rather than from clinical experience. However, she is describing a recognizable phenomenon which may occur to anyone in situations of great emotional stress or confusion. 'Of course', writes Joseph Sandler, who should know, 'there isn't such a *thing* as projective identification . . .' (1988, p. 191). What he means by this is that the account of the phenomenon, something thrown out of one person's mind into another, is metaphorical.

One difference between the psycho-analytic 'projection' and my use of the term 'emotional meaning' is this: that I do think that people, or objects, can develop the capacity to induce emotions in us directly, without the mediation of appraisal, as a result of familiar processes of associative learning. There are good experimental studies, cited earlier in this chapter, which support this.

Another difference between projection, as described by Freud and Klein, and the emotional meanings considered here is that I consider that conferring emotional meaning on emotors is normal and often valuable. Projections are, as Freud intimated in the earliest passage quoted, a way of marking the world and thus providing ourselves with guidance in it. The term 'projection', and certainly the term 'projective identification', have mainly been used for emotional meanings which are in some way distorted or misleading.

One reason for this is that the metaphor of projection is part of a larger narrative in which there are mental contents, a censor mechanism which rates them as being acceptable or unacceptable, and the power of the censor to throw out those mental contents which are repugnant to it. Projection, in other words, is an essential element in Freudian metapsychology, which bears the same relation to psychology as metaphysics does to physics.

Freud, and psycho-analysts since, have therefore been addressing the situation of a person confronted by an emotional meaning which is unpalatable, and assuming that this can only be dealt with by disavowal – or what psycho-analytically inclined psychotherapists think of as restriction to the off-limit area, which is the unconscious mind. Disavowal of emotional meanings may not be as 'all or nothing' as this (see also Chapter 9 for a further discussion). A person may simply avoid the emotor, for example, or may dismiss it. Only in special circumstances do people seem genuinely unaware of the origins of the unpleasant emotional meaning.

Avoidance

Joanne had just received a reminder letter from her accountant informing her that her tax return had to be filed in a week. Every year, she put off doing it. She knew why. It was not only that it was a chore, but there was always a kind of tension in her about it. She wanted to be honest, but there were those occasions when she had been paid cash for little jobs that she had done. It seemed that there would be almost nothing left if she had to pay tax on them. The letter lay on the table like a wasp that would sting her at any moment. She buried it deep into the pile of things that she had to do, and felt relieved when it was out of sight.

Self-deception

Herbert had a terrible row with a colleague about, of all things, the colleague's unwillingness to wash up coffee cups, *ever*. The row went far beyond washing up and things were said that would not have looked good on a personnel report. Herbert did not want to work out the rights and wrongs of it. He treated the colleague like a bomb about to go off, and over time persuaded himself that he did so because she was so aggressive. However, sometimes he remembered what he had said in the row, and knew that one reason for avoiding any close interaction with the colleague was to avoid her mentioning how she felt about him.

Disavowal

Rachel was Herbert's colleague. She had forgotten that she used to quite like Herbert. Now she saw him as an abusive man, all that was worst in men who got into positions of petty authority. He was aggressive, arrogant and uncouth.

She wanted nothing to do with him. If she had to interact with him, she made sure that she kept things at the most superficial level. One of her friends asked her, 'What's with you and Herbert?', and she told the friend just how loathsome Herbert was. The friend was disgusted that such an aggressive man could hold down a management position in an ethical company.

If Rachel's friend had been a psycho-analyst he may well have considered whether Rachel had projected her own aggression onto Herbert. But this would be too cut- and dried a description of what happened between Herbert and Rachel. Both had contributed aggression to their original conflict, and both had yet to resolve who should accept responsibility for this.

There is one other way in which emotional meanings can be made more palatable, and this will be considered in the next section.

Strong emotional meanings

Most emotors have a meaning which is a blend of emotions. The strongest and most durable meanings turn out in practice to be those in which there is a blend of apparently conflicting emotions. This is most obviously true of the emotions associated with sexual desire, which are often blends of excitement and revulsion. Isherwood, for example, wrote that he preferred 'rimming' to all other sexual acts 'because of its grossness' (Isherwood, 2000). Stoller's theory of perversion (Stoller, 1970) makes this one of the most important principles in the durability of deviant sexuality. An unpleasant emotion such as humiliation is experienced in a sexual context and thereby becomes blended with desire. The resulting blend remains exciting. The case example that Stoller gives is a man who, as a boy, was humiliated by two aunts and forced to dress in girl's clothing. In adult life he started to cross-dress again and re-experienced the humiliation, even sought it, but now it was coupled with desire and, an additional blend, the mastery that comes of having been the author of this new humiliation. Stoller describes the resultant emotion blend as 'triumph'. For the client, the emotional meaning of cross-dressing is no longer humiliation, but pleasure, and also, paradoxically, 'relief of humiliation'.

Strong emotors and the fear of extinction

A common feature of many addictive substances is that they are unpleasant. Alcoholic drinks, tobacco and heroin all cause most first-time users to vomit. Instead of arousing disgust at the substance, this seems, in the long run, only to make the habit stronger, as the theory of strong emotors would predict. However, there are other strong emotors which rarely become addictive, even though they combine unpleasantness with pleasure. French cheeses combine a pleasant taste with the smell of body odour. Durian fruit is regarded as one of the most delectable fruits by many, tasting to them like strawberries and cream, but it smells of rotting flesh.

It is often assumed that what makes substances addictive is that they are euphoriant. It might therefore be assumed that French cheeses are not addictive, but that amphetamine is, because amphetamine is more intensely pleasurable than cheese. If addiction were about pleasure, then it would be difficult to explain why anorexia nervosa may have an addictive element, or why a person with an eating disorder may feel so disgusted by their bingeing that they may kill themselves rather than face the consequences of it becoming out of control (Gowers et al., 1994).

Substances or behaviours which become the basis for addictions typically put survival in jeopardy. Rock-climbing, hang-gliding, driving too fast, starving oneself, cutting and self-wounding, asphyxiation with a plastic bag, unprotected anal sex with a stranger, all of these may be activities to which a person might be loosely termed 'addicted'. However, the activities out of the list which become the basis for truly compulsive repetition are those which are also negatively sanctioned. They are activities that are forbidden, taboo or otherwise condemned. These activities risk death or illness, and also risk shame or disgust.

The strong emotors that become the basis of addictions are, I conclude, those in which the unpleasant emotion is connected with extinction of a person's social standing, of their social identity. Weiss has proposed a comparable theory of addiction – control mastery theory – in which he emphasizes childhood experience and the role of shame (O'Connor & Weiss, 1993). As noted earlier in this chapter, Scheff has argued that pride and shame are the primary social emotions which constitute a 'subtle system of social sanctions' (Scheff, 1990). Fairbairn had arrived at a very similar conclusion in his celebrated studies of schizoid personality, or why a person cannot make close personal relationships (Fairbairn, 1946). The metaphors that Fairbairn introduced of the libidinal and the anti-libidinal object can readily be reformulated in terms of shame and disgust, disgust being the obverse of Scheff's conception of pride in oneself (Tantam, 1996a).

These emotions are often cited as obstacles in processing the distressing memories which intrude on everyone from time to time (Spenceley & Jerrom, 1997). Waller and Smith (1994) describe this as 'contamination'. The disgust and shame of being abused transfer to the memory of the abuse, so every time the memory is triggered it overwhelms again by re-evoking the same emotions. Other kinds of historical shame can be perpetuated in the same way, by soaking into symbols and ideas that cannot then be apprehended without also experiencing shame or disgust. This is one reason that contemporary conflicts seem so easily to re-evoke feelings that date back to conflicts many years, sometimes many hundreds of years, before.

Partners in close relationships who argue, like groups who are tied irrevocably together by conflict, may do something similar. If the argument is so conducted that one or both partner(s) risk(s) losing face, the feeling of shame will rekindle memories of past humiliations or shames. Family therapists have sometimes speculated that families play out the conflicts or life histories of previous generations because these humiliations may be vicarious. It seems almost as if people in this sort of conflict do not want to sort it out. As soon as resolution seems in sight, a fresh accusation is hurled. This has led some psycho-analytically influenced therapists to speculate that people may, in this situation, be motivated by unconscious aggression or a death instinct. I think that it is much simpler than this, as we shall see in Chapter 10. Many people will fight almost to the death rather than feel shamed or that they disgust someone else, because these feelings are almost like dying, or at least like being annihilated.

One way of dealing with such powerful emotions is to combine them with some enjoyable or enhancing emotion. Blending shame/ humiliation or disgust/rejection with some strong but attractive emotion may result in a blend which is itself attractive, like blending quinine with sugar-water makes it into the attractive, tonic water.

Foremost among the emotions which make shame or digust palatable is sexual excitement, but more intangible states of well-being may have a similar effect. It may be the enhanced well-being associated with control that makes the inanition of severe anorexia nervosa into a positive experience and prevents the sufferer being disgusted by their physical appearance. Bodily shame or self-disgust may be blended with sexuality, resulting in an enhanced level of excitement: self-asphyxiation is an example.

It is these emotion blends which make 'strong emotors'. Re-evoking the strong emotion can absorb and detoxify more negative emotion. Strong emotors may therefore act as an antidote to disgust/rejection or to shame/ humiliation. It is easy to see why such an antidote may lead to addiction in someone who is susceptible to these emotions.

Emotional meaning and choice

Not everything can be put into words or, even more importantly, put into a register which is compatible with language. Why anyone likes opera, or rock music, or Wensleydale cheese, is indescribable. We can talk about them, and enthuse about our enjoyment of them, even infect others with that enjoyment. But we do not need language to enjoy them ourselves.

Most psychotherapeutic approaches assume some sort of second, covert, process of appraisal and judgement which is not fully verbalized. Psychoanalysts call this the unconscious; cognitive therapists refer to automatic schemata. Many psychotherapists (Muller, 1996) and psychologists consider that this second, 'unconscious process', is not mediated by words at all (Evans & Over, 1997).

Emotional flavour is one possible explanation. In one experiment on unconscious motivation, shoppers bought more French wine when French muzak was being played, and more German wine when the background was German music (North, Hargreaves & McKendrick, 1997). The emotional flavour of the muzak seems to have influenced the shoppers to choose the wine with the same emotional flavour.

This suggests that we choose emotional flavours that suit our mood, or the flavour of our concerns. Indeed there is some evidence for this (Herz, 1997). The relevance of this to psychotherapy is that our actions and our words must all be assumed to have some emotional meaning to the client that is not put in by us psychotherapists but by them. If this meaning is counter to the client's mood or the emotional meaning of their problem, the therapeutic relationship will be less well attuned than if the emotional meaning of the treatment is in harmony with the client's emotions.

Harmonization of flavour and emotional state provides an explanation for a number of other research findings in psychotherapy, which are otherwise anomalous.

Although research studies do support the superiority of some modalities over others for specified problems, the differences are much smaller in clinical practice. Training and experience do not account for much outcome variance either. And a recent study of people with alcohol dependence suggests that, at least in that group, the fit between the type of treatment and the characteristics of the client's difficulties does not account for outcome either (Project MATCH, research, et al., 1998).

Many experienced practitioners think, like Frank (1965), that participation in therapy is a more important contributor to outcome than any particular therapeutic intervention, and that the most important determinant of participation is the fit between the client and the therapist.

Despite these findings, psychotherapists place considerable emphasis on the quality and the amount of training that entrants into the profession receive. Many psychotherapists also assume that it is some characteristic of the client that determines outcome, and that experience and seniority enable a psychotherapy to discern it. So much is this view prevalent that many senior psychotherapists in practice in the UK health service spend most of their clinical time in assessment. But there is little research evidence indicating that the factors on which assessment is often based are predictive of outcome (Tantam, 1995b). There is also considerable evidence that people who are diagnosed with conditions which are often taken to be of poor prognosis for psychotherapy, for example borderline personality disorder, benefit substantially from it.

How flavour applies to these findings is suggested by a study of the outcome of group psychotherapy by McCallum and Piper (1990), which indicates that 'poor prognosis' clients are much less likely to comply with treatment, and therefore to complete it. But those who do complete have as good an outcome as the 'good prognosis' clients who complete. The determinant of outcome is therefore compliance, and not the ability to benefit from the treatment. And it is the flavour of the treatment, and its palatability to the clients, that determines compliance and outcome and not the 'food value'.

Palatability

Parsons, Bales and Shils, in formulating their general theory of action, concluded that action was only possible if objects were cathected, if there was 'an attachment to objects which are gratifying and rejection of those which are noxious . . .' (1951, p. 5). Obviously this is a matter of appraisal. We take an emotional attitude to something. However, our experience is that events or objects have an intrinsic property – the emotional meaning or flavour already described. It is this flavour which makes something repugnant or attractive. Some of our emotional appraisals are so deeply buried in our brains that it really seems that objects are intrinsically attractive or noxious. Babies who pick up a worm will drop it with an expression of distress. Older children will look at a slug and say 'yuk'. On the other hand, a primiparous ewe will eat her own afterbirth.

Most parents remember spoonfeeding and the mysteries of why a baby will sometimes suck food down avidly, and at other times refuse it, spit it out, even regurgitate it, to avoid taking it in. Many terms used by psychotherapists refer back to this formative experience: introjection and projection, acceptance and rejection, assimilation and extrusion are all examples. Babies spit out food when they, or the person feeding them, are anxious, but also when the food itself has an unpalatable flavour or texture. Reverting to the narrative metaphor, events or memories may be unassimilated into a person's life story because the person is so anxious at the time that the event happens that they cannot assimilate it. But events may also remain unassimilated because they are experienced as noxious, and this unpalatability extends to thoughts and memories of the event.

Identity and emotional meaning

Emotors are as much a part of our identity as sentiments. Both are dispositions to particular experiences. Losing emotional meaning therefore has an effect on identity.

Mrs Cox was 82 years old. She had lived in the same house since she had married at the age of 17. Now she was living in an old people's home because she had become physically frail. Her belongings had been either divided up between her children or sold. Most had been sold. There was nothing wrong with her brain, but she had become withdrawn. The nursing staff said, 'We've seen this before. If she gets through the first 3 months she'll be fine, but we're afraid we might lose her'. She said, 'I've lost everything. What have I got to live for? When I lived at home I was somebody. Here I'm just an old woman. I don't feel like myself anymore. I feel that I've ceased to exist'.

'I' experiences involve emotions and are determined by the particular dispositions to react, and to feel, that are characteristic of that person. But identity also includes that person's 'emotors', since these are also determinants of a person's emotions. Emotors are likely to include: my family, my country, my history . . . and all of these, and more, are therefore a part of my identity to the extent that they have emotional meaning.

Identity, and its relation to emotional meaning, emotion and value will be reconsidered in Chapter 5. It is postponed by one chapter because the last key idea that will be needed to consider identity and the practice of psychotherapy is the narrative approach. That will be introduced in the next chapter.

Projective identification and strong emotors

The ideas of Klein, and her term 'projective identification', were discussed in an earlier section of this chapter. It was mentioned there that what was unique about this form of projection was that it was as if some part of a person's self was being projected into the other. As a result, there is a strong tie between the person doing the projecting and the person who receives the projection. This is the Kleinian explanation for the mysterious but generally accepted phenomenon that people who hate each other or fight with each seem sometimes to be in a stronger relationship, more strongly bonded, than people who feel positively about each other.

One possible explanation for this is that intimacy does seem to involve the fusion of both negative and positive emotions, a finding which cannot be attributed to peculiarities of human social development if, as Lorenz suggests, it can also be observed in birds (Lorenz, 1966). Another description of the same phenomenon has been given using an ocular metaphor. Zinkin terms the destructive preoccupation of two group members who dominate a therapeutic group by their constant conflict 'malignant mirroring'.

If projection is the consequence of a person's avoidance, denial or disavowal of the unpalatable emotional meaning, what is the emotional meaning that underlies projective identification?

There are two families of emotions that are particularly concerned with identity. They are the shame family and the disgust family. Both being

scholars working from many perspectives laboured to uncover the hidden regularities of our social relations. Marxists did it in relation to politics and economics; Freudians did it in relation to personal relationships; others have worked on texts and narratives of various, other kinds. Narrative psychotherapists have worked on the discourses of their clients.

The result is the outline of a general theory of narrative structure (Tantam, 1986) which enables insights from a wide range of fields to be applied to psychotherapy. Here is one example. Vladislav Propp, in his ground-breaking study of the Russian folk-tale, concludes that:

1. Functions of characters serve as stable, constant elements in a tale, independent of how and by whom they are fulfilled. They constitute the fundamental components of a tale.
2. The number of functions known to the folk tale is limited (1968, p. 21).

In communicative therapy, it is assumed that when clients give 'indications' of 'madness', what they say should be treated as a disguised message. These disguised messages are often in the form of stories about some person in the client's life. The communicative therapist should always assume that they convey a truth about the client's experience of the therapist, and of the therapist's creating danger in the therapeutic relationship by one of a finite number of 'frame violations' (Langs, 1992).

Both Propp and Langs assume that the introduction of a new character into the story does not mean that a new person is being described, only that the person whom the tale is about is being presented in a new persona. This is an important principle in deciding the preoccupying concern of a client being assessed.

Case example
Mrs Masters was referred to a psychotherapist because she was chronically anxious. Everything seemed too much for her. Whilst waiting for her assessment appointment, she had a mild stroke, although she was only 28 years old. Neither she nor her doctor seemed particularly concerned about this, casually attributing it to her weight (she was 19 stones (120 kg)).

The psychotherapist introduced himself at the start of the assessment interview and checked that she was indeed Valerie Masters (not her real name). He thanked her for completing the history questionnaire, which she had done meticulously, if a bit untidily. She said how worried she had been that she might have misremembered something, and apologized that she did not have time to check all her answers. The assessor skimmed over some of these, stopping to ask her to amplify various points. Uncharacteristically, Mrs Masters had said very little about her father, but became tearful when asked about him. She had let him down, she said. He had expected so much of her, and she had let him down. He died a disappointed man. Talking about her school, she said that she made friends with the pupils, but was always anxious about the teachers. She felt that she would never do well enough in her homework to satisfy them.

This continued throughout her history: every so often a new character would be described with greater emotional force than was usual, and each time she would have felt judged as a failure by this character. What real person were these personae of? There were two possible candidates. Her mother was a home-maker with whom Mrs Masters could find no fault. Everything she did was a bit better, a bit more successful than Mrs Masters had herself been able to achieve, even her affection. Mrs Masters felt that her mother had always loved her, but there seemed to be a reservation in her tone when she said it. Later in the therapy, Mrs Masters was able to admit that there were times when her mother lost her temper with her, and at those times her mother seemed to want to be rid of her.

The other candidate for the judge who was never satisfied was Mr Masters, her husband. Mr Masters was a mild man, a good provider, who never criticized. But he never said anything positive either. Mrs Masters had become convinced that he was disappointed in her, and the more that she rushed around after the children and tidying the house, the more disapproving she thought that he became.

Mrs Masters's concern was to gain others' approval, but she was convinced that this would never be possible when it came to the key people in her life – her mother and her husband. Her story was monotonous because she was so preoccupied with this concern that almost everyone that she mentioned was either a nonentity or a persona of her husband.

Interviewing

Allowing people to tell their stories requires the mental health professional to know how to be a good audience. Listening skills are therefore an essential element of professional skill and they form the basis for many counselling training programmes (Inskipp, 1986). Just listening is rarely enough, and the mental health professional also needs to shape the story. This requires additional skills in the use and timing of questions, prompts and summaries which, together with listening skills, are also essential elements of the skills needed in interviews (Table 4.1). They are often acquired from experience, but are increasingly augmented by formal training. Many professionals assume that they have mastered them by the time that they have finished their training, although studies of experienced family doctors suggest that this is the case with only a minority of them (Marvel, Doherty & Weiner, 1998).

Exercise: how are your interviewing skills?

Explain to one of your clients that you want to test your interviewing skills. Ask them if they would agree to you asking them again about the problem

Table 4.1. Interviewing skills

Listening
  Look at the client
  Look receptive
  Tolerate silence
  Follow verbal cues
  Invite to talk
  Encourage talking with feeling

Questioning
  Use open questions first
  Closed questions to finish

Responding to cues
  Verbally
  Non-verbally (e.g. nods, 'ums')

Paraphrasing and summarizing

Modified from Tantam (1996b).

that first brought them to the doctor, but this time you will be recording it. Explain that a colleague and yourself may review the recording, but that it will then be erased. Make a video-recording if possible. If not, make an audio-recording. If you can find a willing colleague, review the tape with them. Construct a rating scale from Table 4.1 or use a rating scale from previous interviewing training and use this to rate yourself. Make a global rating of your skill on a five-point scale from very poor (1) to excellent (5). Ask your colleague to rate you on this scale. If your combined score is less than 7, consider undertaking an interviewing skills course. If there is a difference of more than 2 in your score compared with your colleague, consider the possible sources of bias in your self-perception.

Constructing a therapeutic narrative

Interviewing people skilfully is a powerful intervention. It may be enough to enable a professional to provide relief by debriefing someone after a disaster, listening to the testimony of someone who has been victimized, or allowing a distressed person to ventilate their feelings.

However, people who come to a psychotherapist are often stuck in a story, and like the Ancient Mariner of Coleridge's poem, telling it does not bring more than temporary relief.

Forthwith this frame of mine was wrenched
With a woeful agony,
Which forced me to begin my tale;
And then it left me free.

Since then, at an uncertain hour,
That agony returns;
And till my ghastly tale is told,
This heart within me burns.

Two factors conspire to make this kind of story less than therapeutic. In psycho-analytic parlance they are termed 'counter-transference' by the therapist of his or her own needs or wishes onto the client, and 'resistance' by the client to the therapist's interventions. However, these terms are rooted in a particular understanding of individual psychology. The same two factors are better understood in a wider context: firstly of the struggle between narratives for dominance, and secondly, of the failure of narrative coherence.

Before considering these factors, it is as well to remind ourselves of where this discussion is leading. The encounter of psychotherapist and client has, as any encounter between people, elements of social interaction which are non-verbal. But it is embedded in a situation which will be narrated – to a supervisor, to a spouse, to oneself. Even if one could imagine a traditional healing ritual which was entirely ceremonial, there would be a story to the ceremony. The narrative of the psychotherapy is the matrix which contains and orders individual elements. We therefore need to arrive at an understanding of what makes a narrative therapeutic before we can examine the individual elements of the narrative, i.e. its beginning in the assessment, its middle in the treatment, and its end in the termination.

The struggle of narratives

The members of the Bakhtin circle, struggling to equate developments in psycho-analysis and linguistics with Stalin's purges of the 1930s, came to the conclusion that the many discourses about the world were in a constant state of struggle with each other. Each discourse served the interests of a particular group, and a group obtained power over other groups by having these other groups accept its discourse. Though officialdom would like to convince us that there was one, 'true', discourse, we should reject this. We should be aware that officials are interested mostly in imposing their rule on others and not in representing life fully (Brandist, 1997). A similar analysis of texts about madness established that the same process applies to narrative as to discourse (Foucault, 1973).

This is not merely an intellectual conclusion. At least one researcher of cognitive therapy programmes in prisons (Fox, 1999) has observed a similar struggle between the offenders' narratives about their violence, and those of the psychotherapists and the prison staff. In such a setting, falling in with the dominant narrative too easily means being coerced and not persuaded. It is questionable how much real change has been achieved when the system itself shows that power matters more than individual values.

One might assume that in everyday psychotherapy, with clients freely coming and going from the clinic, coercion of the client by the therapist can hardly arise. However, even here there is a danger that the therapeutic narrative may be constructed according to the value, emotional meaning, and goals of the therapist simply because of the relatively greater power of the therapist over the client (Bergsma & Mook, 1998).

Case example

William was a shy under-achieving man who referred himself for psychotherapy. The psychotherapist whom he chose was an attractive middle-aged woman who quickly became a source of fascination for him. William underwent a metamorphosis during the early weeks of his treatment and, with the encouragement of his therapist, began to consider getting a girlfriend. Shortly after a particular euphoric session, during which the therapist told him that he was a very attractive man, he became sexually excited in a pub and made a pass at a woman with whom he had fallen into conversation. He felt that she was interested in him, and he stroked her breasts. The woman protested strongly and there was a struggle with bystanders, which led to the police being called.

William's psychotherapist was acting with the best intentions, but her narrative, ostensibly about William, was really about a fiction, a man with a degree of social judgement that William had never possessed. However, such was her power over him that it became the story that he told himself, with unfortunate consequences.

Mental health professionals sometimes assume that what they write about their clients has little impact on the clients themselves. But the letter to the GP, or the summary in the notes, constructs a new narrative about the client which is sometimes considerably at variance with the client's own narrative (Brown et al., 1996). The inclusion of terms like 'personality disorder' or, even more dangerously, 'psychopath', are traps for clients from which it is difficult for them to extricate themselves. It should be remembered that letters to GPs may be read to clients, and will certainly be read by GP receptionists who may know the client or the family, personally.

However, these are remediable problems compared with the difficulty of the therapist who tries to maintain two narratives – one for the client and one for professional colleagues. Pejorative formulations like 'borderline', 'dependent', 'masochistic', 'manipulative' and many others, which are often to be found in professional narratives, inevitably leak into the narrative of the therapy. It is much better, in my view, to grasp this nettle from the beginning by sending copies of any letters about the client, to the client. In fact, this may have a therapeutic effect. In cognitive-analytic therapy, a full written formulation of the client's problems, 'the reformulation letter', is sent to the client usually after the fourth session.

Narrative coherence

Coherence, as it is used in philosophy, means some set of things, typically beliefs, which is both as inclusive as possible and as consistent as possible (Bradley, 1944).

Darren was being interviewed after an affray which had been described by the press as a racial incident. He said, 'I've got nothing against other races. I'm no racist'. Later in the interview he was asked about his interests in the British National Party. He denied being an active member but said, 'They're against immigrants, and so am I. They all ought to be sent home, that's what I think'.

Darren's beliefs are clearly inconsistent, and therefore incoherent. However, had he said he did not care about immigration one way or another, and that it was not his concern that people sought political asylum in the United Kingdom, this too would have been incoherent because his beliefs would be restricted.

Coherence theory has been taken to be a theory of truth (true beliefs are those which cohere with other true beliefs). As such, it is contrasted with correspondence theory, which is that beliefs are true if they correspond to facts. Fisher (1987) proposed that both coherence and 'fidelity', i.e. correspondence to facts, influence people's judgement of when other people are being 'reasonable', and that deciding whether someone or some social product is reasonable is the most important ground on which we accept or reject it. Empirical studies have borne this out. For example, nearly half of the variance of subjects' judgements of the persuasiveness of the 25 test stories that they were told in one study was accounted for by coherence and fidelity (Baesler, 1995).

This chapter has emphasized the narrative approach to psychotherapy – given that psychotherapy has been described as 'an exercise in story repair' (Howard, 1991) – but this still does not fully explain an excursus into philosophy. How, the reader may well be asking, is this relevant to psychotherapy?

One answer is that psychotherapy, particularly long-term psychotherapy, badly needs new paradigms. Freud, Jung and Janet's intrapsychic theories, neuroscientific psychotherapy (Gottschalk, 1990), psychotherapy as applied relationship theory (Derlega et al., 1992), object-relations theory (Greenberg & Mitchell, 1983), communication theory (Ruesch & Bateson, 1951), even emotion theory (Oatley, 1990) – all these have come and whilst none have gone, none have fully succeeded either. One way to generate new paradigms is to return to the mother of science, philosophy, for a new starting point.

Another kind of answer is that appeals to coherence are one of the commonest tropes in the rhetoric of behavioural change. Cognitive psychotherapists ask their depressed clients if they would come to the same conclusion about their worthlessness if they were judging someone else other than themselves, knowing that their clients would not and believing, also, that their clients are right to condemn themselves for holding inconsistent beliefs (Beck et al., 1979). Philosophical consultants use 'Socratic methods' in their work which expose incoherence in the beliefs of their clients in the knowledge that, once exposed, the client will inevitably seek to redress the inconsistency (Marinoff & Kapklein, 1999). Perhaps the most important rhetorical application of coherence has, however, already been alluded to, in the discussion about an integrated self (see p. 67).

Here is how Leo Tolstoy, himself suffering from a generalized anxiety disorder, described the thoughts of the judge, Ivan Illyich, a few hours from the judge's death:

> It occurred to him that what had seemed utterly inconceivable before – that he should not have lived the kind of life that he should have – might in fact be true. It occurred to him that those scarcely perceptible impulses of his to protest what people of high rank considered good, vague impulses which he had always suppressed, might have been precisely what mattered, and all the rest might not have been the real thing. (Tolstoy, 1981, pp. 126–7)

Psycho-analysis might appeal to intentions, gestalt psychotherapy to the closure of unfinished situations, and existential therapy to values, but each of these long-term psychotherapy approaches advocates that the client apply a coherency test similar to that which Ivan Illyich finally applied retrospectively to his life. Ivan Illyich asked whether he had led his life according to the principles he really valued. Psycho-analysts provoke their analysands to close the gap between their desires and their avowed intentions, gestalt therapists suggest to their clients that they complete unfinished business, and existential therapists challenge all of us to live in the full knowledge that we must die. Recognizing our desires, or unfinished business or our fears of death creates a pressure to make our lives coherent with these ends. Nietzsche's formulation of this is the most general: live your life in the knowledge of the eternal recurrence of events, that is in the knowledge that you, and others, will experience this event over and over again in the course of the life of the universe.

Yet another answer to the question, 'Why coherency?', is that coherence is an empirical concept. It is close to the world as I experience it, making no appeal to a hidden hypothetical universe of intrapsychic objects or events, or even unconscious intentions or desires. A sensible person reading a psychotherapist's account of the long-term effects of their work will be struck by the plethora of technical terms. These have a pleasing flavour of certainty and authority, but the unaffected reader will be inclined to ask, 'Why this metaphor, and why not another?' and 'What claim to existence do these things have? Do they correspond to neuronal activity? Do people think in such ways?'.

Here is an example:

> I have often expressed my view that object relations exist from the beginning of life, the first object being the mother's breast which to the child becomes split into a good (gratifying) and bad (frustrating) breast; this splitting results in a severance of love and hate. I have further suggested that the relation to the first object implies its introjection and projection, and thus from the beginning object relations are moulded by an interaction between introjection and projection, between internal and external objects and situations. These processes participate in the building up of the ego and super-ego and prepare the ground for the development of the Oedipus complex in the second half of the first year. (Klein, 1946, p. 293)

This impressive passage contains many of Klein's key ideas, which have such impact on students and experienced psycho-analytic psychotherapists alike. But it is difficult to know how to take it except as a story, a fairy tale about childhood which has narrative truth, even if it does not reflect the psychological processes of the actual infant. And if we take it as a story, why this one?

Splitting, as it happens, can be easily defined as that kind of incoherence which results when two episodes in a narrative have conflicting meanings, even though they have a common subject. Darren's racist declaration cited previously is an example of splitting. It can certainly be helpful to a psychotherapist to observe that a narrative has this kind of inconsistency, but it seems – at least to me – to be advantageous to do this without having to believe in conflicting internal representations, or internal objects.

Similarly, we have all observed when someone seems not to be speaking in their own voice, but in that of someone else, or when someone is making something out to be all about someone else, when we know that it is about the speaker. Does calling the former a consequence of an introject, or the latter a projection, help us to understand them better? It is probably true that it does help us to see that certain narrative themes recur, and that these themes are especially used to infer something about the narrator rather than what is being narrated. But thematic recurrence can be found in the text itself, and invoking an agency like the unconscious as an explanation seems unnecessary.

Simeon was referred, with anxiety problems, to a psychotherapist. They seemed straightforward at first. He had been unemployed, but now bought novelty goods and sold them around the country. He had begun to get panic

attacks on some of his longer trips, and was becoming increasingly chary of travelling any distance from his home town. His first panic attack occurred when he went abroad for the first time. He got drunk, woke up with a hangover, phoned his mother, and then became panicky. His father, who was strict, died when the client was 10 years old. He was an only child, and lives alone with his mother.

The psychotherapist explained the symptoms of anxiety, indicated how a spontaneous panic attack – which might occur, for example, during alcohol withdrawal – could become habitual if it inspired a 'fear of fear', and was confident about the success of a programme of systematic exposure (see Chapter 5). Simeon seemed to accept this information, but then went to see his GP, requesting referral to a cardiologist. The GP complied, and the cardiologist wrote back that the client had a normal heart. For over a year, every formulation and intervention that the therapist tried was met with scepticism, and turned out to be a failure when the client applied it – every one, that is, with the exception of diazepam, which did prove effective.

Simeon was referred to a group which he attended for over 2 years. Few group sessions passed without doctors or psychotherapists being criticized. Occasionally, Simeon would talk about his anxieties, especially about his wife and child (he had by now got married). On those occasions, he would admit that he had overcome his panic attacks to some degree, but would qualify this by saying that he was much more aware of his anxiety than he had ever been. At the next session, Simeon could be expected to be at his most mordant at the failings of the various professionals who had tried to help him or at other members of the group.

The psychotherapist would be the first to admit that he never did understand Simeon. A lot of what Simeon said suggested that he had strong feelings about other people, and that he felt resentful of many of them. He was drawn to selling his trinkets in old people's homes, but spoke disparagingly about elderly people. However, Simeon would have rejected out of hand any link between his behaviour towards old people in general, and his feelings about his elderly mother in particular.

The meagre benefits of therapy for Simeon may be due to a failure of the therapeutic relationship, but Simeon had the same type of relationship with other therapists and doctors who had treated him. It could be because there were technical failings in the treatment that he was offered. However, all experienced psychotherapists, irrespective of how successful they are with some clients, have some clients like Simeon. It could be that he was 'resisting' getting better. The psycho-analytic theory of resistance is that it occurs either because symptoms offer relief from anxiety ('primary gain') or because they have other benefits which outweigh the suffering that they cause ('secondary gain'). Simeon's symptoms included anxiety, and so there does not appear to be any primary gain in them. Simeon received sickness benefit for quite a long period. It could be argued that this amounted to a secondary gain. However, doctors rarely appreciate the humiliation for most people of being unable to work for psychological reasons. Sickness benefit might be a monetary gain, but it is a loss of self-esteem. Anyway, Simeon was not work-shy. Before his anxiety developed, he had worked long and hard selling the novelty goods.

Simeon thought that his actions were entirely determined by circumstances, and his emotions by disease. He rarely spoke of himself as a 'self' in the group. When he did, he had contradictory views. Sometimes he thought of himself as a 'mug', at other times as a survivor. If, as the introduction to this chapter suggests, the self is the leading character in the story that each of us has about our actions, then Simeon's story was fragmentary and incoherent. Or, to put the matter in commonsense language, both Simeon's account of himself and his personality were 'mixed up'.

A person's ability to provide a coherent narrative is related to their ability to extend the narrative to assimilate adversity, and therefore to their resilience. Contrary to psycho-analytically influenced theorists and to some behaviourists, early childhood influences are not the most potent influence on narrative coherence. Catastrophe at any time of a person's life may lead to the world becoming an incomprehensible place, and to the degradation of a person's narrative about themselves and their future. On the other hand, if adverse experience can be fitted into a coherent narrative, it is less likely to lead to persistent psychological sequelae (Peterson & Biggs, 1998). Narrative incoherence has been shown to correlate with having an ambivalent relationship to one's parents (Pearson et al., 1993), and to a lack of secure attachments (Main, 1996). The latter two are both factors that correlate with relationship problems in adult life. A correlation has also been noted in men between a lack of narrative coherence, and the tendency to 'externalize', i.e. to attribute problems to outside factors rather than to personal agency.

All of the associations in the previous paragraph applied to Simeon. He was unable to come to terms with his panic disorder: it did not fit into his account of himself as an unemotional and hard-boiled man. Simeon had an ambivalent relationship with both of his parents. His separation anxiety when he first went abroad suggests a life-long propensity for anxiety. We have already noted his tendency to externalize.

Externalization, or the closely related projection and lack of psychological mindedness, are facets of narrative incoherence. Another expression of being 'mixed up' is that the self narrative is split into interwoven but separate strands: Stiles (1999) has called these 'voices'. An extreme variant of this is when a person considers that they have multiple personalities. This may be a recourse that is more accessible to women, who tend to be more narratively and linguistically able than men. However a person tries to manage being mixed up, the consequence is the same. Any conversation that they have about themselves draws only on a partial narrative, from which the reasons for many of their actions or emotions are missing. The psychotherapist trying to address these missing reasons loses his or her audience. The therapist and the client are at cross-purposes.

Simeon's meagre therapeutic response does not have to be attributed to an intentional or an unconscious refusal to hear the truth about himself. It is more that words did not seem to Simeon to fit his very mixed feelings about himself and his experience. Without having the words, he could only converse in a fragmented way and therefore could not build a coherent narrative about what was happening to him. We should note that this is not an original formulation. Bion (1988) wrote about 'beta elements' leading directly to action without being metabolized by language into 'alpha elements', and the same theme can be found in many other psychotherapy theorists.

It is important to distinguish between not having the words, and not having the vocabulary. It is sometimes argued that psycho-analytic and narrative approaches emphasize verbal fluency too much. These critics say that psychotherapy consequently disadvantages people with a below-average education, or a learning disability. In my experience people with learning disabilities, if they have any language at all, put it to work to understand themselves and other people. It is quite possible to construct a therapeutic narrative with someone who uses only the simplest words so long as these words are able to be applied across the whole range of experience. The problem of narrative incoherence is not an absence of words, in fact wordiness may be used to describe incoherence, but a restriction in their application. Something as simple as a lack of verbs may render a narrative incoherent (Haberlandt & Bingham, 1978).

Splitting and narrative coherence

Simeon's narrative was described in the previous section as incoherent and it was noted that it was split into several strands: for example, he accounted himself as both a mug and a survivor. 'Splitting' is a term that is also used by psycho-analysts who attribute it to divisions in the self resulting from having to deal with a carer with two faces. Fairbairn, for example, imagined a mother who was at one moment loving, and at the next, rejecting. He thought that the child would split the mother into two people, a libidinal and an anti-libidinal object, and would split him- or herself into two as well. There would be a libidinal ego which responded to mother when she was loving with love, and an anti-libidinal ego which would respond to the rejecting mother with fear, withdrawal or anger.

Splitting apart incompatible narrative strands, and splitting of the ego, are not very different when it comes down to it.

Zena had had a very hard life. Her mother, Roma, had been the victim of a hard destiny. She had married a man who beat her, and then deserted her. Roma had hit the bottle for a while, and Zena had to go into care because of her mother's neglect. Then Roma had successfully sued to have Zena back. There was no doubt in Zena's mind that she was a very caring mother, but she was very inconsistent. When there was a new man in her life, she was happy and did not drink much, although the men always drank enough to make up for that. When she was alone, she clung to Zena, but sometimes got so depressed that she lapsed into a sort of stupor, when she was just not there for Zena or anyone else.

Zena did not know the extent to which this had affected her. She, too, was very inconsistent in her attitude to others. If things were going well, she could be friendly, but she would often lapse into a black mood and could be curt or even hostile. Friends had known her invite them around to her home, only for her to refuse to let them in when they arrived. It was not just that she was inconsistent over time, but that she seemed to have a very black-and-white view of people. She loved some people, and hated others, with no apparent reason for either extreme. She would tell one friend how much she trusted them, and disliked another friend, but would think nothing of reversing these judgements if she was speaking to a different person. This habit of Zena's had started many a row between her friends, and one or two had become permanent enemies.

Some friends said, 'I think Zena's got a split personality. Sometimes she's one person, and sometimes another'. Other friends said, 'The trouble is that Zena doesn't know whether she's living a comedy or a tragedy. When she's happy, she talks about her life as if it was a story by P.G. Wodehouse, but when she's miserable, she speaks about her life with a Raymond-Carver-like gloom'.

Some of Zena's friends were influenced by psycho-analysis, so explained her splitting on the basis of her split personality though, like most lay people, they did not bother with the fine distinctions that psychotherapists would make between 'dissociation' and 'splitting'. Others took a more literary approach. Neither group argued with each other because they recognized that each was describing the same thing – one in terms of the narrator and the other in terms of the narrative.

The therapist's responsibility for the narrative

People go to psychotherapists, as has been mentioned several times already, because they are mixed up. Arrangements must therefore be made as clear and unambiguous as possible, and this includes the therapist doing everything possible to foster the development of a coherent therapeutic narrative. This may not be easy. Even so apparently simple a matter as using verbs instead of nouns, noted just above to be one characteristic of a coherent narrative, may require special effort. In fact, therapists tend to do the opposite when they theorize, turning verbs into nouns (Schafer, 1976). This is doubly strange as more coherent narratives are more persuasive (Baesler, 1995).

Therapists generally make the greatest contribution to narrative coherence if they can develop the habit of plain speaking. Plain speaking does not mean blaming (or praising) and respects the client's intentions, which are usually to try to resolve a problem. However, it does not pull its punches about the consequences of a person's actions either.

Case example
In a family therapy session with Rod and his parents, Jim, Rod's father, turns to the therapist and says: 'He might say that he's getting better, but what he hasn't told you is all the queer things he does. A week or so ago, he went into this room and chucked everything out – calculator, clock, the lot. He said that the room was too cluttered'. Rod has had meningitis, and is left with a low tolerance of anxiety, an intolerance of change, a need for order, and impulsivity. The therapist knows that many young men with a disability feel humiliated by it, and react by becoming over-sensitive to criticism. He says to Rod, 'I suppose you suddenly felt it was all too much, and you wanted to have less to deal with. You probably didn't calculate the value of the things that you were throwing away, you just felt the urgency of needing to have some order in your life. It's difficult to see your father's side of things at the moment, because you think he's criticizing, but you probably know where he's coming from. He doesn't know how you felt. He just worries about the cost of replacing the things that you threw away'.

Very few people that a psychotherapist meets are deceitful or trying to sabotage treatment. Very many of the people that the psychotherapist meets will be ashamed of not being able to sort out problems themselves, and probably guilty because they will feel that they could have done more. They will be half-expecting to be accused of failing and it is very important that the psychotherapist does not go along with this narrative. People do often make mistakes, and these may contribute to their emotional problems. But they do not intend the mistakes or the consequences. Criticism may wake people up to bad intentions, but only makes people more defensive about mistakes.

Narrative types in psychotherapy

On particularly auspicious evenings, my father would ask me if I wanted to play a game and, if I did, whether I wanted to play chess or draughts. Chess was definitely the superior game in terms of seriousness. Chess was to train the mind, but draughts was fun. There was an intensity to chess, composed of

Table 4.2. Narrative structures in psychotherapy

Psychotherapy	Components
Trauma	Assessment; formulation; contract
Symptom relief	Assessment; formulation; contract; procedure
Predicament	Assessment; formulation; contract; resolution; reformulation; ending
Addiction	Assessment; formulation; contract; relinquishment and releasement; reformulation; ending
Relationship	Assessment; formulation; contract; re-narration; reformulation; ending

equal portions of the fear and of the triumph of winning. The starting conditions of both would be the same, two players on opposite sides of a board with 64 alternately light and dark squares, but the values, emotional meaning and action of the two were quite different. Once committed to a game, the structure of the two games was also quite different. When I was young, before I had fully grasped the rules of chess, games would sometimes come to a premature end because I lost my queen in a silly way. There were the usual arguments when my father remembered a rule that he hadn't told me yet, which usually happened when I had just made what I thought was a rather good move. Once I knew the rules, games went better.

We have already noted that a well-structured therapeutic narrative is one that follows the general principles of narrative composition, and that is as coherent as possible. The therapeutic narrative also needs to instantiate the shared values of the psychotherapist and the client, carry a palatable emotional meaning, and further the actions of the client. In practice, psychotherapists do not 'construct' narratives in a self-conscious manner. M. Jourdain (Molière, 1670) declaimed: 'Par ma foi! Il y a plus de quarante ans que je dis de la prose sans que j'en susse rien'. Working psychotherapists construct narratives without having to think any more about them than M. Jourdain had to do about speaking prose. It is often only when the narrative goes wrong that attention is paid as to why (see Chapter 10).

There are a limited number of narrative structures in psychotherapy, composed from a limited number of elements (see Table 4.2). Assessment is common to all of them, and has been considered in the previous chapters. Formulation and contract are also components in every type of psychotherapy. They are considered in this chapter. Symptom-relieving procedures are considered in the next chapter, resolving predicaments in Chapter 8, relinquishing addictions and perversions in Chapter 9, and renarrating relationships in Chapter 10. Ending is considered in Chapter 11.

Formulation and reformulation

The formulation is the narrative of the client's difficulties which leads on to a contract with the client. The reformulation is the narrative of the client's difficulties, and how the therapist and client have worked on them. It may lead on to a contract review. Both formulation and contract are essential to psychotherapy. If they do not occur explicitly, they will be implicit in both the client's and the psychotherapist's mind. Some psycho-analytically orientated psychotherapists value a lack of explicitness because it allows for misunderstandings, which they term 'transference', to develop, and these give valuable information about a person's character. However, experience suggests that there are many other opportunities for glimpses into character and, anyway, it is not clear how much the behaviour of someone in such an artificial situation is typical of their behaviour elsewhere.

Formulation

The formulation narrative will be couched in the psychotherapy genre to which the therapist belongs. This does not mean that any story will do. A therapeutic story must be narratively coherent, consistent with the client's and the therapist's values, impregnated with palatable emotional meaning, and able to lead to action which is appropriate to the client's concerns.

Case example (from Perczel-Forintos & Hackmann, 1999)

Background
Jane was the younger of two adopted girls who, at 16 years old, needed dental treatment and was given two injections of local anaesthetic into her gums. She was given these without warning and without consenting to them. She felt shocked, frightened and numb afterwards. At 18, she planned to go on holiday to the tropics, and was advised to have immunizations. She realized that she was frightened of having an injection, and went to see a psychologist who treated her needle phobia by behavioural methods. She felt fine when she was waiting for her injection, but as soon as she saw the needle being prepared for her, she panicked and wanted to leave the room. Her father held on to her and she had the immunization under restraint. Subsequently, her phobia was much worse and she had weeks of anxiety before a blood test or an immunization. She was referred to a psychologist again when she was 20 because she was starting to worry about having a baby, which she thought would involve blood tests and injections.

Formulation (taken from the paper, but put into the first person)
Jane, you definitely have injection phobia. In fact, you meet the standard criteria (DSM-IV criteria were used) for this disorder. But we note that it is not the blood

or the pain that you are afraid of, unlike many people with injection phobia. And we also note, even after the exposure treatment which stopped you being frightened of watching other people being injected, you still wanted to run away when it was your turn. We are also struck by the fact that the two occasions of being injected which you remember both involved you being out of control of the situation. In the immunization clinic, your father actually restrained you. When we asked you to say what you thought when you remembered that scene, you said a lot about feeling powerless and vulnerable. If we had to put your thoughts into words, it would be something like this: 'If I depend on other people and let them control me they might let me down'. What we would like to do is to help you change this thought into: 'When I am pregnant, injections and blood tests will be good for me'.

Three points are worth noting in this account. Firstly, the focus of the treatment is given by the diagnosis. This is generally true of phobias, but is not true of other psychiatric diagnoses. Secondly, minimal personal historical information is given. Thirdly, the proposed treatment plan has something of the same emotional meaning of the phobic situation: do what we tell you, because it's good for you. It is perhaps fortunate that the therapist involved was a woman, otherwise we might suppose that Jane would have found the emotional meaning of the therapy too unpalatable.

Evidence suggests that, although cognitive-behavioural treatment is more rapidly effective in the treatment of phobias than client-centered therapy or psycho-dynamic therapy, both of these latter approaches are as effective in the longer term (Teusch & Bohme, 1999). The evidence about other approaches is not yet available, but there is no reason to suppose that there would be a difference. It is therefore worth considering how other approaches might focus on Jane's problem.

Case example (cont.)

Alternative focus for Jane's problem
Psychodynamic: 'We are struck by the fact that all the situations that you have mentioned involve men, and also by the fact that you are particularly frightened of penetration. Although this is penetration by needles, we wonder if you are also frightened about the consequences of having intercourse with a man'.

Existential: 'The situations that you have mentioned all involve settings associated with illness and death. You were brought face-to-face with these anxieties, as all of us have to be, but with the realization that you were alone with your anxiety. You received no understanding of your fears, and no comfort, from those around you at the time. It is true that we are all alone when we finally face death, but this is a hard truth for which many of us need the experience of life to prepare. It has overwhelmed you for the moment, but let us discuss it together and see whether you can confront it without turning away'.

Client-centered: 'You told us about your fear, and you also told us about how various men have ignored it. You have told us that these men seem more interested in you not making a fuss than in really addressing what's bothering you. We would like to offer you the chance to explore what else may be bothering you'.

The point of setting out these different stories about Jane's problem is not to show which one is right, but to indicate how, even in the formulation, a narrative is being constructed which will both inform and restrict the treatment. This narrative may be written down – in a letter to the referrer, or in a reformulation letter – but it is never finished. In fact, there is usually, in longer-term treatment, a case for reviewing it and reformulating before the end of the treatment. Sometimes, this leads to a quite different emphasis.

Reformulation

Although Jane's therapists started out undertaking cognitive treatment, they (fortunately) did not stick slavishly to it. They felt that there must be a reason for Jane reacting so strongly to the two incidents, and they asked her: 'When, in your life, do you first remember having experiences like those?'. We may suppose that they were expecting Jane to talk about her adoption, but she spoke about her first sexual relationship. Readers might wonder why this relationship had not been discovered in the assessment interview, but perhaps Jane did not feel ready to trust the therapists with the information at that stage. That would have been a pity because a great deal might have been discovered about how Jane experienced her world if the relationship could have been systematically explored. Did Jane tell her mother, and not tell her father? If so, why was it concealed from her father? Why did Jane embark on a sexual relationship so early in her life? How old was her boyfriend? Did he leave her for someone else, and was that person known to Jane? Did her boyfriend comment critically on her teeth, and is that why she went to the dentist? These are some of the questions that immediately arise.

Case example (cont.)

Further background
Jane had her first sexual relationship when she was 14 years old. She and her boyfriend often had rows, but even so she was gob-smacked when he told her that he didn't want to see her any more. She felt that she would never trust anyone again or, at least, any man again. She felt lonely and empty without her boyfriend, and was determined never to allow anyone else to get such of a hold over her.

Reformulation

'Jane, we understand better how you feel now. We do not know about the circumstances of your adoption, but we do know that some adopted children feel that they did not matter enough to their biological parents, and that they were abandoned by them. Whether or not you feel like this, it does seem as if your traumatic first relationship, which you had begun with such trust, led to you feeling that you had misplaced that trust. The only way that you could get through it was to tell yourself that you would never make yourself vulnerable to a man again, and yet within months you had a further traumatic experience at the dentist. You must have felt then that you could not protect yourself against being hurt. We suppose that this was the source of your fear, and your subsequent experiences of injections have only confirmed it. Fortunately you have managed to keep this fear of your own powerlessness under control in other situations, but perhaps you have only been able to do so by keeping unusually tight control over these situations. In clinics, and during pregnancy, you cannot avoid giving some control to other people. But we think that there are people you can trust more than you think, and that you know that yourself now that you have talked about the relationship breakdown for the first time. We also think that you may now be much less anxious when having an injection. So let's check that out.'

Reformulation allows correction of the course of the psychotherapy. It establishes whether the factors which the therapist thinks have been therapeutic are the ones that the client also values. It also enables a review of the treatment contract.

Contracting

There are a surprising number of considerations which apply to the treatment contract (Table 4.3). In practice, it is probably best to reach some explicit agreement on all of them. This may not mean discussing each of them. It may be enough to set out the policies of the unit in the initial letter to the client, and ask the client to bring up any matters which concern them. However, the onus is clearly on the psychotherapist to have ensured that consent is obtained if, that is, the psychotherapist intends to be a collaborator with the client.

It should be noted that few psychotherapists only have a contract with the client. Many also have a contract with an employer or a third-party payer, some might have a contract with a court who has ordered the treatment, and students have contracts with their training organizations. Wherever necessary, these conflicting interests should be declared to the client.

Table 4.3. Elements of a treatment contract

Elements	Considerations
The focus	Taking account of the client's preoccupying concern
The relationship with the therapist	Combined treatment approaches, e.g. group and individual, individual and marital
	Prescribing medication and giving psychotherapy
	Undertaking physical examination and giving psychotherapy
The type of treatment	What suits the client
	What the therapist is qualified to give
Who will carry out the treatment	Particularly important if it is not the assessor
How long the treatment will be	May need to specify review periods
What the treatment is expected to bring about	Wanted and unwanted effects
Who is responsible for the treatment working?	
Who brings up treatment failure for discussion?	
Treatment cost	Effect on other relationships
	Time as well as money
The limits of treatment confidentiality	Limits of discussion with supervisor
	Legal responsibility to divulge
	Clinical governance
Consent	Special issues raised by children; clients who are incompetent
Record keeping	Access to records
Research	
The ethical framework under which the treatment is being carried out	Each psychotherapy organization may have its own codes
What the client should do if they wish to complain	

Issues in third-party contracts

Three issues about third-party contracts come up repeatedly. These are: (1) collecting information of relevance to the organization, (2) the duration of treatment, and (3) reporting on outcome to a third party.

Collecting information of relevance to the organization

Social services, psychology departments, community teams, psychiatric units and many other settings in which psychotherapists work will require information to be collected from clients. The impact of this needs to be considered and, wherever appropriate, discussed with the clients themselves.

Mental health professionals may be required to make a diagnosis according to accepted international criteria. Trainee psychiatrists may be required to ensure that their clients are not physically or mentally ill. Psychologists may be concerned to provide quantitative evidence of a client's distress or disability by using questionnaires. Certain background information may be required by good professional practice. Most professionals will have to obtain demographic information required by client management, quality assurance, and audit systems.

Time and cost prohibit the client from being interviewed by several people, each of whom is responsible for eliciting different information. If clients are referred by a medical practitioner, the psychotherapist can expect that physical assessment has been carried out. If there is any doubt, it is advisable to suggest that they contact the referrer again. A formal psychiatric history is not so easy to combine with an assessment of the client's concerns. For one thing, both are time-consuming and, taken together, are usually too time-consuming.

One solution is to use questionnaires as a means of collecting the information that might be required. This method is used by many psychotherapists who find it works well. It has the intrinsic disadvantage that it could impede access to psychotherapy by people with poor English, with a learning disability, or with impaired literacy. These, and other, advantages and disadvantages are discussed in detail by Mace (1995). An example of a questionnaire that has been used over a number of years is given in Appendix I.

The questionnaire can be used to provide systematic information, and the assessor can then discuss aspects of the history which seem particularly important. As noted in an earlier chapter, this gives important information about values, concerns and the attribution of emotional meaning, as well as embedding the client's current problem in a developmental narrative.

The duration of treatment

What do counselling and psychotherapy in general practice, community nurses in mental health teams, junior psychiatrists who rotate from firm to firm, and psychotherapists employed by third-party payers like health insurers and employee assistance programmes, all have in common? They are limited in the duration of the treatment that they can offer.

Short-term contracts are widely considered by psychotherapists to be anathemas. Clients may have more mixed feelings about it. Many clients expect psychotherapy treatment to be time-limited, and many who are offered open-ended contracts simply drop out of treatment when they feel that they have had enough. The indications are that the longer the treatment, the less the gain (Howard et al., 1986), with 50% of people considering that they have achieved their goals after eight sessions.

Many more people are eligible for psychotherapy than receive it. It is inevitable that some form of rationing has to operate. It is debatable which is more just – some clients receiving unlimited treatment, or many clients receiving limited treatment. Personally, I lean towards the latter.

There is a sharp distinction between the situation in private practice, and working in a health service (DeBerry & Baskin, 1989). Rationing is almost inevitable in the latter. The psychotherapist cannot but accept these limits, and the contract with the client therefore needs to be agreed on the basis that only limited treatment will be available. One compromise position is that clients are offered a finite number of sessions, typically from four to six, followed by a review. The review may result in the client being offered further sessions, but in some settings this can only happen if agreement is obtained from the case-manager or third-party payer. If the case-manager is knowledgeable and client-orientated, this system works reasonably well in practice. The only disadvantage is that neither the client nor the therapist has the luxury of being able to stretch out with no concern for the passage of time.

Reporting on outcome to a third party

Courts increasingly often sentence people to psychotherapy or counselling. Courses, too, may require that students complete a period of personal therapy. Naturally, probation officers and course coordinators would like to know whether or not the psychotherapy has produced the hoped-for changes. Psychotherapists should consider these situations carefully, but in practice, it is almost never in the client's interests to report on the outcome of the therapy. Whether or not psychotherapists should even say whether or not their client is continuing in treatment is a matter for careful consideration and will depend on the agreement made with the client and third party before treatment was begun.

Issues about the treatment contract with the client

The relationship with the therapist

The therapist and the client need to conduct their work in a safe relationship. In practice, this means that clients and therapists cannot also be friends, business partners or lovers. Any reader doubting this might want to look at some of the books on the subject which contain case-histories of what can go wrong (e.g. Bond, 1993).

The metaphor that many psychotherapists use is that there needs to be a boundary around the therapeutic relationship. 'Boundary violations', like having sex with a client, are more common than many professionals would like to admit, and when they occur, they can be profoundly emotionally distressing to the client. However, it is the more subtle boundary problems that are more common and may more easily be overlooked. Very often they can be tackled by having a clear agreement with the parties involved about how sensitive matters like confidentiality will be handled.

Boundary concerns arise if clients are being seen by the same therapist individually and in a group (a common practice among some group psychotherapists), or being seen individually and with their partner. One common approach is to agree that anything that is brought up in the individual session may also be brought up in the group or marital session.

When a suitably qualified practitioner prescribes medication and gives psychotherapy to the same client, boundary problems can also arise. The relationship of a prescriber to a client is often very different to that of a psychotherapist to a client. There is a danger that problems in the therapy will be disguised as requests for, or offers of, more medication, for example. Wherever possible, it is probably best that prescription is left to another doctor.

This boundary between two medical functions is even more important when it lies between psychotherapy and another medical function, physical assessment. Physical examination is only kept from being intrusive or sexual because it is so 'clinical', with all that word implies. Psychotherapy is not clinical. Physical assessment in a psychotherapeutic context is too open to misuse or misinterpretation for it to be a useful or ethical practice.

The type of treatment

Psychotherapy should not be a Procrustean bed, with every client being fitted into the therapeutic mould of the psychotherapist. Clients who want symptom relief have a right to receive it, even if the psychotherapist is more comfortable with exploratory therapy. Psychotherapy is a small and specialized field, and practitioners can therefore be expected to be experienced enough in at least two or three approaches to be able to carry out whichever of them suits the client best.

However, psychotherapists should also be wary of being all things to all clients. No psychotherapist can be qualified to provide all types of therapy. If the psychotherapist comes to the conclusion with the client that the right treatment for the client is one which he or she is not qualified to provide, this should be openly discussed with the client and the client advised how to get in contact with a psychotherapist with the required qualification.

Assessment and treatment carried out by different psychotherapists

As psychotherapists become more experienced, they spend more and more time in assessment, and less and less time in treatment. This is a pity since there is little evidence that experienced psychotherapists are any better than inexperienced ones at predicting who will benefit from treatment (Tantam, 1995b). It does, however, mean that clients of a psychotherapy department or centre are likely to be seen by one psychotherapist for assessment, and by another for treatment. In community psychiatry, about a third of clients do not attend their first appointment with a new clinician (Tantam & Klerman, 1979). This means that a third do not show up for a first assessment, and that a further third that attend the assessment will drop out before attending the first treatment session with a new therapist. Asking the proposed therapist to attend the first assessment interview (if the client consents) reduces this additional drop-out rate substantially, and is a practice I recommend.

If a different therapist carries out treatment, the first treatment session should be used as a new assessment, even if the treating therapist sat in on the earlier assessment. This is for two reasons. Treatment contract needs to be between the therapist and the client, and not negotiated by the assessor on behalf of the therapist. The second reason is that assessment is just as much about the client assessing the therapist, as about the client being assessed. Clients need to consent to their therapists, and this cannot be an informed process unless there has been sufficient social interaction between the two of them.

The duration of treatment

The vexatious matter of treatment duration has already been considered once in this chapter, from the perspective of the agency paying for the treatment. Clients pay in terms of time and emotional commitment for their treatment, even if they do not pay in money. Some clients, particularly once they have become friends with their psychotherapist or the fellow-members of their therapy group, may enjoy therapy and not want to give it up. However, this is exceptional. Most clients want the briefest treatment compatible with the treatment aims. Indeed, people waiting for an appointment for a psycho-therapy assessment anticipate being in treatment for a much shorter period of time than do their assessors.

Treatment duration should be determined by how long it will take to attend to the agreed focus of the client's difficulties. The average length of treatment required can be estimated precisely if the client has a condition like agoraphobia, where there is a clearly effective treatment and many outcome studies. However, even in the case of agoraphobia, symptom relief may not be possible until previously unsuspected or unreported alcohol misuse or a chronic marital problem is relieved.

Therapists may feel reluctant to negotiate brief contracts, either because they feel that the client's problems are so great that a brief contract would be an insult to the client, or that brief therapy is too superficial. However, the evidence is that short-term psychotherapy can be useful for many conditions, for example opioid dependence (Lerner et al., 1992) and even personality disorder (Winston et al., 1994). Experience also suggests that clients are less likely to drop out of treatment if they are offered short-term treatment contracts initially.

In practice, it is best to suggest to almost every client entering individual psychotherapy or every family beginning family therapy that there are four or five sessions of treatment, followed by a review. The treatment focus of these four or five sessions will be determined at the assessment interview. It may be to resolve the symptoms that concern the client, with the expectation that the client will be discharged after the initial four sessions. To go to the other extreme, the focus of these sessions may be to identify more clearly some of the patterns of relationship difficulty that would need to be resolved in long-term treatment. In the latter case, even though there may be an expecta-tion that the client will stay in treatment for a substantially longer period, I normally suggest a further review after 12 sessions. This enables the client and the therapist to review what progress can be made once the 'honeymoon effect' of the treatment is starting to wear off.

Reviews at 4 weeks, and re-reviews at subsequent intervals, establish a culture of quality monitoring. If either the client or the therapist thinks that the treatment is not helping the client, then the review is an encouragement to be open about it. Review sessions are also a good opportunity for the client and the therapist to agree any necessary reformulation of the client's concerns and the treatment focus. Knowing that time is limited also means that both therapist and client are highly motivated to address the preoccupying con-cerns. Sometimes a reminder by either party that time is passing can bring the other person back on track.

There is a turning point in many psychotherapies when something new enters into the client's reckoning which starts the process of resolution of the preoccupying concern. Resolution may not follow straight away. There may often be a long process of working through the changes of beliefs, values and emotional meaning that follow from the turning point. This can be easy and rewarding work in psychotherapy, but it is questionable whether it is necessary. If the client can work things out for him- or herself, perhaps with the help of friends and family, that is likely to increase their confidence more than being assisted by a psychotherapist. Termination should not be left until preoccupying concerns have been resolved.

What the therapy is expected to bring about

I remember once a lively discussion with the council of a senior psychoanalytically inclined psychotherapy organization in the UK. They were dissociating themselves from the umbrella body of psychotherapy in the UK, the United Kingdom Council for Psychotherapy. Their first objection was to the code of ethics. This states (see Appendix II, 1.2) that: 'All psychotherapists are expected to approach their work with the aim of alleviating suffering and promoting the well-being of their clients . . .'. The psychotherapy organization objected to the health orientation of the definition of psychotherapy. Psychotherapy could, they said, be justified if it increased self-understanding or had an educational role, without any effect on well-being or distress.

It is true that people may embark on psychotherapy as a form of exploration in which it is the process of discovery that matters, not whether or not the discoveries have a practical application. These people are not looking for anything in particular. In fact, trainee psychotherapists, for whom exploratory psychotherapy may be an important element of training, may be relieved not to find any significant personal difficulties. Exploratory psychotherapy which has no practical purpose other than exploration should not be belittled, but it belongs to other leisure pursuits which a person might pursue to enhance or increase their understanding of themselves.

Therapy derives from the ancient Greek word, 'therapei-a'. The original meaning of therapei-a is 'service', for example to the gods, where it has the connotation of worship; to a lord, also connoting flattery; or to parents, also connoting respect (Anonymous, 1999). Service continues to be an important element of the role of the psychotherapist, as the group psychotherapist, Foulkes, recognized. However, the English word 'therapy' now has the single meaning, 'The medical treatment of disease; curative medical or psychiatric treatment' (*Oxford English Dictionary*). Confusion can only come from the widening of the term 'psychotherapy' beyond the boundaries set on one of its roots, the word 'therapy'. Fortunately, there is another word, 'analysis', which does apply to exploration. It means, *inter alia*, to trace things to their source, and to discover general principles underlying concrete phenomena (taken from *Oxford English Dictionary*). Psycho-analysis, group analysis, existential analysis and transactional analysis are all common applications of 'analysis' to exploratory psychotherapy.

It makes good practical sense to use 'analysis' rather than 'therapy' when exploration or training is the issue. However, we are not quite out of the woods if we use 'treatment' as a synonym for therapy. Treatment means how we conduct ourselves towards another person, and can apply equally to the client and to the therapist. We might say, for example, that a client treated us badly because they failed to pay their final account. Unless the context makes our meaning clear, it is necessary therefore to add some qualifier to 'treatment' to show what we are speaking about. But the qualifier is not easy to come by. If we say, 'medical' treatment, does this make psychotherapy a hand-maiden of medicine? Are we 'medicalizing' our clients, or going overboard for the medical model? If we say, 'psychological' treatment, we avoid this trap but introduce another. There is a very real danger in many European countries that psychotherapy becomes a branch of psychology. In the UK, there is an equally strong tradition of psychotherapy being an independent profession. Psychological treatment would seem to pre-judge this debate.

Readers might think that all this concentration on wording has no real practical importance. But this would not be true. The splits in the field of psychotherapy, and the lack of cohesion in its theory and in its practice, are direct consequences. Let us look at one last example. Treatment, when used in a medical context, has the synonym, 'remediation'. Defining psychotherapy as 'the professional application of remedies for mental suffering' seems to me as close to a good definition as one is likely to get. However, it will not be acceptable to many psychotherapists because it incorporates a presumption that psychotherapy improves something. Almost all psychotherapists would accept that psychotherapy changes something, but many would not accept that the change can be specified or evaluated. Both of these latter steps are required to show that improvement has taken place.

There are clearly dangers in committing oneself to improvement: fixing things before they are broken, for example. There is a more subtle danger in having the responsibility of improving something about someone else since improvement readily turns into making a person more acceptable to other people. To guard against both of these dangers it is essential that improvement is based on consent – consent on what would constitute improvement, and on what needs to be improved.

Case example

Anna had become progressively more withdrawn until she was mute. She remained in this state for almost 3 years until she was referred to a specialist centre. A diagnosis of depressive stupor was made, but she made little improvement with medication. The family situation was investigated, and it emerged that Anna's state dated from the time when her mother-in-law had become frail and, at Anna's husband's insistence, had come to live with Anna and her family. Family meetings were arranged and at one of these meetings the therapist stood behind Anna and spoke for her. The therapist said that Anna felt that she had no role in the family any more, and that it was time that a place was found for her in the family again. The meeting at which this was said turned out to be the last meeting that the family attended. They failed to keep subsequent appointments, and Anna killed herself some 3 months after discharge from hospital.

When the therapist takes it upon him- or herself to know what improvements are required, things go wrong. But this is not to say that psychotherapy is not about improvement, only to say that it is about consensual improvement. Determining what improvement should be concerned with, what plan is needed to secure improvement, and what will constitute improvement – all of these determinations must be made by the psychotherapist and the client working together.

Anna's case also indicates that psychotherapy has unwanted effects. It is sometimes argued that these are very unusual, and that psychotherapy is a treatment which has no greater adverse effects than placebo. After all, it is argued, what harm can there be in talking to someone? Placebos themselves have adverse effects. Their use may, for example, delay diagnosis. But, if it is true that psychotherapy has no greater adverse effect than placebo, it follows that we should strongly suspect that psychotherapy is a placebo.

In fact, Anna's case, and others like it, indicate that psychotherapy may have adverse effects, some of which may be fatal. Although the frequency of such severe adverse effects may be too low for it to be practically necessary to warn clients of them, the frequency of relationship breakdown is high enough for it to be necessary to advise clients of the danger of this. The greatest risk of this occurs in the longer-term, more exploratory treatments. These involve the greatest intensity of personal relationships between therapist and client. Frank admission of a person's dissatisfactions with their personal relationships are also most common in longer-term therapy. Group psychotherapy offers the further danger that one member may become personally or sexually involved with another. Although most group therapists explicitly advise against such meetings or other contacts outside the group, they often occur.

The risk of relationship breakdown or sexual experimentation may be increased in clients of therapists who value 'authenticity' particularly highly, i.e. therapists with a humanistic or existential orientation. This is not because such therapists are less committed to an ethical framework than their colleagues. The experimentation is not between therapist and client. It is because authenticity, a concept first introduced by Heidegger (1927), takes no account of social ties but relates only to how clearly a person can contemplate their own fate. The pursuit of authenticity, unmitigated by other values, makes throwing up one's place in the world seem virtuous if it opens one's eyes to the world as it really is. However, such masterful behaviour can be self-deceptive, too (Deurzen, personal communication). All psychotherapy must be a compromise between values rather than a wilful assertion of them.

Two other adverse effects of treatment are common enough to merit consideration. Dependence may lead to a client losing confidence in his or her own coping techniques and abandoning the people who, before therapy, might have helped him or her to overcome problems. It may lead to a crisis at termination when a client is suddenly faced with having to replace coping techniques involving the therapist. Dependence may be particularly likely in treatments which strip clients of ideas or things which strengthen their identity, treatments which provoke severe anxiety, or treatments which heighten the power differences between client and therapist, particularly if the therapist presents his or her power as unreservedly benign. Particular types of group therapy, body therapies and psycho-analysis may all have this effect.

Psycho-analysts sometimes argue that dependency is desirable in the early stages of therapy because it encourages regression and the discovery of unresolved problems in parental relationships. Positive transference, according to these psychotherapists, always involves an element of dependency and regression. In practice, there is no evidence about whether or not outcome is improved by the development of dependency. The induction of dependency is a crucial stage in recruiting people to religious cults, and is associated with their loss of autonomy. It seems more likely that it is an effect of psychotherapy which should be minimized rather than encouraged, and that clients who are at risk should be warned that this is a recognized adverse effect.

The final adverse effect to be considered is the construction of false memories under the influence of the psychotherapist. Finding the past coming back often happens in therapy, particularly in those psychotherapies which emphasize the influence of the past on the present. The value of this is uncertain. Folk wisdom suggests that 'some things are best left forgotten'. On the other hand, many psychotherapists cleave to the surgical principle that an unprocessed memory is like a foreign body. If the wound closes over it, if, that is, it is forgotten, there will inevitably be sepsis which will lead to greater trauma than if the foreign body were removed at the beginning. Many psychotherapists are minded to try to unearth buried memories on the principle that they may be the foreign bodies that are causing the client's current problems. Hypnosis, which increases recall, may be used, as may more active techniques of suggestion.

The fallacy of both the 'best forgotten' and the 'foreign body' approaches is that the recall of autobiographical memories is like the discovery of a buried recording. What is remembered about the past is, however, more like a narrative about oneself and one's experiences than like a film. Each time that the narrative is rehearsed, it is refreshed but it may also be changed. If something new enters the narrative then this, too, is incorporated into the memory. If, for example, the psychotherapist says, 'When your father came into the room, what was his expression like?' and the narrative context suggests that the father was looking lustful or devious, this may become a memory. Such memories are indistinguishable from any other memory. Neither vividness, nor emotional arousal, nor level of detail distinguishes a false from a veridical memory. Likelihood is a double-edged tool. There are as many dangers of ruling a person's memory as false because the perpetrator is a friend, or a colleague or a person above suspicion as there are dangers in being credulous about fantastic memories of satanic abuse or the cannabalism of babies. It should always be remembered that false memories are not made up – they are believed to be true.

Falsification of memory is less likely to occur if a person has never forgotten an incident, i.e. if they have sufficiently regularly re-narrated it. When there is a long gap, during which a person has no memory for an event, the possibility of falsification becomes much greater. A working party of the Royal College of Psychiatrists in the UK recently concluded that '. . . when memories are "recovered" after long periods of amnesia, particularly when extraordinary means were used to secure the recovery of memory, there is a high probability that the memories are false, i.e. of incidents that had not occurred' (Brandon et al., 1998, p. 296). This statement may suggest more certainty about memory than is justified. False memories are not restricted to recovered memories, nor is it possible to say what proportion of recovered memories are false. Further details about the arguments can be had from the associations on both sides of the divide.

Brandon et al. (1998) suggest that psychotherapists should do what they can to avoid implanting false memories. Loftus (1997) concludes from current research that the falsification of memory can be reduced by: (1) not making demands on a person to remember, (2) not asking someone to imagine what might have happened, and (3) not telling someone to ignore whether or not they think a memory is real. Hypnosis increases the production of memories, apparently without altering the ratio of true-to-false memory. It is not a means of discovering the truth, nor is it more likely to implant false memory unless it is coupled with one or more of the factors mentioned by Loftus.

I like to challenge my students to think differently about the past. I say that, contrary to commonsense ideas, the present cannot be changed, the future can be changed, though with difficulty, but the past is the easiest to change. In speaking about the past, what I really mean is our memory of it. Psychotherapists should accept that memory falsification is a potential adverse effect of treatment and should treat clients accordingly.

Who is responsible for the treatment working, and who brings it up if it is failing?

Psychiatrists and other doctors rightly feel responsible to their clients for making the right diagnosis and prescribing the generally accepted treatment, but they are well aware that there will always be a proportion of clients who do not respond. These 'refractory clients' may need further assessment and special treatment. Sometimes the psychiatrist may need to admit that he or she has failed to help them. But he or she has not failed in their duty of care to the client. Indeed, it is usually the knowledge base of psychiatry that has proved inadequate, and the psychiatrist has not failed personally at all.

In psychotherapy, to a much greater extent than in medicine or psychiatry, the therapist's personality and ability to make a relationship is part of the active treatment. It is therefore more tempting to think one is responsible for the outcome of the treatment. As in psychiatry, one is responsible for doing everything that one can to understand the client's concerns and formulating a treatment plan that is appropriate. There is also a responsibility to keep appointments, to provide suitable rooms, to see clients without unnecessary interruption, and so on. Finally, there is also a responsibility to prescribe oneself in an appropriate way: that is, to use appropriate therapeutic methods. However, given all these caveats, it is not the therapist's responsibility to make the client better. Indeed, it is not the therapist's responsibility to make the client do anything, or to get them to do anything either.

Similarly, it is not the client's responsibility to get better, although clients do have responsibilities which increase their chances of getting better. These include keeping appointments, not deliberately deceiving the therapist, and doing their best to stick to agreed contracts.

Failing to improve is a catastrophe that can happen to any client. Catastrophes should never be taken lightly, but nor can they be reversed. Keeping someone on in treatment because they are not improving is compounding a mistake: if they are not improving with the treatment that the psychotherapist is providing, then the client needs to try something, or someone, else.

The reason for continuing with treatment is that the client's concerns are being ameliorated, however gradually. Sometimes it makes practical sense to say to someone that treatment will end if they are not improving, but will continue if they are.

What are the limits of treatment confidentiality?

Confidentiality is important to both psychotherapists and their clients. However, there are many factors which make it less than absolute. Students, trainees, counsellors and psychotherapists in many modalities are required to have supervisors with whom they discuss cases. Information about clients may also be required by employers, and this may increase as employers take on the burdens of clinical governance. Detailed records may not be kept about clients in some settings, and in these settings it may not be considered appropriate to send assessment information to referrers. In health care settings, both detailed records and letters are expected. These may be read by people other than the addressee, such as administrative staff, secretaries, receptionists and other health care workers.

All information about clients in psychotherapy is potentially sensitive. Psychotherapists and administrative staff should therefore be trained to deal with enquiries from third parties, which may include lawyers or alienated partners, without releasing confidential information. Even divulging whether or not a person is known to a psychotherapy department may be a breach of confidentiality so far as that person is concerned. However, this absolutism should be tempered with good sense and good manners. Some third parties, for example the referrer, may have a right to some information.

Psychotherapists have no special professional privileges in law. They attract the same penalties for refusing to disclose as do any private citizens. Courts may require that both they and their records are subpoenaed, and not only in relation to criminal cases. One party in a divorce case may require a psychotherapist or counsellor to give evidence about the other party, or be in contempt of court. It is less clear whether there is ever a duty on psychotherapists to initiate disclosure. Jurisdictions throughout the world vary, and legislation is changing. In the UK, the gradual adoption of the European social charter, with its attendant right to privacy, is likely to change the law further.

Case example

Robert was born as a woman but had gender reassignment treatment. He came for psychotherapy partly because of his difficulties in adjusting to being a man. He had started a relationship with Julie, but had not yet told her of his history and was unsure about her likely reaction. She had quite homophobic attitudes, and he was afraid that she would think that their's was a lesbian relationship. Julie was appointed as a temporary cleaner in the psychology department, and Robert became preoccupied by the thought that she would find his records and discover the truth about him before he had a chance to tell her himself.

The duty to disclose arises in two situations: where child abuse is suspected, and where disclosure might prevent a serious crime against another person. Practising psychotherapists should be clear about what is expected of them by their employing institutions and by the law of the land. Wherever possible, any proposed disclosure should be discussed with a supervisor or, failing that, with a senior colleague before any action is taken. Psychotherapists with professional indemnity may discuss their proposed actions with advisors employed by the company or association providing the indemnity insurance. The psychotherapist should do everything possible to persuade the client to disclose, and should only be responsible for disclosure if the client refuses. If the client does disclose under coercion, the psychotherapist can still be taxed with breaching confidentiality, but at least the client has the chance of managing the disclosure.

The general ethical principles governing disclosure are, on the one side, the breach of contract to the client and the likelihood that clients will not disclose facts to psychotherapists which are essential for their treatment to be successful, and on the other side, the benefits of preventing abuse to a child, or serious harm to another person. The latter may include an innocent person being punished if the psychotherapist withholds evidence from the psychotherapy with the actual offender. It may sometimes be argued that the longer-term interests of the client are better served by disclosure if a crime is prevented for which they would have to pay the penalty. This argument would be stronger if it did not assume that the psychotherapist sometimes knows the client's interests better than the client does him- or herself.

Where the psychotherapist draws the line between disclosure and confidentiality may depend on his or her particular practice. A forensic psychotherapist would not be able to work unless his or her clients were sure that they could report their violent or sexually violent thoughts without fear of being arrested. However, psychotherapists outside the forensic sector rarely have clients who are paedophiles, and, it is doubtful whether non-paedophile clients would be put off disclosing information because their psychotherapist would draw the attention of the authorities to paedophilia.

What is clear is that clients should normally be told about the limits of confidentiality before they accept their treatment contract, especially if there are special considerations, for example supervision or the possibility of publication of case material. Many psychotherapists do not currently do this (Dsubanko Obermayr & Baumann, 1998).

Special confidentiality considerations arise in group and family psychotherapy. Here, it is a matter for the group members to agree the principles that they wish to follow, and for the group to respond if a group member is unwilling to adhere to them. Most groups agree in the first or second session that personal information exchanged in the group will not be discussed outside the group. However, many group members do discuss other members with partners or close friends, even so.

Psychotherapists working with families need to respect the family's own principles concerning confidentiality. Families will have, for example, restrictions on discussing the sexual life of parents with their children, and any sexually mature children will also expect that their sexual life can be conducted in private. It will rarely happen that the therapist believes that a family secret should be disclosed, even though one or more member(s) of the family wish(es) it to remain confidential. The same principles of disclosure to a third party also apply to family disclosures, and the precautions of consulting a supervisor or peer, previously discussed in relation to third-party disclosure, should also be followed before disclosing in a family. It is also usually worth meeting with a family member or members who are in on the secret to request that it is they who disclose it, and not the therapist.

If a psychotherapist is publishing a case-history, then confidentiality can normally be maintained by omitting key information. Failure to do so adequately may lay the psychotherapist open to a complaint. Leaving out key information may not be enough to conceal from the subject of the case-history that it is their case which is being written up. Unlike other readers, the subject will know that he or she has consulted the author of the case, and what precise problems were reported. If the subject has not consented to publication, he or she may be affronted to have the case discussed in public print. He or she may also take exception to the conclusions of the psycho-therapist.

Consent

Much of the foregoing discussion of confidentiality has assumed that clients can give valid consent. Psychotherapists may work with children or people with learning disability in whom this might be in question. It will rarely be the case that clients can benefit from psychotherapy and yet be unable to give any form of consent. Clients should therefore always be consulted when it is possible to do so. However, the next of kin or 'best friend' of a child or a person with learning disability may also have a justified wish to be consulted. Normally, the client will be happy to accede to this, and some clients may ask that someone else is consulted, in which case their wishes should be respect-ed. In all these situations, it is important to establish with the client what will be said to the friend or family member. Very often, clients may consent to someone else being consulted, but not to them being given all the informa-tion in the psychotherapist's possession. Situations in which the psycho-therapist is required to approach a parent or other person to obtain consent to a psychotherapy procedure, but the client does not consent to the ap-proach, will be rare. If one does occur, the psychotherapist should discuss it with a supervisor or a peer.

Publication presents other special problems about consent. When consent to publication can be obtained, there is no problem. Many journal editors require written consent from clients whose cases are being reported. How-ever, when the therapist has lost touch with the client, for example when it was a client who was treated many years before, it is not always possible to obtain consent. Moreover, the value of case illustrations in psychotherapy is different from that of many case reports. Retrospective analysis of case reports may be part of an empirical study. Disguising case reports may therefore falsify future research (Tantam, 1995c). This is not true of illustrations which are required to be true in spirit, but not in detail. I take the view that disguising case illustrations is justified, as long as the fact that these are illustrations and not reports is made clear. I also take the view that consent does not need to be obtained to publish case illustrations so long as they are sufficiently disguised that they are not recognizable by the person or persons on whose case or cases they are based. However, this view has not been tested in a complaints hearing or other tribunal.

Record keeping

Clients should be made aware what records are kept and who has access to them. The very detailed and personal information that is often collected by psychotherapists may not be appropriate or relevant to other medical records. In many health settings, it is therefore common to keep psychotherapy records separately. Records about staff members are also often kept in a secure place to which only a limited number of staff members have access. In most countries clients have a legal right to read any records made about them, although not necessarily copies of information provided by others about them. Procedures will normally be in place to enable access, and to assist clients in interpreting what they read in their records.

It is a good discipline for all professionals to write only what they would not object to their client(s) reading. There seems little justification for private comments about personality or mendacity, or for all the other pejorative observations that health care professionals are sometimes inclined to make. If a client gives unreliable information or if their behaviour is threatening, this should be in their records, but supported by evidence.

The very detailed records that are often kept by trainees may not be appropriate for more experienced psychotherapists. However, psychotherapists and counsellors are sometimes inclined not to keep records at all. This is a head-in-the-sand approach to the ethical problems raised by records which cannot be condoned. Sometimes clients ask that certain items of information should not be put in the records. The psychotherapist needs to remember that the records belong to him or her, and not to the client. The client's wishes should always be considered, but the final consideration is what the psychotherapist thinks should be recorded.

Audio- or video-recordings of psychotherapy will normally be made only for specific purposes, and will usually be destroyed afterwards. Special consent needs to be obtained, and most organizations and professional associations publish guidance (e.g. for the guidance of the General Medical Council, see http://www.gmc-uk.org/n_hance/good/aud_vid.htm).

Research

Research into, and audit of, psychotherapy is highly desirable. Psychotherapists sometimes argue that research changes the relationship of the client and the therapist. This is undoubtedly true, but that is no reason to assume that it is changed for the worse. As long as it is the treatment that comes first, and as long as research is ethical and carried out only with the consent of the client, there seems to be little objection to it. For many years, I have sent out a notice before seeing clients for assessment, stating that they might be approached about participating in research. No-one has ever refused assessment for this reason, or ever taken issue with the notice itself.

The ethical framework under which the treatment is being carried out

In an increasingly litigious world, disputes are more likely to be resolved by appeal to a tribunal. All psychotherapists can therefore expect to receive complaints about their work. Each complaint should lead to an audit by the psychotherapist, of the circumstances that led up to it. Very often these will include a breakdown of communication between the client and the therapist, for example a letter or telephone call from the client that has not been answered.

Impeding a complaint may simply harden the potential complainant's resolve. Psychotherapists should therefore be as ready as any other professional to give information about how to complain, and to whom to complain. It may be appropriate to have a notice about this in the waiting room, too. A complaint is likely to be upheld if the psychotherapist has been negligent or has breached the relevant codes of ethics or practice. The basis for upholding a complaint of negligence in psychotherapy is only just being worked out. Codes of ethics and practice are much better established. Unfortunately, there may be many codes that apply. Which of them is considered may depend on who is hearing the complaint. Many psychotherapists have membership of several professional organizations and any of them may deal with a complaint, as may any of the psychotherapist's employers.

In practice, this situation is not quite as bad as it might seem. There is considerable agreement about the principles of ethical psychotherapy (see, for example, the code of the United Kingdom Council for Psychotherapy).

Termination

Termination of treatment may be distressing, it may have after-effects, and it may be unwelcome. All of these issues are discussed in more detail in Chapter 11. Termination should be anticipated at the beginning of treatment, and included in the therapeutic contract. It is a fundamental right of clients to withdraw from treatment. The therapeutic contract should not legislate against this, although it may sometimes be useful to specify that a limited number of further sessions should normally take place after the decision to end the therapy, to enable the consequences of the decision to be worked through. It is always desirable that the decision to end, and when to end, is made jointly between client and therapist. However, the circumstances when therapy will be unilaterally terminated by the therapist also need to be spelt out. For example, how may therapy sessions can the client miss, without notifying the therapist, before they are considered to have withdrawn from treatment? Many therapists would say that this should be the same as the notice period following a client's decision to withdraw, and that 4 weeks is about the right time period.

Psychotherapists may assume that they will always be there. However, this may not be true of psychotherapists with a chronic health problem, psychotherapists who are very elderly, or psychotherapists in circumstances which may require them to relocate. Trainee psychiatrists are often in the latter category. The possibility of treatment being ended prematurely should be faced before treatment starts, and what will happen if it does should be part of the therapeutic plan.

5

Narrating the self

Story-telling does not stop when we move from public to private domains. Narrative therapists observe that we tell ourselves and our partners stories, too, and sometimes they tell us alternative stories. These stories deal with ethical issues primarily: who was responsible, whether what was done was good or bad, caring or negligent. As Harre has argued, they position us in relation to other people (Harre & Gillett, 1994). Just as importantly, they give us the opportunity to show that our actions are consistent with our values. It is rare for such stories to be more than episodes, sometimes quite trivial ones. They may be about why we omitted to get the car serviced, where we were at 10 o'clock last night, or why we were less than kind to our daughter. However, each of these episodes will have raised questions about our relationship with someone else, with the values that govern that relationship, and our ability to cleave to those values.

I may not have got the car serviced because I rarely use it, and I leave it to my partner to sort out. My partner might conclude that taking responsibility for the things that we hold in common is not high on my list of values, or that, even if it is, I allow myself to be governed by other concerns. My story about this episode might be focussed on this issue, emphasizing perhaps those special considerations which might reinstate my partner's confidence that we share the same values. I might, for example, emphasize stress at work as one reason for unusual forgetfulness.

Petitions for divorce on the grounds of cruelty used to be made up of stories about episodes just like these. The overall effect was to create the character of the respondent as someone whose whole way of conducting him- or herself was such that any reasonable person would be discountenanced by it.

William was feckless, and his father could not stand it any longer. His father had been an army officer and since then a company director. He was used to high standards. William's father had a pretty good knowledge of people, and he knew that some were weak and needed to be shored up by authority. But he did expect that with a bit of backbone provided by someone else, everybody should be expected to adhere to certain basic standards of conduct. Since

William's mother had left, and incidentally almost given up contact with William, William's father had the sole responsibility for his son. His son would not get up in the morning. He could not get a job, and he was completely reliant on his father for the simplest things. But the worst thing, according to William's father, was that William lived in a Walter Mitty world. Like Mitty's character, he made up stories about himself. He told some people that he was a well-known football player, other people that he had this or that job. Sometimes he wrote letters to himself, describing his achievements.

William had Asperger's syndrome, and therefore had a profound difficulty in grasping the unspoken in social situations. He could not read faces for clues about attitudes or feelings. He was only able to interact successfully with people who were much younger than himself, who treated him like a contemporary. His father said that he would deny that there was a problem, and he did not really see much point in William being assessed at all. William was completely lacking in insight. He just could not help being completely insensitive, his father said. What was so unfair was that people not only turned against William, which was understandable according to his father, but that they turned against him, William's father, too.

The doctor told William the story of Walter Mitty: of a man who lived with a woman who made him feel quite inadequate. Walter could not argue with his wife's perception of himself, but he could not bear it either. So he made up stories about the life that he would like to have led. The doctor said that he understood Walter Mitty doing this, because in his real life, Walter Mitty felt so unimportant and powerless. The doctor wondered if William also felt like that. William did and, startling his father (it was a joint interview), said that he knew it made people angry when he told them yarns, and that he wished that he didn't have to. But what he could say to people at the age of 26 years, when they asked what he was doing? William felt that it was just too miserable to say that he lived at home with his father, that he was unemployable, and that his mother wanted no more to do with him. The doctor could only agree.

William used stories to create a character with the values by which William would have liked to live. However, the stories could not stand comparison with his real life, and quickly collapsed. William's true story, according to his father, was a sort of moral incapacity. The story that William told when he was called upon to tell the truth was of someone grieving the absence of abilities and rewards that he saw in others, but it was also a story about living with someone who did not value him.

Narrative therapists argue that there is, implicit in each episode of our life, a plot and characterization that belongs to a larger story: the story of our lives.

Plot

Imagine writing your own obituary. If this were the starting point for an existential exercise, the workshop leader would expect that the very process of writing the obituary would make each person think of how their present life measures up to it. The life-story is not merely a description. It has a rhetorical force. We might want our life-story to be of a certain kind. We might want it to be as successful as that of our parents, or as noble as the life of our favourite historical character, for example. Or we might want our life-story to be a warning to others. Victims of war-time horror get relief from telling their story to others because it gives it a purpose. They can testify to the horrific acts that they have seen (Weine et al., 1998).

Each life-story has a plot which encompasses the events in a person's life. It is through the plot that we gain a sense of a person being the agent of their life. Of course, contingency throws events and limitations in their way, but that is what makes the story interesting. No-one reads 'riches-to-riches' stories, but lots of people feel vicariously satisfied by a 'rags-to-riches' story. The twists and turns of fate are what brings out a person's resourcefulness. Even more importantly, they bring out the values of a person. Few people would steal if they were not in want. It is being in want that brings out a person's real values about property and about theft.

Character

A person's life tells a story about the person themselves – about their character. However, narrative therapy asserts that these stories do not just describe who we are. They also constitute who we are.

Roger grew up in a rural area of Northumberland. He worked in a factory for a while in the local town, but felt dissatisfied with his life. He wanted to have some authority, to be someone. He decided to apply for training as a pharmacist because he was interested in drugs. In fact, his interest was not merely professional. He smoked cannabis regularly, and occasionally used amphetamines, too. The access to drugs was an exhilarating aspect of pharmacy training. He was able to steal tablets on a regular basis, and used them recreationally with a group of acquaintances. However, he was caught quite quickly. He was relieved to be treated leniently and completed his training under supervision.

Twenty years later, when he went to see a psychotherapist, he was a university lecturer in pharmacy. He had a strong sense of the values of his profession, and was somewhat shocked that he had been allowed to complete his training. 'It would not have happened these days', he said, 'but then, it wasn't serious drug taking, just experimentation.'

Roger had absorbed the values of his profession, and now looked back at his youthful self with some criticism, if not downright rejection. Becoming a pharmacist had meant that he had adopted some professional values as his own, and he could no longer think with quite such equanimity of himself stealing drugs.

It is not just occupying a position in society which changes character. Life-events might, too. The kind of life-event that has received most attention in this respect is trauma, especially trauma in childhood, which is associated with long-term problems in feeling secure in relationships and in being able to rely on the world to be a safe place. The consequences for character are subsumed by some people under the rubric of 'borderline personality disorder'.

Kim's father was a social worker, her mother a cleaner. There were several daughters in the family, but Kim was born with a speech impediment and, from the outset, this had irritated her father. He would hit her when she cried and, if this did not work, would lock her in the toilet for hours on end. His manner to her changed as she got older. There were times when he would be very kind to her. Kim felt relieved at first when he was like this, but it soon became apparent that he wanted to have sex with her and that kindness was just a way of seducing her. She went along with it because she felt that she had no choice. She has always been teased at school. At the age of 14 years old, another child threw a piece of broken glass at her which cut her face. Kim picked up the glass and grazed her face with it some more. She felt calm after doing this, and repeated the cut when she got home, but this time on her wrist. This began a regular habit of deliberate self-harm. Kim could never trust anyone, especially men. Whenever a man became interested in her, she became frightened and the incidence of her deliberate self-harm increased. The more he persisted, the more she felt that she needed relief. She began to use sleeping tablets regularly, often buying them illicitly. Overdoses of these tablets joined cutting as one of her regular means of deliberate self-harm.

Many private and professional conversations are about the degree to which character can be attributed to circumstance. Often, this is presented as a binary opposition: either it is one, or it is the other. In stories, when characters do things, we consider both that they are responding to circumstances and that they are responding in their own way. When Sherlock Holmes, Conan Doyle's fictional detective, undertakes some inexplicable examination of an apparently insignificant object, Lestrade attributes it to his rival's eccentricity and to what we would now call 'attention seeking'. Watson is wiser. He is inclined to think that Holmes is responding to some particular of the circumstances of the crime that will turn out to be important later. Watson almost always turns out to be right. Psychotherapists are wise to take heed of this dictum of Kierkegaard: 'Most men are subjective toward themselves and objective toward all others, frightfully objective sometimes – but the task is precisely to be objective toward oneself and subjective toward all others' (1967, journal IV, para 4542).

Kim was normally guarded with her psychotherapist, but in one session she said that she had just had a busy week. She described going out to two successive hen parties, and obviously had a good time at each. The psychotherapist was so used to dealing with despair and hopelessness on Kim's part that he rather unkindly said that he was pleased to see that she could enjoy herself, too. Kim said that she normally never went out, and then clammed up. At the next session, she was even more distant than usual, but did tell the therapist that she had cut herself on two occasions and also taken an overdose since her last visit.

The psychotherapist felt put out. 'How can one work with someone who is so determined to be unhappy?', he thought. He felt that Kim's character was to blame. Only much later did he begin to think that he might have done something to provoke Kim. He thought about how she would have experienced his remark about being pleased with her. He remembered that such remarks by her father would have been provoked not by his concern for Kim, but his desire to exploit her sexually. He remembered that Kim had been to hen parties and knew that she would have been bombarded there with sexual innuendo and questions about her own sexuality. Perhaps there had been something seductive about his comments that he had not wanted to see, and perhaps even this hint was enough to alert Kim, with her senses tuned by ill-usage, to danger. Kim only knew one escape from that sort of danger: to become the aggressor, herself.

The assumption that others are to blame but that we are merely the victims of circumstance is one of the tenets of attribution theory, discussed in more detail in Chapter 10.

'Me'

Therapists have often tackled character from the point of view of the characteristics of the self.

The first uses of 'self' by psychotherapists were reflexive. Freud spoke of self-analysis without intending the analysis of some part of a person called 'the self'. Goldstein (1939) wrote similarly about self-actualization. However, Carl Rogers began to use the term 'self' in a free-standing fashion, as if 'self' were an entity. Rogers subsequently claimed that his clients made him do it. As he said in an interview: 'I was really forced to examine self and forced to define it for myself, because my clients in therapy kept using that term in all kinds of significant ways. They'd say, "I think I've got a pretty solid self underneath this kind of phony existence" or "I'd be terribly afraid of getting to know my real self"' (Evans, 1975, p. 14).

At some time during the course of the twentieth century, it has become possible to have a self, not just to be oneself. It has become possible, even mandatory, to create a self to present to the world, even in intimate situations. This self is, to use Cooley's memorable phrase, partly a 'looking glass self' created by one's 'reflection' in the facial expressions, responses and reactions of other people. It may also be – and this is the twentieth century discovery – a creation or, to use the theoretical framework which will become more important later in this book, a narration. If the narrated self is 'me', 'I' may be the narrator, but so may 'you' or 'them'. What I say about myself may be influenced by what other people have scripted for me, what they expect, the 'ideal self' of Rogers.

In the fairy tale of Cinderella, Cinders is kept in the social position of a poor relation. Her self-image is consistent with this position, and this provides the dramatic irony of the plot. The reader knows that she is entitled to a high position in society, but Cinders has no aspirations to it. It is only her fine bone structure, manifest in her tiny feet, which reveals her aristocratic origins.

In the modern fairy tale invented by Patricia Highsmith in the Ripley series of novels, Tom Ripley has exactly the social position for which his parents have prepared him, but he feels entitled to much more. He is a piano tuner, but dreams of being a concert pianist. He is a confidence trickster, but feels entitled to the same social position of those he impersonates. He creates a new persona, a new 'me', which is one of these elite. It turns out to be surprisingly easy to do. He takes on the identity of someone he murders. However, one difficulty remains – how to deal with the tensions between his own values and those of the comfortable and well-educated self that he has created.

Had Cinderella sought psychotherapy, the therapist may have suggested family therapy and opened up issues of scapegoating and questioned the skew in the family power structure. Or, alternatively, the therapist may have taken on Cinderella in individual therapy, and questioned her need for approval by her step-family and how they used this need to maintain her in a much lower position than her native abilities and endowments would seem to justify.

Given that how I seem to others is partly a creation, it becomes possible to have a 'false' self (Winnicott, 1988). Indeed it becomes a social responsibility to present oneself in a socially acceptable fashion (Goffman, 2001). Subsequently, self has been reified into a thing which can become disordered (Kohut & Wolf, 1978), be multiplied and, most famously, be divided (Laing, 1960). Robert Musil's novel, *The Man without Qualities*, describes the tyranny of too much preoccupation with this reflected self.

Ulrich has a vague but pressing wish to be someone of importance, but is trapped by the reactions of others. He confides to his cousin, Diotima, that:
The feeling of having firm ground afoot and a firm skin all round, which seems

so natural to other people, is not very strongly developed in me. Just cast your mind back to when you were a child – how everything was a soft shapeless glow. And then as a young girl whose lips were scorched with yearning. In me at any rate something rebels against the notion that what is called mature manhood is the peak of such a development (Musil, 1980, p. 344).

Ulrich contrasts the unselfconsciousness of the child, and the directedness of desire, with his own state, which is never explicated in the passage but which is the obverse of the 'mature manhood' that Ulrich elsewhere attributes to Diotima and their mutual friend, Arnheim. Unlike Arnheim, Ulrich suffers from an excess of self-scrutiny and a deficit of self-direction. It is noticeable in the passage quoted that Ulrich succeeds in describing himself without ever using the word, 'I'. One might say that Ulrich is all 'me', and no 'I'.

Attribution theorists have questioned the commonsense assumption that there is a self at all. Nisbett and Ross (1980), in a sustained critique of character rather than situational judgements, point out that 'individuals may behave in consistent ways that distinguish them from their peers not because of their enduring predispositions to be friendly, dependent, aggressive, or the like, but rather because they are pursuing consistent goals using consistent strategies, in the light of consistent ways of interpreting their social world' (1980, p. 20).

Social psychologists' views of consistency do not, however, correspond to commonsense notions of it.

Rowena was facing a difficult decision. Her husband had told her that he was having to work late at work every night for 2 weeks because of a big project. She didn't believe him.

Their marriage had been taking a turn for the worse for a long time. Rowena had developed pain on intercourse, and their love life had almost dwindled to nothing. At first, Roger had seemed frustrated by this, but recently he had seemed relieved. She suspected that he was having an affair. She talked it over with her psychotherapist. Should she confront him, or should she pretend that nothing was happening? The psychotherapist's inclination was towards confrontation, but all Rowena's instincts were against this. She said, 'I've read that if the wife is just there for her husband, very few of them actually leave. They've too much at stake. But if I confront him, I'll force him to make a decision when he's not ready for it. I'm no good at making people sorry for me, and he'll just get angry and go off'.

Rowena decided to say nothing, but the following day she received an odd phone call. It was from a woman who asked for Roger, and then said that she must have got the wrong number. Rowena, on an impulse, said, 'Don't ring off. I know you're having an affair with my husband. I just want to know why, that's all'. They had a long conversation. Later, Rowena asked her husband, when he came home, if he knew what that call was. He broke down and told her that he was so relieved to get it off his chest. It was his boss who had come onto him. He had just given into temptation once, and now she was tormenting him. Could Rowena forgive him? Rowena said that she couldn't and that she had already packed his overnight things. He could leave straigh away and find a hotel. As she told her psychotherapist later, hearing another woman talk about her husband had made her realize how she had come to despise him. It was actually a relief to see him leave the house.

The psychotherapist might have told Rowena that she had been very inconsistent: in that the first week she had said that she would never question whether or not her husband was having an affair, and in just the following week she had directly asked the woman she suspected whether or not she was having an affair with him. Rowena would have denied it. She would have said that the circumstances were completely different.

Rowena, as it turned out, actually thought that she had proved to be stronger and more indomitable than she would have believed possible of herself. And she had. If the psychotherapist had quite correctly pointed out that Rowena had simply been influenced by circumstances, and that her husband and she would never have separated had the other woman not phoned, Rowena would have felt attacked. She could remember screwing up her courage and using all her character to ask the questions she had.

For most people, the experience of having a strong and consistent character does not imply that one acts independently of circumstances or that one always acts in the same way in different circumstances.

The difference between the commonsense understanding and that of the scientist is that the latter is orientated towards the causes of behaviour. The scientist wants to know what, if any, aspect of behaviour causes behaviour. There are causes of our actions which would be considered to be part of character. There are temperamental characteristics which are probably inherited (Tantam, 1988). There are also traits of character which may be established during early or middle childhood, and be relatively enduring thereafter, for example empathy (Tantam, 1995a). But these are, as Nisbett and Ross argue, of relatively little effect.

What matters to the ordinary person is not what causes behaviour, but what reasons a person had for acting as he or she did. And, completely contrary to our intuitions, these reasons are fixed retrospectively (Tantam, 1999a). What an ordinary person, whether client or therapist, means by being consistent is that the reasons that are fixed retrospectively for an action are consistent with the characterization of the actor.

In George Eliot's *Middlemarch*, Will Ladislaw is deeply in love with Dorothea Brooke but conceals this from himself and, to an extent, from the reader. One way that he conceals it is by flirting with the wife of one the local doctors, Lydgate. Will is a laconic, apparently uncommitted, man who laughs off most of life's unpleasantnesses. One day, Dorothea finds him with

Rosamund and assumes that he and Rosamund are lovers. Suddenly he is confronted with his reflection in Dorothea's eyes and he is enraged. He turns on Rosamund viciously.

> Explain! Tell a man to explain how he dropped into hell! Explain my preference! I never had a PREFERENCE for her, any more than I have a preference for breathing. No other woman exists by the side of her. I would rather touch her hand if it were dead, than I would touch any other woman's living.
>
> Rosamond, while these poisoned weapons were being hurled at her, was almost losing the sense of her identity, and seemed to be waking into some new terrible existence.

The reader is confronted with this very different view of Will, but instead of concluding simply that he is inconsistent, the reader's mind flashes back to Will's previous appearances in the novel. Could his character have been as passionate as this all along, with the passion concealed behind a world-weary veneer? Most readers of the book conclude that – yes – Will is a deeper and more passionate person than he previously seemed. These readers simply alter their assessment of Will's character and apply this altered assessment retrospectively.

Lesser writers risk losing the reader's belief in the narrative when they insert such a *bouleversement* into a story. The reader might think, 'That doesn't fit with what Will said on page x', or the reader might simply think, 'People don't act like that'. The reader will, in other words, apply the same criteria of narrative conviction that were introduced in the previous chapter – fidelity and coherence.

Narrating a self that is convincing to others

As in art, so in life. We impinge on others as characters, characters that we can justify and, as Goffman described, present in a favourable light. The closer our relationship with another person, the more likely it will be that our character, and not our actions, is the subject of scrutiny. Examples of this happening are considered in Chapter 7 in a discussion of conflict resolution.

Whether they want to know whether we can be relied upon as a business partner or as a spouse, other people need to know whether they can trust us. The greatest impediment to trust is unreliability. Even completely selfish people can be trusted, if they are reliably selfish, as long as the person trusting them can ensure that it is always in the selfish person's interests to cooperate.

The commonsense tests of unreliability are the same in life as in art. A person's actions are expected to be in character, and that character is expected to have a coherence, an integrity, that makes it a whole. In fact, the demands of coherence are slightly greater even than that. The account of a person's character has to be coherent with their own accounts of their own character if that person is to be accepted as being like others, and therefore likeable to others. The narrated self, the 'me', has to be valid both with respect to other characteristics of the person and with respect to requirements of membership of the social group.

Psychotherapists may formulate this using metaphors of 'outside' and 'inside' a person, and in terms of identity. Such a psychotherapist might say that my identity, my 'self', is formed from the internalization of other people. Internalization might happen like this. I love and respect my mother very much and I therefore like myself when I behave like her. Gradually these behaviours which I like about my mother become integrated into my self: I have internalized my mother. However, to be a member of a group I must also be identified with it. I must act in a way which shows that I am a member of this group, and not of that group. Perhaps I have to wear a uniform, or speak with a certain accent, or have certain opinions. My identity must therefore encompass my identification.

Psycho-analytic psychotherapists give a central place to the causes and consequences of an incoherent self, although they describe it using the same metaphor that runs through most of Freud's writing – as a conflict between autonomous psychic agencies. One advantage of this metaphor is that it shows up the close link between interpersonal conflict and narrative coherence. This can be illustrated by a second extract from Middlemarch.

Narrative example

Mr Bulstrode, the banker, has a pivotal place in Middlemarch society. No-one likes him, everyone smarts under his religiose reproofs, but no-one dares to challenge his position in society. His life is led according to the values that he preaches: intolerance, strict religious observance, and conservatism. Much of the period which the book describes is, for Bulstrode, a struggle for ascendancy over his fellow townspeople which focusses on the building of a new hospital. However, he has a past of which he cannot be proud, and out of this past comes a stranger to Middlemarch, Mr Raffles. Mr Raffles is a drunkard and, in his cups, tells scandalous stories about Bulstrode. If this were all, Bulstrode's new identity might have weathered the scandal. Many people in Victorian England had a few shady secrets in their past. But Bulstrode has Raffles in his power and fails to intervene when his housekeeper gives unlimited opium and brandy to Raffles as a treatment for his acute liver failure. Raffles dies, and Bulstrode has a sore conscience but feels relieved. Relieved, that is, until he attends a town meeting where he hears Mr Hawley address the meeting in the following terms: 'It is our united sentiment that Mr Bulstrode should be called upon – and I do now call upon him – to resign public positions which he holds not simply as a tax-payer, but as a gentleman among gentlemen . . . I don't say that Mr Bulstrode has been guilty of shameful acts, but I call upon him either publicly to deny and confute the scandalous statements made against him by a man now dead, and who died in his house – the statement that he was for many years engaged in nefarious practices, and that he won his fortune by dishonest procedures – or else to withdraw from positions which could only have been allowed him as a gentleman among gentlemen.'

Bulstrode had moved to Middlemarch, a small market town apparently far from London, probably not unlike Eliot's native Nuneaton. He had been taken there as a respectable man of property, and over the years this identity, this self, had become established. It was consistent with many of Bulstrode's life-long values of thrift and industry. Bulstrode had developed himself into not just a successful man, but a sanctimonious man. No-one, except perhaps his wife, liked him, but he could not be rejected without Middlemarch society rejecting the values that everyone in it stood for. Bulstrode exploited this by becoming a sort of Protestant conscience for them all. Then came the discovery that Bulstrode's narrated self was not faithful to the values of his criminal past, and that his behaviour in private, to Raffles, was not coherent with his public behaviour. He had, for example, shrugged Raffles off to Caleb Garth as an old business acquaintance.

The failure of his self-presentation enabled hidden hostility to explode into open conflict between himself and the truculent auctioneer, Hawley. The result was that Bulstrode was shunned from Middlemarch society and had to move away. Eliot describes the anguish for Bulstrode of the collapse of his narrated self.

[Bulstrode had] 'The quick vision that his life was after all a failure, that he was a dishonored man, and must quail before the glance of those towards whom he had habitually assumed the attitude of a reprover – that God had disowned him before men and left him unscreened to the triumphant scorn of those who were glad to have their hatred justified – the sense of utter futility in that equivoca- tion with his conscience in dealing with the life of his accomplice, an equivoca- tion which now turned venomously upon him with the full-grown fang of a discovered lie: – all this rushed through him like the agony of terror which fails to kill . . .'.

Bulstrode might have been down, but he was not out. The shame and self-disgust that he dreaded did not come about, partly because of his intrinsic strength. Mr Bulstrode's temperament was unchanged:

Through all his bodily infirmity there ran a tenacious nerve of ambitious self- preserving will, which had continually leaped out like a flame, scattering all doctrinal fears, and which, even while he sat an object of compassion for the merciful, was beginning to stir and glow under his ashy paleness.

But his social position was irrevocably altered. Bulstrode had been excluded from the ranks of the gentlemen of Middlemarch.

Eliot knows full well that there are always two stories about actions in the interpersonal domain. One is a story about individuals, and one is a story about groups. She therefore writes in two registers: a private one, in which her characters introspect and reflect on each other's intentions and sentiments, and a public one, in which they are described in relation to each other, as being able to command affection or dislike, and as occupying a position or place in society. For a detailed description and analysis of sentiments as tendencies or dispositions to react with certain emotions, see Frijda et al. (1991). However, it is worth noting that George Eliot's intention was to deepen the contribution of character over situation. She was one of the artists who has created the current folk psychology tendency to attribute behaviour to character, an assumption that is increasingly questioned by philosophers and social psychologists who find little evidence for the kind of consistency that would support more than a weak conception of identity (Harman, 1999). Many of the characters in the book – Bulstrode, Rosamund, Garth, Celia Brooke – are portrayed by the same tune in both of these registers. What they do is who they are, and vice versa. Bulstrode experiences himself as a man with a strong will, little influenced by sentiment. His social standing is a mirror image of this. He is a self-made man, who occupies a near-dominant position in Middlemarch society and who is accustomed to the respect, but not the affection, of his neighbours. Garth is honest, confidential and kindly. He is loved by his neighbours, although not much respected, and is never calumniated once in the whole novel.

Each of these men, Bulstrode and Garth, express their will and their sentiments directly in their actions on the world. Any conflict within their characters is also played out as a conflict between their actions. Garth comes across as such a steady character because his actions are all consistent with each other. It is this which gives such a strong sense of coherence to his narrative. He can be secure in others' affection and esteem precisely for this reason. There will never be any discovery that could threaten his sense of self-worth.

Caleb Garth is an idealized figure, a rustic version of the holy fool who so intrigued the Victorians. Bulstrode is much more realistic. He is a man whose character has to be maintained by a degree of what Goffman (1956) called 'face-making'. He had taken pains to hide his earlier, murkier past when he came to Middlemarch. It was only the reappearance of the wretched Raffles, who had known him in a much more humble character, that his face was threatened, and ultimately lost. Looked at developmentally, there is a conflict between Bulstrode's character as a younger man and the character that he assumed in middle age.

The conflict is also played out in cross-section, although this time in the public rather than the private register. There are many in Middlemarch who oppose Bulstrode and not just on issues, but because of this character. These 'had a strong suspicion that since Mr. Bulstrode could not enjoy life in their fashion, eating and drinking so little as he did, and worreting himself about everything, he must have a sort of vampire's feast in the sense of mastery'. Bulstrode tries to contain these conflicts by controlling others through, for example, small private loans. 'In this way', comments Eliot, 'a man gathers a domain in his neighbours' hope and fear as well as gratitude; and power, when once it has got into that subtle region, propagates itself, spreading out of all proportion to its external means'.

Bulstrode was an anxious, unhappy man, only too conscious of his uneasy relations with others. He told himself that what he did, he did for the glory of God. But, 'He went through a great deal of spiritual conflict and inward argument in order to adjust his motives, and make clear to himself what God's glory required'.

The significance for psychotherapy

- There is no opposition between individual and group accounts. They are two stories about the same thing.
- Being a coherent self, being trusted, and securely belonging are all facets of one situation.
- Similarly, not being coherent, a self-presentation that is not faithful to one's biography, being seen to be unreliable, and being uncertain about belonging or not belonging at all are all facets of one situation. This is a situation with a history. Adults who were treated inconsistently by parents, sometimes wanted and sometimes rejected, have less coherent narratives about their lives than adults who were treated either consistently positively or consistently negatively as children (Pearson et al., 1993).
- Values are important characteristics of a 'me', which can lead to a person either being accepted or being rejected.
- People's values distinguish them as characters. Both Bulstrode and Garth had values which were different from those of their neighbours. Bulstrode's values aggravated other people, and Garth's exasperated other people. These differences were sufficient to create a separation of Bulstrode's and Garth's characters from that of their neighbours. Enough to establish an identity for them. But they were sufficiently coherent that this separation was small, and on bigger values there was no separation. Bulstrode and Garth were both a part of a larger entity – Middlemarch society. However, when Bulstrode was discovered to have different values, values which allowed him to let another man die to save his reputation, a much greater separation was created between Bulstrode and his neighbours, and he was rejected from that society.

• A therapist does not have to have the same values as his or her client, and he or she may put pressure on the client's values, for example by inviting the client to reflect on them. But outright rejection of the client's values leads to rejection of the client.

Boundary and salience

Bulstrode's character might meet the DSM-IV criteria, but to say that he had a narcissistic personality is no more definitive a description than it is to say that he was a man determined to establish a new and better identity, or that he was an outsider defeated by the hostility and suspiciousness of strangers of a small rural town. Each of these elements is necessary to our grasp of Eliot's conception of Bulstrode, and none are sufficient. However, it is true that at different times one or other of them becomes salient. Indeed, one of the riches that makes *Middlemarch* a special novel is that one may read it in one mood and experience it as a commentary on English life, and in another mood, as a human tragedy of hubris and nemesis, humility and reward.

However, if each of these accounts is true of Bulstrode, which one should the psychotherapist prefer? In practice, it seems right sometimes to side with someone who feels excluded, when the psychotherapist might privately agree that this is unfair or inappropriate. At other times, exclusion seems the best opportunity for differentiation and development. Or the psychotherapist might want to bring out the contribution of the person themselves to being excluded; that, too, might cut both ways. Some clients may not be owning up to the consequences of their action, but the psychotherapist might conclude that others have already suffered enough for it, and are right to ask for a fresh start.

A useful and influential metaphor for dealing with these problems is that of the boundary. A psychotherapist working with a client who wants to be closer with others will work to dissolve the boundary between the client and those others. When psychotherapists think that a person needs to be empowered, they may help that person to strengthen their boundaries. This may happen in family therapy, and in group psychotherapy. Agazarian, for example, believes it is important at some stages in the life of therapeutic groups to strengthen minority sub-groups which develop in order that there may be a more equal conflict between them and the remainder of the group. This, she believes, leads to a deeper resolution of group issues (Agazarian & Peters, 1983).

The concept of boundary is a useful one in psychotherapy, and it has taken firm root, principally in psycho-analytic psychotherapy but also in widely different approaches, for example in psycho-synthesis (Kowalski, 1993).

Many papers have been written about borderline phenomena and borderline personality, about boundary violations, and about setting limits. There is an assumption that people with borderline personalities have weak or diffuse identities, and tend not to be able to respect other people's boundaries. Their boundaries, so the metaphor goes, are both extensive and open. Kernberg has been one of the most cogent theorists who have concluded that such people can best be helped by other people placing boundary markers for them in more appropriate and more defensible places, that is, by setting limits (Kernberg, 1984). Whitaker (1985) writes of people whose boundaries are too close. To continue the territorial metaphor, she imagines them as having too little buffer zone around their core identity, and so a therapeutic intervention that is too active penetrates them too deeply. Just this act of penetration, which Foulkes called a 'plunging interpretation', may cause more harm than any intrinsic value of the interpretation itself. Douglas Adams has invented a narrative version of this same human situation. The 'Total Perspective Vortex' was created by a physicist who was angry at his wife. She had chided him for his lack of understanding of what was important in life. So, like a truly meddlesome psychotherapist, he created a vortex which would show her true place in the scheme of things. She saw it, and died. The vortex became the preferred galactic method of execution. Any person placed in the vortex experienced themselves in their objective relations to everything else in the universe. Only Zaphod Beeblebrox, whose ego was at least as big as the cosmos, could survive it.

The boundary fable draws great strength from its roots in tribalism and territoriality. 'Us and them', 'ours and yours', are very basic apprehensions of our social and physical environment. For the young mammal, there are strangers who are potentially threatening from whom the infant runs away, and carers whom the infant runs towards. Panksepp, Knutson and Pruitt (1998), in summarizing current research on the neurochemistry of emotional development in the mammalian brain, conclude that there are six separable systems: seeking/fear/attack (one system, centering on the amygdala), separation distress, play, sexuality, nurturance and dominance. These systems interact. For example, dopaminergic activation increases approach behaviour, but whether or not this results in attack depends partly on the activity of serotonergic neurons. Animals that have been socially isolated have lower brain serotonin, and are more likely to attack than animals which have been housed with conspecifics.

They go on to consider how different blends of these systems subserve the two fundamental dimensions of social behaviour – competition and cooperation. Competition in male mammals is, they note, over two things: sexuality and territory. Female competition is over pups and nest-sites. Competition is initiated by the more dominant male, but its progress may activate the fear/attack, sexuality or play systems.

Both cooperation and competition involve setting an appropriate distance between two conspecifics. The attachment, play, nurturance and sexuality systems all tend to reduce distance and open boundaries, while the fear/attack and dominance systems tend to increase distance and close boundaries. Later in life, all mammals recognize familiar others, who might elicit grooming or affiliative behaviour, and strangers, who might elicit hostility or attack. Territorial animals may attack, or threaten to attack, any other animal that crosses over the boundary into their territory. We observe these behaviours all the time. When presented with a challenge to our identity, it is easy to imagine ourselves being invaded by a threat or confronted by an alien presence.

Boundaries, shame and disgust

If we try to apply the boundary concept in practice, it can sometimes seem confusing. We each of us need a boundary to be able to individuate, but if it is too impenetrable we experience ourselves as isolated. As we get older, we discover that our individuality is not our greatest asset. In fact, holding on to our values may stop us discovering that our greatest asset is that we are members of a universe of values and ideas. To prepare for death, we have to allow our boundaries to dissolve to the point where it becomes almost satisfying to relinquish our identities.

Societies need boundaries to maintain their culture and for practical reasons. But the boundary always excludes someone, and the society is often impoverished as a result. Societies which have taken in large groups of migrants have often benefited from the skills and ideas that they bring, but the society also changes.

Psychotherapy organizations often confront this issue. They are driven by a relentless dynamic to set, and then to increase, membership requirements. But the more stringent the requirement, the more homogeneous the membership, and the less adaptable the organization becomes to change.

Psychotherapists have very different views about whether or not their organizations should be catholic or closed. Clearly, therefore, the identity 'psychotherapist' does not have this as a central value. Or, to put it in a more natural way, psychotherapists are not called on to rule whether or not this person should have different values, or that organization should have different membership criteria.

What concerns psychotherapists directly is well-being, emotional health and a healthy capacity to make relationships. The boundary concept does not directly address these issues, however much its adherents invoke the analogy of biological systems and the well-known dicta of general systems theorists (von Bertalanffy, 1974).

What matters to people themselves is their standing in relation to others, which they know not by reference to a boundary but to their own feelings, in particular their feelings of anxiety, shame or disgust.

A person who feels sure of their bond with others feels proud. If this bond becomes threatened, they feel anxious. If the bond is broken, a person feels self-disgust or shame.

Bulstrode, the Middlemarch character already discussed, had a strong, almost indestructible, 'I'. He experienced the dread which comes with rejection and denunciation, but did not accept that he deserved other's condemnation. He was able, therefore, to prevent himself becoming ashamed, and even if his social self was destroyed, he was able to carry on narrating his life. He was able to carry on with plans to deal with the situation, particularly after he had established that his wife would remain loyal to him. He had sufficient inner resources to leave Middlemarch and start again.

Clients who drop out of treatment, or who withdraw in a group, may, like Bulstrode, have experienced rejection of themselves and their values, and be staving off the experience of shame or self-disgust. Provoking conflict may also be a way of hiding shame following an experience of rejection.

Case example

Dr Myers was the head of a large, international professional association. It had been his brain-child, and he had worked tirelessly to promote it. This had involved many foreign trips, meeting influential people throughout the world and persuading them of the importance of the profession that he represented. As the years went by, Dr Myers's personal life became less and less important to him, and his travelling more and more important. He knew that he had many qualities that made him an ideal ambassador. His association's success seemed to him to be his own success. When he arrived at a ministry of health in some foreign country, he expected to be treated with some respect, and he was. This was his due, he thought. He became impatient about accounting for his movements, or his expenditure. The association should recognize, he thought, that he and only he was responsible for its success and should trust itself completely to him. After all, he subscribed to the same professional ethics as everyone else.

There were rival groups within the association, however. They disliked Dr Myers's assumption that only he could represent their profession. They were angered by his skimpy reports to the Board, by the lack of detail in the accounts, and by Dr Myers's use of charm or coercion instead of reason when dealing with an opponent.

These opponents were ill-organized until they managed to persuade two of Dr Myers's fellow officers to support them. A motion was put forward to amend the statutes and to limit Dr Myers's independence. A special general meeting was called, and battle commenced. The statute issue was quickly forgotten when Dr Myers accused his fellow officers of wanting to take control of the association and locate it in their own country. He described them as 'riddled with envy' and 'wanting to destroy everything that they could not control'. They were 'narcissists', he said. Support for Dr Myers came from the developing countries where he had spent most of his time recently, and who found his plenipotentiary style reassuring. The support for his opponents was more divided. There were a small group of countries who strongly supported them, but they, in turn, were distrusted by many other national delegates.

One delegate said that Dr Myers was the only possible chief executive because the association's head office was in the country in which he was the undisputed leader of his profession. To move the head office would be to change the dominant language of the association, and therefore to change its identity. Some said that it was time to change it. Others said that to change its identity, which was not yet fully established, would be to destroy the association. One said that if the association's identity changed, neither he nor the group that he represented would be able to stay in it. Another said that she and her group would leave if the association did *not* change.

There was intense anxiety generated by these remarks. Dr Myers walked out in a rage, and many delegates followed him. It seemed that the association was splitting into two.

The effacement of the 'I': catastrophic reactions

Dr Myers had experienced the potential loss of something that he valued highly, something that was central to his social identity. Rather than accepting other people's criticisms and resigning as a way of hiding his shame, he kindled a conflict which took the focus away from him.

But other people less robust than Dr Myers or less socially supported may not be able to limit the attack on themselves to an attack on their 'me', their social presentation of themselves. The attack may be an attack on their 'I', their core being.

What happens when invalidation of someone's life-story goes beyond the story itself and becomes an invalidation of the narrator? People who are ashamed simply want to hide. They can no longer account for their experience. Like Hamid in Chapter 3, they may feel that they no longer have an identity.

In these circumstances people may resort to catastrophic reactions, to what psychotherapists sometimes call, 'primitive defences'. Becoming enraged and attacking anyone or anything may be one such defence (Dunnegan, 1997). Families (Dutton, van Ginkel & Starzomski, 1995) and nations (Scheff, 1994) with a shared shame may become locked in intractable conflict. Alternatively, people may efface themselves and look up to the very people who have destroyed them, a phenomenon known to Kleinian psychotherapists as 'identification with the aggressor' (Klein, 1948).

The more intensive that psychotherapy becomes, the more risk there is of shame or disgust becoming evoked. We shall therefore return to catastrophic reactions in Chapter 10, the chapter concerned with long-term therapy.

However, the next chapter takes us back to the much less dangerous ground of symptomatic treatment where issues of shame or disgust may arise because of the stigma of having a psychological problem, and not (at least, not normally) because of the relationship with the therapist.

6

Procedures for gaining relief

John was advised to seek psychotherapy by an occupational health nurse at work. He went to her at the instigation of his manager, following an appraisal. The manager had told him that his subordinates had complained that John was irritable, colleagues felt that he was not pulling his weight, and, to top it all, his performance was also deteriorating.

John was unable to account for these changes at first, but as the assessment interview continued, he admitted that he found travel more and more difficult. As a result, although he did more than his fair share in the office, he often tried to avoid work that required travelling. He knew that this was not good, and he had begun to worry constantly about it. The travel problem increasingly became the focus of the assessment interview. John said that he would worry for days if he had to make a long rail trip and that he would hardly sleep at all if he had to fly. He had taken to having one or two stiff drinks before travelling, too. When actually on a train, he would be OK if he could bury himself in something, but as soon as he started to think about not being able to get out in the event of an accident, his anxiety mounted. When it became really severe, he could hardly breathe and had thought in the past that he might have a heart attack. Recently, he had to get off the train before he arrived at his destination, and was only able to continue travelling after several drinks. His wife suspected him of meeting someone, and he felt too ashamed of what he took to be his weakness that he did not disabuse her.

John's case shows how relieving a specific symptom may be the key to resolving a complex situation. John's symptoms were of agoraphobia. His anticipatory anxiety, panic disorder, alcohol abuse and social dysfunction could all be seen as flowing from it. This is certainly how John saw it. His preoccupying concern was to rid himself of this unaccountable and un-wanted problem, although his shame about it had prevented him from stating this explicitly to anyone before the psychotherapist.

Symptom relief is an important procedure in psychotherapy when some-one is distressed by something about their mental or interpersonal life which seems faulty, and which they would like to correct. It is only really successful when there is a distance between what a person thinks of as themselves, or their body, and the symptom: when, that is, the client's concern is about their problem, not about themselves. The parents of a young woman with an eating disorder may think of her as having abnormal symptoms, such as carbohydrate avoidance, and if the young woman also thinks of herself this way, a symptomatic approach would be appropriate. But it is more likely that their daughter would think of herself as engaged in a more diffuse struggle to establish her own identity, and a symptomatic approach would be meaningless to her.

As with all other aspects of psychotherapy, it is important that the therapist is not dogmatic. Sometimes, surprisingly complex problems can respond to a symptom relief kind of approach. At other times, an apparently simple symptom is like the small entry wound made by certain bullets which disintegrate after impact. This symptom is the superficial manifestation of a wound to the self which needs exploration and healing. Fear of eating in front of others, fear of vomiting, disabling nostalgia, chronic pain of unknown aetiology, obesity, lack of energy, violent temper, primary impotence and morbid jealousy are all examples of symptoms which usually turn out to be indicative of more diffuse emotional difficulties. None of these symptoms is usually responsive to a symptom relief approach. This should not deter the psychotherapist from working with a client who wants to take this approach, but it does mean that the therapeutic plan should emphasize outcome monitoring, and the use of reviews to change the focus of the treatment if symptom relief is failing. Moreover, clients who want the relief of one of these symptoms should be warned that this may not be possible.

Table 6.1 lists some symptoms which have been shown to be relieved by psychotherapy. The approaches that have been consistently shown to be the most effective in symptom relief are behavioural and cognitive therapy. Other approaches do not target symptoms so directly, although they may have as much effect in the longer term (Roth & Fonagy, 1996). The treatment of choice is the one that is most compatible with the client's perception of his or her difficulties. Addis and Jacobson (1996) reported that depressed clients who found a behavioural approach helpful at the beginning of treatment complied with homework requirements, and did well with it at the end. However, clients who thought that their depression was the result of life-problems were not so satisfied with behavioural treatment and did better with an approach which tackled the way that they thought about themselves (cognitive therapy). Clients who thought that their depression was because of a relationship problem did not do so well with cognitive therapy or behaviour therapy. It is important to remember that, whether a relief approach will be palatable or not, depends on the client's own values and aims, and the emotional meaning of the symptom.

All the symptoms in Table 6.1 may lead to referral to a psychotherapist

Table 6.1. Some symptoms for which relieving procedures are available

Disordered emotions	Anxiety, panic, generalized social anxiety
	Depression
	Rage
	Shame
	High 'expressed emotion'
Disordered ideas	Delusions
	Dysmorphophobia
	Suicidal thoughts
	Fear of dying
	Fear of disease
	Worries
Disordered experiences	Hallucinations
	Dissociative disorders
	Flashbacks/post-traumatic stress disorder
Lack of skills	Poor conversational skills, e.g. social phobia
	Memory impairment
	Language and speech problems
	Unassertiveness
Disordered biological functions	Sleep disorders
	Lack of energy
	Stuttering

because they are 'distressing', and because the distress may be making the symptoms worse. Distress may be crudely defined as negative emotional arousal. It includes angry frustration, as well as misery, anxiety and fear. It is what makes people cry, and induces doctors to prescribe sedatives. Most clients feel less distressed than usual whilst seeing a psychotherapist. This is because of the non-specific, distress-relieving factors which are normally present in therapy. These factors are also important in relieving distress in other settings, such as a home visit, a liaison visit or in the emergency clinic.

Non-specific distress-relieving factors

Catharsis

Aristotle, challenged by Plato to explain why tragic plays attracted audiences, proposed that tragedies induce fear in those audience members who identify with the characters whose disasters they see portrayed, and pity for the characters, too. Both are, in Aristotle's view, unpleasant emotions. However, Aristotle supposed that in effective tragedy there is a sudden change in the expected outcome – a shock or peripeteia – which results in a sudden increase in both emotions which is so great that the pity or the fear pour out and are 'purged'. This Aristotle termed 'catharsis' after the medicinal purges that were well known to Greek physicians. Breuer and Freud (1950) applied Aristotle's account of the effects of watching tragedy to the effects of psychotherapy. However, they noted that it was not enough to pour out emotion. It is sometimes supposed that the intensity of the emotion is the important element, and some psychotherapists use emotional intensification for that purpose. However, whilst it is true that spontaneous intensity is some clue to the centrality of an emotional meaning, rehearsed or forced emotional intensity is not.

It is not only the emotional build-up in the audience that the tragedy induces. The plot also canalizes the release of emotions, too. The important element of catharsis is that the emotion that is expressed has a desirable effect. Breuer and Freud termed this 'the need for psychic change'. Strong emotions about people have the aim of changing social relationships. They are not a kind of energy which accumulates, but they do increasingly dominate a person's attention. Distress about some human situation, if it fails in its aim of altering a human situation, at the least persists, and at worst becomes enhanced. Speaking and being heard is one of the most important ways of altering a human situation, but that requires that the listener may be changed by what is being said. The alteration may not always be for the better, either. Encouraging people not to 'bottle up' their emotions is only good advice if disclosure does not lead to indifference or rejection. Diary studies of quotidian experiences of strong emotions and their resolution show that disclosure to a partner may sometimes lead to acceptance and resolution of the emotion, but may sometimes lead to rejection (Macdonald & Morley, 2001).

Catharsis therefore requires:

(1) the arousal of a strong emotion
(2) its intensification
(3) the expression of the emotion
(4) the belief that another has been moved by the emotion expressed

The other person may not always be physically present. Speaking at a grave, praying or writing (Smyth, 1998) may all have a cathartic effect. Sometimes catharsis requires something more than simple understanding. For example, the survivor of a horror wants the listener to be a witness, to remember what he or she has been told. The psychotherapist has, therefore, not only to allow or facilitate the intensification of emotion, and be understanding when it is finally expressed, but also to be alert to the request that may lie behind it.

Rowena was a successful secondary school teacher who had become head of her subject in the previous year. However, she was currently off sick with symptoms of depression. The ostensible reason was a disagreement with the head teacher which had become acrimonious, but this did not seem enough to

explain the depth of her unhappiness. During the course of the assessment, Rowena began to talk about her stature. The assessor had noted that she was short, but Rowena felt tiny. She remembered an incident at a family get-together when she had been asked to sing. She had refused, but one of her uncles had lifted her easily onto a table. The family had clapped and she felt herself to be an exhibit. She did sing, and felt more like a freak than ever. The memory was vividly recalled in the assessment and she recounted it, shaking with feeling. There was a moment of fellow-feeling with the assessor, who had also felt a freak as a child. He respected Rowena's struggle to break free of these family expectations, and he told her that he recognized her success in doing so.

The next week, Rowena said that she had been thinking almost constantly of her childhood experience of being an object of pity or condescension. It had been a powerful theme in her adult life. She felt able to surmount it for the first time. She intended to arrange a meeting with the head of her school and sort out their disagreement, which she did, and make a successful transition back to work.

Witnessing

Catharsis as a cure for physical disease is not only recommended in ancient Greek medicine. It is prevalent in many other parts of the world, including equatorial Africa. The idea is simple. Disease is caused by something noxious, and creating a flux washes it away. The idea is so seductive that it is just as readily applied to psychological disorder. It is supposed that psychological problems are also caused by a build-up of bad feelings, but that creating a flux of feeling washes them away, too. In practice, people often do feel exhausted after a powerful emotional outburst, and may then describe themselves as relieved.

Catharsis has a sister concept, that of 'bottling up'. 'Bottled up' emotions are supposed, by many, to be particularly damaging, but also to be particularly susceptible to catharsis. 'Bottled up' emotions are emotions that are denied social expression. Denying someone else your feelings is a way of cutting off that other person. It seems probable, therefore, that 'bottling up' feelings is more threatening to other people than it is to the person who is doing the bottling.

Catharsis and bottling up go together and seem to reinforce each other's rightness. They both seem particularly applicable to acute stress disorder: what is known to the media as 'shock'. Shock is assumed to happen when a sudden, traumatic event causes such an effusion of emotion that a person cannot express it. The nearest equivalent in physical medicine is a haematoma.

So strongly has this paradigm suggested itself to people that it has become common to offer preventative counselling to people who have been exposed to shocking events in the expectation that this will allow the outflow of emotion before it accumulates and causes longer-term damage. In practice, asking people to talk about a shocking event seems, if anything, to make their longer-term emotional adjustment worse, not better (Hobbs et al., 1996).

Although there are many other studies that have reached the same conclusion as Hobbs et al, there are some studies of selected individuals where good outcome has been shown. One reason is that the outcome does seem to be better if a person seeks out 'de-briefing', as one of the commonest cathartic approaches is termed. However, the most important element in 'de-briefing', even if this is sought out, is unlikely to be catharsis, but 'witnessing'.

Two linked features single out both acute and post-traumatic, or chronic, stress disorders: (1) the trauma is not simply remembered, but is re-experienced again and again in the form of intrusive flashbacks (Selly, 1997), and (2) the affected person experiences a range of dissociative phenomena.

Dissociative phenomena – not attending, having memory problems, experiencing sensations and perceptions which are not obviously linked to the present but may be linked to the trauma – are indications to the lay person that the trauma has been 'too much'. They fit in neatly with the cathartic model because they seem to indicate that a person's ability to process the trauma has been exceeded, just as in a haematoma the body's ability to lyse the clot is exceeded by the clot's tendency to swell.

Dissociation is not in itself pathological (Heber et al., 1989), but it does seem to be associated with a diminished ability to deal with trauma, at least in western populations (Kolk et al., 1996). One reason has already been suggested in Chapter 5: that dissociation is associated with diminishment of identity. Instead of 'me' being a functioning, reliable presence in the social world, it becomes disorganized and unreliable, prey seemingly to factors outside my control.

Telling other people about the traumatic experience, and telling them why it was traumatic, is an important way of repairing the narrative about 'me'. It seems that in each of us there is a role as witness which makes sense of disorganization and helplessness, if we can just get our communiqué out to others. The very fact that a person is demoralized may be a strength if they can pass on to someone else that demoralization is an understandable and appropriate reaction. Allowing the survivors of trauma to testify is more than catharsis, because it requires that other people make themselves open to the testimony. If they can, then witnessing can provide relief where de-briefing does not (Weine et al., 1998).

Reassurance

Reassurance is an over-rated means of relieving distress. When mother goes to the window and says to the child who is terrified that she has seen a face there, 'There's nothing to worry about. There is nothing there', this might reassure the mother, but it does not relieve the child's distress because the child knows there is something to worry about. If there is nothing outside, then the cause is something else. But a child knows that fear does not usually arise *ex nihilo*. Reassurance involves listening and taking seriously.

A new, and very worried, father consulted his family physician about his first child's colic. The child had very loose stools, the colic had begun after weaning, and the child was convinced that his son had coeliac disease. The family physician said, 'You are right. It could be coeliac disease. If you like I can refer your son to the paediatrician straight away. But very often these problems turn out to be something much less worrisome – an intolerance of orange juice, for example. What would you like me to do? Refer him straight away or wait for a bit, perhaps while you try him without any orange?'. The father's anxiety had diminished considerably whilst the family physician spoke and he felt comfortable about deciding to wait. Everything settled down when orange juice was omitted.

The family physician took the father's anxieties seriously, and debated them. The possibility that there were less anxiety-provoking, alternative explanations was introduced as information for the father, who felt more in control as a result. His anxiety abated, but at no point was he told that he was over-anxious or that he should stop worrying.

Hope

Hope is inspired by a feeling of calm competence in the psychotherapist, and a sense that the psychotherapist has hope. Clients are not fooled by false hopes, although they may pretend to be, to avoid upsetting the psychotherapist. An absence of hope can also be crushing. When a psychotherapist does not think that he or she can help a client, it is important to be clear that this is a failing on the part of the psychotherapist, not the hopelessness of the client's case.

Normalization

There may be initial outrage that the external world is so little changed by a bouleversement in one's personal world, but this quickly gives way to a relief that routines continue unchanged, that life goes on. Taking a history, however slowly and gently, of a distressed person may prove to be intrinsically comforting if it conveys the sense that, however terrible the disaster that the person has experienced, they can still function effectively as a social actor.

Relaxation, breathing control and imagery

These three interventions form the basis for many first-level 'anxiety-management' approaches, and are often used by self-help groups. There are many manuals describing them which are readily available and so the details will not be discussed here. Relaxation training, guided imagery and meditation all produce a mild sense of well-being in susceptible subjects, probably as a result of changes in opioids (McCubbin et al., 1996). The rationale for their use in anxiety is that the well-being will offset the anxiety, and so reduce it.

The rationale for breathing control is slightly different. People disposed to panic have an anxiety response to acidosis, the so-called 'suffocation alarm' (Bouwer & Stein, 1997). They therefore tend to hyperventilate with anxiety, but this reduces $p_a co_2$. Clients with panic disorder are particularly prone to doing this. Over-breathing produces de-realization in some panic clients, and in others, who are able to drive their $p_a co_2$ even lower, it causes muscle pain, including chest pain (Kopp, Litavszky & Temesvari, 1997). This may then fuel fears of incipient heart atttack. Breathing re-training is designed to break this cycle.

Studies do not support a strong specific effect of any of these interventions in relieving symptoms, however. When they are used in a self-help programme, it is more likely to be other factors, such as increased social support and self-exposure, which are the effective techniques.

Distraction

Like each of the other distress-relieving factors that have been discussed, distraction is only effective if it follows on from recognition of a person's concern. However, unlike other distress-relieving techniques, distraction works not just for distress but for other symptoms as well, for example sensations like tinnitus or pain, or thought-based symptoms like worries.

Distraction is often advocated by carers and health professionals, but is rarely acknowledged to be helpful by the person with the symptom. A closer look at worries helps to understand why this is so. Worries are triggered by a perception of threat, and worriers are more likely to perceive threats than non-worriers (Tallis & Eysenck, 1994). However, one study of students suggests that everyone experiences intrusive, potentially distressing thoughts quite frequently; the main difference between worriers and others is in the response that these worrying thoughts elicit (Freeston et al., 1991). This study indicated that three main responses were used, listed here in increasing order of frequency of use: 'no effort', 'attentive thinking' and 'escape-avoidance'.

When people enjoin someone else to 'think about something else', they are referring to this experience of effortless response to a worry. They remember an occasion like the following.

An example of a transient worry
Ann is working at home when she gets an e-mail from her section leader to say that there has been a discrepancy in her expenses claim. Ann feels anxiety and starts to worry about what the discrepancy might be. Did she leave out some bills? Had she over-inflated her mileage?

Just then she notices the subject of the next e-mail, which is: 'Do you need a holiday?'. She reads it – it is about cheap holidays in Cyprus – and thinks about how good it would be to go away, and rehearses going to the travel agent and booking. She has been successfully and effortlessly distracted from her worry about the expense account (although not gone, it may spontaneously occur as she lies in bed that night).

Had Harry, Ann's husband, come into their office at home at the moment that Ann had just read the first e-mail, she may have told him about her worry. His best strategy to distract her would have been to acknowledge her worry, but then to raise some other topic of particular interest. However, if he had said, 'Just think about something else', she would have to make an effort to switch her attention. As soon as she made this effort, distraction would become impossible because distraction cannot involve effort. Only two courses of action would have been open to Ann. Either she could have said, 'But, Harry. You just don't understand, this could be serious', or she could have said, 'I'll try to stop thinking about it'. The former rejoinder is an expression of the 'attentive thinking' strategy. Ann perceived the worry as sufficiently serious to need thinking about. The second remark is an assertion of Ann's agreement to use escape-avoidance. However, escape, as Freeston et al. (1991) noted, is associated with further worry.

This discussion has led us into an area that is central to symptom relief. Many people, professionals included, who have to deal with someone who is preoccupied by a psychological symptom tell them to try to pay attention to something else. This approach never helps, and may make matters worse. There are at least four reasons for this failure:

(1) The injunction to stop thinking about the symptoms is interpreted as being unkindly meant, and more an injunction to stop upsetting the other person.

(2) The sufferer thinks that the symptom is important and needs attention.

(3) The sufferer feels that if they do succeed in escaping, it is only because the symptom has proved too strong for them, and they wait fearfully for its return.

(4) The sufferer thinks that if they stop paying attention to the symptom, something even worse might happen.

Distancing

Many of the symptoms considered in this chapter have force because they seem to have acquired autonomy. They, rather than the client, rule their appearance and disappearance. In relation to anxiety, this phenomenon is sometimes termed the 'fear of fear'.

Ultimately, only a change in a person's narrative about themselves can overcome the power of the symptom. This happens not through controlling the symptom, but through changing a person's experience of themselves to take account of their lack of autonomy. Everyone discovers, sooner or later, that they are at the mercy of contingency. Overcoming this realization is achieved not by fortifying the self, but by releasing the need for supremacy (see Chapter 9).

In the short term, some people who have strong imagery can learn, although slowly and with difficulty, to distance symptoms which cause anxiety. For example, frightening images can be put into frames so that they look as if they are on television rather than being 'real'.

Other distancing techniques include: (1) questioning, for example whether hallucinations which are announced as the voice of God are real, by querying the evidence that they are real, rather than by just accepting it, or (2) insisting that a vivid flashback does not just stop, but should continue.

Relief of future symptoms

Anxieties, worries, low mood, concerns about physical appearance – all of these are nearly universal experiences. They come and they go, commanding only our fleeting interest. Only those experiences which take hold of our attention and will not let it go get called symptoms. These experiences have, to use the glue metaphor so common in psychotherapy, an adhesive quality which prevents us from shrugging them off. Simply trying to tear one's attention away from them is, as noted in the previous section, as harmful as pulling something off one's finger that has been accidentally stuck on with superglue. The bond needs to be dissolved first.

Details of the treatment of specific symptoms and syndromes by psychotherapy can be found in a number of recent books, for example in *Clinical Topics in Psychotherapy* (Tantam, 1998). In the remainder of this chapter, I shall consider some of the principles that each of these approaches has in common. Three of them have already been mentioned in the previous section, in the reasons why making an effort to ignore a symptom does not get rid of it. They are: avoidance, salience and undoing. Before considering them further, it will be worthwhile to look more carefully at assessment and, in particular, at the cognitive diary.

Diaries and homework

The art of psychotherapy is to question the unquestionable. The art of cognitive-behavioural therapy is to hook the client into questioning the unquestionable, too. When a person hears a voice saying, 'He is damned', it is difficult to question its provenance and very easy to believe the condemnation. Similarly, when a person feels that they are going to die during a panic attack, it is difficult for them not to feel that there must be something that is seriously wrong, otherwise they would not feel that way. Even when the symptom may not seem so self-evidently pressing to the psychotherapist, it has usually become so to the client.

Mrs Rogers had cut her wrists several times, and had recently taken a potentially lethal overdose of her antidepressants. She did not want to die and leave her family, she said. But she could not stand her tinnitus. It drove her crazy. People told her to ignore it, but she couldn't. As soon as it started up, it just maddened her. She felt she must stop it, in any way that she could.

When a symptom becomes as intrusive as Mrs Rogers's tinnitus had become, it dominates the person's life. Just the advent of the symptom is enough for them to feel incapacitated. The first step in the psychotherapy is to establish what makes the symptom so salient. A useful way to do this is to ask a person to keep a diary of their symptoms. Many more or less complicated variants of this exist. Some psychotherapists use printed diaries or forms. I ask my clients to buy an exercise book, to rule each page into four columns and to head them 'Time', 'Symptoms', 'Situation' and 'Thoughts'. I suggest that the client completes the diary each day, normally at more or less the same time, which will often be in the evening. We agree on which symptoms to monitor, and sometimes write these under the heading 'Symptoms'. This, in itself, may lead to an interesting discussion about which symptoms are linked, and which are independent. It may also lead to a discussion about which symptoms the client most wants relief from, and an agreement that not all symptoms can be tackled simultaneously. Each time that such a discussion takes place, the client experiences more of a sense that the symptoms are not 'incubi', but indications of problems that can be solved. Completing the diary puts the symptoms into a context, and helps this process further.

It is important that the diary, like all homework that clients are asked to do, is taken seriously by the therapist and that the client is expected to take it seriously. Few people manage the diary without a hitch in the first week, but after this clients who are going to do well with the approach usually complete a page for each day, as requested, and do not leave columns blank, again as requested. Therapists differ about how they use the diary in a session. It is my practice to read it through with the client in the first part of the session, drawing attention to any aspects that I think need discussion. Each column might yield useful information.

Table 6.2. The symptom diary of Mr Perkins for Wednesday 6 April

Time	Symptoms (chest pain, shortness of breath, tension)	Situation	Thoughts
7 a.m.	Felt a bit tense	Waking up	How will I do today?
10 a.m.	Bit short of breath	Looking at order book	What will happen if I can't work?
2 p.m.	Very tired	Just finished sandwich at my desk	So tired
9 p.m.	Worried	Thinking about having an early night	What will happen in the night?
1 a.m.	Very short of breath with terrible pain in my chest	Woke up like it	Nothing, really

Timing of symptoms

Case example

Mr Perkins, a married engineer, had been, in his own words, overdoing it. There was a decline in the automotive industry, and his small company, which supplied parts for vans, was struggling. He heard about a fellow businessman who had collapsed at work one day, and died. He discussed it with his wife, and she told him that he could not continue to work as he had been doing, and that they both needed a holiday. All seemed to go well at first, but he could not fully relax and woke regularly at night. One day, he had an episode of chest pain lying on the beach. At first he thought that it was nothing, but when he got home, he found that he was tired every afternoon and that he could hardly lift the machinery that he would not have thought twice about lifting previously. He went to see his doctor, who examined him and sent him for an ECG, which was normal.

His family doctor prescribed antidepressants, and these had helped a bit. He had also borrowed a relaxation tape from his wife, and had tried to relax regularly every night. However, as soon as he felt himself relaxing, he would immediately tense up and become panicky. He was referred to a psychotherapist. Table 6.2 shows his symptoms for the first Wednesday of his first week's diary. The psychotherapist noted that Mr Perkins's worst symptoms seemed to occur at night. He agreed. He said that he had not slept well since the break-ins at the rugby club. It emerged that another stress on Mr Perkins had been his occupation of the role of secretary to the local rugby club. He had wanted to give this up for many months, but no-one else wanted to take it on. Then there had been a series of nights when he had been woken to say that the alarm was going off in the club building, and he had to go out to attend to it. He had never really got back into a good sleep pattern since then.

The next week Mrs Perkins came with her husband, and asked if she could see the therapist. The therapist asked Mr Perkins what he thought, and Mr Perkins thought that it would be a good idea. So Mrs Perkins came in with her husband at the beginning of the session. She said that her husband had told her that he and the therapist had been talking about Mr Perkins's sleeping problem. She wanted to tell the therapist how it was at night in case her husband had not said. The therapist was concerned that this might be some attempt by Mrs Perkins to take over the treatment, or to infantilize her husband, but Mr Perkins nodded. He seemed relieved that his wife would say what he couldn't. 'Doctor', said Mrs Perkins, 'You should see him. He wakes up and thrashes around. He wakes me up immediately with his moaning. He looks so terrified, almost like he's going to die. I have ever so much difficulty in calming him down. It takes us almost an hour sometimes. I give him a warm drink, and sit him up, and rub his chest. Usually though it's only when he's walked around the room for a while that he gets better'.

Mrs Perkins had tears in her eyes, and clearly felt deeply for her husband. When she had gone back to the waiting room, her husband admitted that he had somewhat understated his night-time anxiety. The therapist, too, was feeling a bit shaken. Did Mr Perkins have some paroxysmal cardiac arrhythmia, or perhaps orthopnoea? He asked some questions relevant to heart and lung function. However, this had already been carefully checked out by the family doctor and Mr Perkins's answers to the questions were not consistent with a physical disorder. The psychotherapist suggested that Mr Perkins might have got into the habit of anticipating the phone calls about the rugby club, and therefore started to wake up at night in anticipation. Mr Perkins agreed. The therapist then pointed out that, although Mr Perkins had written something in the 'Thoughts' column for every other entry, he had not written anything when he had noted that he had woken up with anxiety.

Mr Perkins had seemed very pensive since his wife had left. He now said that he hadn't really liked to think about it but, well, what passed through his mind at night was the statistic that he had read that most men die of a heart attack in the early hours of the morning.

Further discussion made clear that Mr Perkins was sure that he had coronary artery disease, and that sooner or later he would wake up in the night unable to get his breath and that he would then die. He tried hard to exclude this thought from his waking life. He just could not imagine taking any more time off, and anyway, what could he do about heart disease? So he tried not to think about it, but somehow the tiredness and the tension were increasing inexorably.

The therapist now had a plausible explanation of the genesis of Mr Perkins's anxiety. It went something like this. Mr Perkins had been feeling stressed about work, and the alarm calls at night had added to this stress. More importantly, they had induced the habit of anxious waking at night. The death of another man in a similar situation to Mr Perkins had raised in Mr Perkins the idea that he, too, might die of a heart attack. The holiday had reinforced this because of the episode of chest pain, which may easily have been a consequence of unusual over-indulgence, but which Mr Perkins had attributed to his heart. Throughout this period of anxiety induction, or incubation, Mr Perkins resolutely avoided giving the thought that he might have heart disease any serious credibility except at night, when it flooded him so much that he could think of nothing else. The result of this avoidance was that his preoccupation with his heart had become increasingly salient, and he was constantly testing it, for example by seeing how well he could lift heavy machinery.

The therapist discussed this way of looking at the problem with Mr Perkins, who disagreed with some particulars. For example, he did not think that his night-time symptoms began because he was thinking about his heart. However, he did accept that there really could be another explanation for his symptoms, and now, when he felt discomfort in his chest at night, he thought that it was more likely to be a result of stress than a heart problem. He was not becoming so distressed by his nocturnal symptoms now and thought, in fact, that he was on the way to being cured. The therapist warned Mr Perkins that he might for a long time have a propensity for worrying about his heart. He should not expect that to be cured, exactly. But the therapist was glad that there had been a definite improvement and did think that this was likely to be sustained.

Thoughts

Mrs Angstrom had twin sons, both rather headstrong. Her husband was a quiet man who kept his thoughts to himself increasingly during their marriage. She had always been an anxious person, but over the last year, since one of her sons had crashed his car, the worries had become impossible. She felt that she had not had a single good night's sleep. The more she worried, the more her sons seemed to be devil-may-care. She tried to complete a diary but she worried so much about not writing down the wrong things, that she had to abandon it. The psychotherapist therefore asked her to go through exactly what went through her mind when she was most worried.

Mrs Angstrom told the therapist that could never sleep unless her sons were both home. If they were out in the car, she would first think about their route, and all the possible hazards on it. She would try to determine whether they would have been drinking, and the weather conditions and consequent state of the roads. Then she would imagine the worst that could happen to them. This would make her more anxious, but she felt that she had to persist with it.

Somewhere she had read that bad things happen when you least expect them. She had the idea that if she thought of all the possible bad things that could happen, she could in some way actually prevent them, because they would not be unexpected. But then the images of her sons actually getting hurt frightened her even more. She felt so frightened, in fact, that she thought that something must have happened. She had always been a very intuitive woman: perhaps something terrible had happened and had been communicated to her. She wondered what she should do. Should she try to ring her children? Should she ring the police to find out whether an accident had been reported? Just then, she heard her sons come in, and she felt quite angry that they had disturbed her night so much.

Mrs Angstrom used thoughts to try to undo any possible harm. Worry for her was a kind of protection against the recurrence of her son's accident. She willingly accepted the anxiety it brought her if it protected him and his twin. But when she told them how much she had worried about them, they were not grateful, but angry. She felt so confused about it all. All she knew is that she was more upset and for longer than she had ever been before.

Situation

Lorraine Rolls was, she thought, happily married but she did have, well, a bit of a problem with her mother-in-law, Daphne. She was a lovely woman, but ever so slightly bossy. The emphases were Mrs Rolls's own.

Mrs Rolls's problem was bulimia nervosa. She said that she thought constantly about food, and constantly had to wage a war on her tendency to over-eat. She hated vomiting. It hurt her so much, and it was so disgusting. Yet she felt that it was the only way that she could control her food intake sometimes. If she did not vomit, she would blow up like a balloon, and her husband would hate that. He often said that he liked petite women.

Mrs Rolls was asked to keep an 'eating and symptoms' diary. Table 6.3 shows one page from her diary.

The therapist suggested to Mrs Rolls that this had seemed a day in which she had been criticized heavily. She began to cry, saying that her mother-in-law always seemed to find fault with her, and that her husband always took his mother's side, and never hers. She always felt that because her husband looked up to his mother so much, she should try to understand her point of view, too. So she never argued, but she did find it hard. The therapist asked her to describe this day more fully. Could she remember how it felt? Mrs Rolls could. She always dreaded Daphne's visits. She felt that Daphne, who never seemed to have had any weight problems, would be watching what she, Mrs Rolls, ate like a hawk. It was therefore particularly frustrating that Mrs Rolls always seemed so hungry on these days. On this particular Saturday, Daphne had arrived just after Mrs Rolls had finished breakfast. Here the therapist pointed out that Mrs Rolls had

Table 6.3. The eating diary of Mrs Rolls for Saturday 9 June

Time	Symptoms (including vomiting) and diet	Situation	Thoughts
8 a.m.	Felt a bit tense	Waking up	Daphne coming
8.30 a.m.	Small bowl of cornflakes with skimmed milk, tea	Breakfast on my own	Got to avoid bingeing today
1 p.m.	Diet bread, low-fat potato salad, slice of ham with fat removed	Lunch with husband and mother-in-law. Daphne told me that I looked a frump because I had not done my hair	Got to stick to 300 kcalories
2 p.m.	Some biscuits	Husband showing his mother the new car	I can't stop myself
4 p.m.	Being sick	Mother-in-law just left. Husband shouted at me because I wasn't nicer to her	Such a relief to get rid of it

eaten a very abstemious breakfast. Had she felt hungry after? Mrs Rolls thought not. The hunger had started at about mid-morning. Daphne had started criticizing as soon as she walked in the door, and Mrs Rolls had felt her stomach churn and realized that she was really empty inside. Lunch had been an agony. Mrs Rolls knew that she should try to stick to her diet, especially in front of Daphne, but when Daphne had made the remark about her hair, it had seemed almost too much. Her husband had nodded, as if he agreed with his mother. She thought that she would have to leave the table. Her stomach actually knotted up. When she was clearing up, while her mother-in-law and her husband were off somewhere together, she felt she had to have something just to ease the pain in her stomach. She ate one biscuit and then another until she realized that she had eaten a whole packet. As if this wasn't enough, she had actually opened another packet, of chocolate biscuits, and eaten that, too. She felt disgusted with herself. She caught sight of herself in the mirror, and thought that she was actually fatter than she had been before, and that her mother-in-law would probably notice it. She worked so hard to hide all this and to be polite when her husband and Daphne came back that she felt a little better, because she thought that she had succeeded. Then her husband shouted at her, and she felt so guilty that she had let him down. She felt so nauseated that she thought that she might have been sick even without putting her finger down her throat. But that is what she did as soon as she could get to the toilet and be unnoticed.

The therapist thought it was important to listen to this account without comment, since comment would almost be taken as criticism. However, she now pointed out that the diary had a flaw in it for which she, the therapist, wanted to apologize to Mrs Rolls. There was no column for emotion. What might Mrs Rolls have put in that column, had the therapist been thoughtful enough to provide one? Mrs Rolls looked puzzled, and the therapist said, 'Well, take lunch-time. This is a situation in which you are being criticized, unfairly probably and certainly inappropriately since you are in your own home and your mother-in-law is just a guest. And your husband, instead of taking your side as you might reasonably expect takes his mother's side. This is a situation of considerable irritation and many people would have felt very angry. In feeling angry, they would have experienced their stomach knotting up with the effort of not losing their temper. You had this same feeling in your stomach. What emotion went with it?'.

There was considerably more discussion after this, but this was the crucial point in the therapy since Mrs Rolls could understand that the emotion that belonged to this situation was anger. She had been brought up not to show anger, but to see another person's point of view. Yet her relationship with her husband had been full of frustration ever since they were married, and not only because of her mother-in-law. The salience of her feelings of emptiness, and therefore hunger, reflected the pervasiveness of her frustration. The therapist explained that, although Mrs Rolls used vomiting to try to keep herself looking good for her husband's sake, it actually increased the likelihood of bingeing because it made the hunger worse by emptying her stomach and increasing the motility of her bowel. (The therapist might also have said that vomiting was itself an act of aggression, but decided that such an interpretation would be taken as a criticism by Mrs Rolls who was already looking as if she was wondering whether the therapist was telling her off.) Subsequent sessions focussed much more on Mrs Rolls's frustration, and her bingeing and vomiting diminished markedly.

Common features in symptomatic treatments

Dealing with emotions
The symptoms for which people want relief are associated with strong, unpleasant emotions. Psychiatrists tend not to be very discriminating about these, tending to lump them all into 'dysphoria', anxiety or depression. Differentiating between different emotional states is fundamental for most psychotherapeutic approaches, but psychiatrists may be right in not thinking

it so important for symptom relief. For whether the emotion is disgust, shame, fear, anger, regret or longing, all of which may be associated with symptoms, the sufferer and their circumstances are more likely to determine how the emotion is handled than the nature of the emotion itself.

It is the nature of emotions that, as discussed in the Chapter 3, their flavour tends to spread and permeate thoughts about the emotion, and actions that the emotion has caused. Longing for a lost child may not only be evoked by thinking of the child, but by thinking of the last time of having a thought about the child, or by looking at a photograph of other children, or even by being in the same place where the longing was last felt.

How people handle thoughts and actions which evoke unpleasant emotions depends on their temperament, and on some of their assumptions about emotion. In a paper that I wrote some time ago, I contrasted three ways of handling shame which I called 'shame-proneness', 'mortification' and 'brazenness' (Tantam, 1991). Mortification occurs when a person is constantly mindful of their shame, and yet feels incapable of relieving it. Like someone who fiddles with a wound and prevents it from healing, they do not take any steps to deal with their shame, but yet do not let it rest, either. People who have become brazen seem proof against shame, but at the cost of insensitivity and sometimes callousness. Their avoidance of shame results in a blind spot. Shame-prone people, on the other hand, are supremely sensitive to shame and embarrassment. Their mission in life is to do whatever they can to prevent it occurring and, if they cannot prevent it, to assuage it.

The reader is invited to re-read the paragraph, substituting disgust, or longing, for shame. I think that the reader will be satisfied that the same terms apply. Mortification with longing, for example, was recognized in the nineteenth century by the name 'chlorosis' (Loudon, 1984). This exercise will probably also have made the reader realize that mortification, brazenness and shame-proneness correspond to avoidance, salience and undoing respectively. In fact, with the proviso that for 'unconscious' one should read 'hidden', they also correspond to the defence mechanisms of suppression, reaction formation, and reparation described by psycho-analysts (Laplanche & Pontalis, 1973). There is a reassuring consensus that psychotherapy practitioners have recognized such regularities, although there is an important difference in how they choose to deal with them.

The persistence of emotions implies either that the emotion is constantly being rekindled, or that it is not being relieved (or both). Symptomatic treatments emphasize the former, while other approaches, to be discussed in later chapters, emphasize the latter. Relief of emotion normally requires some action which, for many of the social emotions which are of interest to psychotherapists, normally means some action in a relationship. The paradigm of an action in a relationship for a psychotherapist is revealing something to someone that has previously been hidden, for example telling someone you can trust about the shameful secret that has previously been so mortifying. Revelation is a potentially dangerous procedure since it may lead to rejection or condemnation. Creating the right circumstances for allowing revelation, and ensuring that revelation is most likely to lead to greater intimacy, is an aspect of psychotherapy that is considered in Chapter 10.

Symptomatic approaches concentrate on the ways in which an emotion may constantly be fed and therefore kept at an uncomfortable and disabling level of intensity. Naturally, it may be fed by external circumstances. As in the case of Mrs Rolls, chronic difficulties in a relationship may constantly refresh an unpleasant emotion. When this happens, the client is likely to opt for a therapeutic approach that does not assume, as symptomatic approaches do, that their emotions are inappropriate or 'maladaptive', but is one that targets these circumstances. Most often, the problem will arise from a conflict in a relationship which leads to a person being in a predicament about how to proceed. Psychotherapeutic approaches to these predicaments are considered in the next chapter.

The symptomatic approaches considered in this chapter are particularly appropriate when the client and the therapist consider that the symptoms, and the emotions that go with them, are not appropriate to their situation. This approach to symptom relief assumes that symptoms are maintained or exacerbated by faults in the processing of emotions and that relief can best be achieved through finding and fixing the faults in the process. Folk psychology and religion are replete with methods of fixing emotional faults. They include spiritual exercises, aesthetic contemplation, physical activity, change of scene, rest, taking up an interest, alternative healing practices, shopping, finding a guru or a role model, and changing one's appearance.

Some of the methods of fixing faults may, however, be counterproductive. Avoidance and denial have already been mentioned. Suppressing upsetting thoughts, as noted above, just seems to make the thoughts more insistent. Even more likely to refresh rather than diminish an emotion is the adoption of measures to avoid harm 'just in case'. Washing rather more thoroughly, ringing up to check someone is alright, and taking one's pulse when there is some discomfort in the chest, seem harmless but actually give strength to the emotion to which they are a reaction.

Perhaps the single most important ground rule for dealing with emotional disturbance is to learn that emotions signal problems but they do not signal solutions. The anxiety will still be there even when a person reflects on their chest pain and decides that it is not angina, or looks at their hands and thinks that there is no significant likelihood that they are carrying some disease on them. The mistake that many people seeking relief from symptoms make is to think that the symptom will go when they stop feeling so distressed. In fact, it is the symptom, or the belief or the behaviour, which has to change first and only then will the distress gradually fade. This means that people must take some steps to change their actions or beliefs before they feel comfortable or relieved of their emotions.

Actions, beliefs and appraisals which exacerbate symptoms

Cognitive approaches to fixing faults in emotions are based on two observations. The first is that emotions include beliefs or attitudes which are potentially open to conscious reflection. The second is that emotions result from perceptions of happenings which are also influenced by beliefs or attitudes.

Some of the beliefs that sustain emotional distress have already been considered in this chapter. Lorraine Rolls had the belief that expressing anger could only be destructive, and as a result she was regularly emotionally disturbed by her husband and her mother-in-law without being able to counter their attacks. Mr Perkins believed that he was going to die from coronary artery disease, and this belief led him to interpret everyday physical symptoms catastrophically. Mrs Angstrom believed that she was responsible for her sons' safety and as she had no way of discharging this responsibility was constantly guilty that she was failing and was often casting around for better ways of doing the impossible.

The methods of challenging abnormal beliefs that have been found to work for the beliefs that underlie emotional disorders have also been found to work for other symptoms that are exacerbated by distress. Hallucinations are an example. The distress, and therefore the impact, of a hallucination depends on the provenance to which it is attributed. One of the most distressing hallucinations that I have ever encountered in clinical practice was of an elderly woman who had immigrated from Poland via a Russian detention camp.

Mrs Powlinski's war-time experiences were horrific. Now she heard the sound of her daughters' screams. For reasons that she did not understand, her daughters had been kidnapped and replaced by doubles. However, she could still hear them by some mysterious means. In fact, it was what she heard that gave her the evidence of what happened. With screams like that ringing in her ears, she could not doubt that something terrible was being done. And she also heard male voices that she knew must be their torturers.

Changing beliefs like those of Mrs Powlinski or Mr Perkins is not easy as they appear to be supported by evidence, such as Mrs Powlinski's auditory experiences and Mr Perkins's chest pain and tiredness. Even no evidence might be evidence.

Miss Power had been a hospital technician, but had lost her job after developing severe anxiety symptoms following a road traffic accident. Soon after returning home, she had received a letter from the hospital and had the thought, 'What if there are some germs on this letter, say from an infected client? What if I might catch them?'. She went off immediately to wash her hands, and over a period of a few months had begun to wash her hands every time that she saw a picture of a hospital, if she passed a nurse in the street, when she went to places like chemists where nurses might go, if she had put her washing into the machine, which she did increasingly frequently, or if she heard the words 'illness' or 'disease' spoken. When asked whether she had ever had an infection that could be attributed to any of these causes, Miss Power said, 'No, she hadn't', and that was because she had taken so many precautions.

Much of the evidence is emotional. As already noted, it is of three types: salience, avoidance and undoing. Salience reflects the intensity of the emotion. Its use in evidence is the basis for the adage, 'There's no smoke without fire'. The fact that a person feels a strong emotion in association with a belief is taken as evidence that the belief is justified, and therefore true. The cognitive approach seeks to challenge the belief without challenging the emotion. Confrontation does not do this. Nor does dismissal. Telling someone that something is not very likely makes no difference: they know that it's not very likely that they should have become so distressed, but they have.

The recommended approach is to create a distance between the emotion and the belief, and then to brainstorm some alternative means so that the belief can be tested. Mrs Powlinski had difficulty with this. She had heard people scream before, and they were being tortured. Nor could she think that her distress could be attributable to any other cause. And if I wanted further proof – well, there were her daughters – or at least, the people who were pretending to be her daughters. She knew that they were fake. She could not tell me how exactly, but a mother knows. They were different. Not her real daughters at all.

Mrs Powlinski was, of course, deluded and the therapist was unable to create any space for alternative explanations of her experience. Mr Perkins was less convinced, and when the therapist explained about anxiety leading to over-breathing, and then to chest pain and a feeling of being short of breath, Mr Perkins was able to consider that that could be a possible alternative explanation. He objected to this at first because he had felt so tired during the day, and because he did not think that he would get so agitated unless he was really ill. However, the therapist explained that anxiety could not only have physical effects, but was sometimes so strong that it felt as bad as some of the worst physical conditions.

Mr Perkins was asked whether there would be some way in which the two possibilities – whether he was having a cardiac crisis or anxiety – could be tested. He had heard that people with heart attacks get worse if they move about. Perhaps he could try some physical jerks? The therapist thought that this would not be a fair test as, if Mr Perkins was having heart problems, physical jerks would be dangerous and he doubted that Mr Perkins would want to undertake anything that put his health at risk. The therapist told him that if it was anxiety caused by a breathing problem, it would improve if Mr Perkins could slow down his breathing. If it was a heart problem, this would have no effect, either for good or for bad. Perhaps the therapist could teach Mr Perkins a breathing technique which he could use, and perhaps he could also teach it to his wife so that she could help him to do it. The Perkins agreed and when Mr Perkins was proficient he was asked to rate his symptoms on the following night on a scale of severity before and after using the breathing technique. In fact, this particular experiment was a failure because Mr Perkins's symptoms had already improved so much that he had already stopped thinking that he had heart disease, and his symptoms were much better.

Emotions also become salient if a person looks out for situations which generate that emotion, and dismisses situations which go against it. Depressed people can remember that they had happy memories, but cannot recount them with any detail. Suspicious people catch other people's eyes, and report that other people look at them the whole time. Anxious people are easily startled and perceive more threats in their environment as a result. Overcoming this kind of appraisal bias requires explanation and education about the effects of emotions on perception. Indeed, giving the client a model of why their condition has developed, what might be maintaining it, and how they can test this hypothesis, is an important element in all cognitive therapy.

This general tendency to perceive evidence which seems to support an emotional attitude is not the only way that perceptions can contribute to symptoms. Mental imagery may be provoked by emotional upset but may also cause it. Beliefs can be tackled by reason because they belong to the realm of reason. Disturbing imagery is best tackled in its own realm, too.

Case example

John had lost his daughter, Julia, after a long battle against cystic fibrosis. He was devastated. All his energy had gone into prolonging her life using antibiotics, chest physiotherapy, support and trying to beat the doctors at their own game. He had never really thought that she would die, but now she had. About one week after her death, he dreamed that he had seen her face as it was just before she died, blue and distressed as she fought for oxygen. He felt anxiety and, if only he could admit it, revulsion. The image recurred on subsequent nights, and then he began to see it in the day time. He fought against it, but deep down believed that it was possessing him because he had failed her. It occurred so often that it interfered with his work, and he felt constantly anxious.

The psychotherapist taught John some relaxation and breathing exercises. When he was proficient at these, the psychotherapist asked him to relax and then to summon the image into his mind. John was reluctant to do this, having than the client. So every time that the client avoids thinking about their feelings, they are adding to their belief that those feelings are more than they can cope with. A person may come to this conclusion even if they intend to avoid something just out of convenience, or they say to themselves, 'It's just as easy to order food over the phone as it is to go to the supermarket'. Covert avoidance, in which a person hedges their bets for example by using a mental ritual just in case, may similarly undermine confidence.

Forbidding these behaviours is a form of confrontation that is not likely to work. The usual approach of the cognitive therapist seems more effective: to help the client to question whether these procedures reduce anxiety, or whether, as the therapist expects, they ultimately make it worse.

A rather more difficult challenge may be posed by actions that are thought to be essential, like Mrs Angstrom's worrying, to avert some future catastrophe. Mrs Angstrom thought that she had to get to the bottom of her worries because if she stopped worrying before that, there may have been something that she could have done that she had not thought of. But she could never get to the bottom. The more she worried, the more there was to worry about. She could find no terminal point when her fears were quieted. Instead they grew worse. This means of dealing with emotion has been called 'undoing' because people grapple with the emotion as if they could find its basis and resolve it. They may be motivated by an intolerance of anxiety or doubt, and a need to find certainty. They may be concerned that if they do not get to the bottom of their feelings, they will have left something undone which will cause harm to others.

Undoing, an intolerance of doubt, and a doomed sense of responsibility are particularly characteristic of obsessive–compulsive disorder. Intrusive thoughts may be of violence or harm to others, and these seem especially important to eliminate or avoid. The compulsive element of the obsessive–compulsive disorder may be sustained by the fear that, unless it is performed, some catastrophe will follow. However, there is a habitual element to it, as there may be in worrying, and in hypochondriacal rumination which may become independent of any beliefs or emotions. Relieving these symptoms may need to take into account the addictive nature of some mental operations and symptoms. But this will have to be considered in the next chapter.

The crucial role of meaning

Time was when behavioural therapists and psycho-analytic therapists vied for the territory of psychological treatment. Psycho-analysts anathematized behavioural therapists for treating people as animals, as mere emitters of behaviour rather than makers of meaning. Behavioural therapists countered this with the accusation that psycho-analysts did not seem concerned to always fought to suppress the image, but did so. The therapist asked him to describe the image, which John did, in horrific terms. The therapist then asked John to try to keep the image as clearly in his mind as possible, whilst imagining what would happen to Julia's face as death approached. Would she be frightened or would it be a relief after her long struggle? Would death welcome Julia, and make her safe? Would it be good for her not to have to fight for breath, as she had been doing for so long? John looked into the face that his mind had conjured up. It did seem to soften, and become calmer. John had been there, at Julia's death. The therapist asked him to keep the image of Julia's face in his mind as clearly as possible, and then asked, 'Where is she looking? Is she looking at you, John? Is it a look of love? Does she think that you have done everything that you could for her? Does she want you to remember her with pain, or with tenderness?'. John's gaze continued to be inwards but tears formed in his eyes, and then rolled down his cheeks. His daughter had looked on him with love at her last moment.

John was asked to repeat the exercise at home, and over 2 weeks the image gradually faded. John expressed some regret when it had finally gone, because he felt that he had lost Julia a bit more. But his relief far outweighed this regret.

John's difficulty was that he had stopped his internal 'film' at its most horrific moment, before it could be resolved. This had the same effect as a couple who break off an argument at its most vitriolic point, or a person who wakes from a dream or loses a memory at its most frightening moment. John had been a wonderful father to Julia, and she had clearly felt warmly towards him. The therapist was sure that there was a resolution to come, and felt confident therefore in asking John to continue with his 'film' until he experienced it.

Hypno-psychotherapy and neuro-linguistic programming include many other techniques for dealing with images, especially those that do not seem so replete with emotion. Many of them involve image modification, which may be especially useful when, as is so often the case with fear, the client feels that the image is in control. Possible types of image modification include zooming out or zooming in to the image, inverting it, introducing a new person into it, putting a frame around it, or challenging some particularly intense aspect of it.

Testing beliefs about treatment and self-treatment

Avoidance and undoing are consequences not just of the emotion, but of the coping strategies that a person has adopted to try to control it and which, paradoxically, have actually strengthened it. Avoidance means, in behaviour therapy, that a person does not unlearn the association of anxiety with the avoided situation. Cognitive therapy adds an extra dimension to this. Avoidance means not only that a situation is being avoided, but that an emotion is being avoided and this can only mean that the emotion is stronger relieve distress but were much too interested in making things complicated. Fortunately, these polarizations are disappearing. It is clear that there are unconscious processes in emotion, and that they do involve conscious appraisal, even if it is not of the symbolic kind that psycho-analysts suggest. It is also clear that talking to an anxious person about what they fear can lead to a conscious reappraisal of the level of threat which will subsequently alter automatic processes of threat appraisal (Mansell, 2000). However, when this does not happen, the therapist needs to question why. It may be that the threat has not yet been fully understood, or that the intensity of the symptom is too great, and some other symptomatic intervention also needs to be used. But if the therapist has tried all the symptomatic approaches that seem appropriate and palatable, and yet the symptoms still persist, it may be time to question whether the client has concerns other than symptom relief which need to be addressed.

These concerns are considered in the following chapters. They include: symptoms which arise as a result of the risks or physical consequences of an addictive behaviour (Chapter 7), symptoms which occur as a result of a predicament such as a long-standing marital conflict (Chapter 7), and symptoms which result from problems in relationships more generally (Chapter 10). Clients may deny having concerns in any of these areas, however, and then the therapist must face his or her own limitations. It is important at these times for the therapist to consider whether he or she has contributed to the client becoming stuck (Chapter 11) and whether he or she can get the therapeutic relationship unstuck. Sometimes, after all these avenues have been explored, the only practical thing to do is to admit defeat. Perhaps another therapist, of another flavour or with another value system, will do better. After all, we're all of us, only human.

7

Resolution: finding out what's doing this to me

In the previous chapter, persistent and disabling emotion was considered from the point of view of the client who found it useful to consider it to be an emotional malfunction or the consequence of a habit. The treatment approaches considered in that chapter had many values in common with medical practice. Indeed, many practitioners combine these approaches with drug treatments. These shared values include attributing problems to illness or pathology rather than to personal agency, emphasizing the causes rather than the reasons for things, and minimizing responsibility for anything but being a good client. Additional values inherent in symptomatic and motivational approaches include social cooperation, and the priority of the future over the past. Family members, if they are involved, are recruited as therapeutic assistants and they, and the therapist, are seen as helpers. Whatever has happened in the past, there is optimism and potential relief or change in the future.

The symptom-relieving approaches considered in Chapter 6 assumed that neither past emotional experiences nor current interpersonal conflict was relevant to the therapy. If we wanted to use metaphors of emotional flavour, we could say that symptom-relieving approaches are sweet rather than salty (if conflict is the salt), and sour rather than bitter (if the past is the gall).

Many people, including many therapists, consider that a psychotherapeutic approach that takes no account of interpersonal conflict is too saccharine, and that the past must be faced, however bitter it might be. This is not to say that these values are right, only to say that if a person holds them, the therapeutic approach needs to be compatible with them. Many people seeking assistance with a mental health problem who consult a doctor or a mental health professional, let alone a psychotherapist or a counsellor, believe that the problem must, in some way, be linked to their relationships with others, and to be 'telling them something' about those relationships. For people who take this view, ignoring the past, quietening down their bad feelings, and assuming that everyone else is just trying to be helpful is exactly the opposite of what they want.

When people want to sort out a problem, or to get to the bottom of whatever has brought them to the psychotherapist, it almost always turns out that the solution involves considering their relationships with others. How they present this problem may be quite variable. Sometimes a person may say in the first assessment interview that they don't want just to feel better, they want to know why they are feeling bad in the first place. At other times, a person embarks on cognitive therapy or some other symptomatic approach, but it is clear that their motivation to succeed in it is defective. They have found out through trying to eliminate their feelings that it is more important that they resolve them.

A person may also present their problem in relationships directly as the cause of their difficulties, although this is probably more common in private than in health service practice.

Mrs Horton and her daughter had lived with Mr Roberts for almost 10 years. It had started as being a relationship of convenience to some degree. Mrs Horton had split up from her daughter's father and had struggled both emotionally and financially. Mr Roberts had seemed kind and was willing to share his home with both Mrs Horton and her daughter. However, he was a passive man and where his partner wanted strength, he gave only passive-aggressiveness. She asked her GP to refer her to a psychotherapist because she could not sleep properly and was taking time off from work. However, she was clear that this was because she felt at an impasse. She had met another man, who seemed everything that she wanted and that Mr Roberts could not give her. But he was an unknown quantity emotionally. She knew that he was well established and that he wanted her. But she was not sure that she could rely on him. Mr Thompson, her new man, wanted her to move out to her own place as a preparation for them building up a relationship. But she would have to give up her home and, more importantly, many of her own things that she had bought over the previous 10 years, because Mr Roberts was a vindictive man and would want to get his revenge.

Mrs Horton found herself in a predicament: should she risk her, and her daughter's, future security, or should she remain in her present relationship but lose a man who seemed as if he could give her so much more satisfaction? It was her failure to resolve this predicament which she knew was causing her insomnia and other emotional difficulties, that made her consult a pychotherapist.

Mrs Horton's predicament involved a motivational conflict. This is typical. Most predicaments involve a person believing that they have to make a decision which will affect their relationships, and yet finding all their potential choices equally unattractive (or more rarely, equally attractive). Even when the predicament is about work, or sport, or a religious affiliation, it will usually be found that the source of the difficulty is how other people will react, and what effect the choice will have on relationships with others.

A person may constantly find themselves in predicaments with different people, and in different spheres of their life. When this happens, the client will often experience the same predicament in the course of the therapy and in relation to the therapist. The therapist, too, might find him- or herself in a predicament in relation to the client, and may sometimes think that this predicament is of the client's, rather than of their own, making. Therapy which becomes a predicament is the concern of Chapter 11. In this and the next chapter, we shall consider shorter-term therapy, in which the focus of the treatment is not on the therapeutic relationship, but on one particular predicament in one particular relationship or relationship type (with the children, or with boyfriends, for example).

Interpersonal, exploratory, dynamic, analytic . . .

It will be obvious why the term 'interpersonal psychotherapy' has been applied to the therapy of social relationships, although the term was introduced for a therapy originally intended to help people to mobilize the social support that they might need to alleviate depression (Klerman et al., 1984). Interpersonal therapy drew on many of the values of symptomatic treatments like cognitive-behavioural therapy. It was a treatment designed to fix something that was wrong, although it used the then-current social psychology of personal relationships rather than emotion theory as its basis. Interpersonal psychotherapy should probably, therefore, be considered to be an applied relationship theory, and be included in the later section. However, it is a term which has migrated to cover psycho-dynamic or psycho-analytic therapies, being taken in some quarters to be preferable to these older terms.

Many psychiatrists at the turn of the century had recognized that people might act, speak or think in apparently opposing ways at different times. Kraepelin had observed the ambitendency of people with dementia praecox, and Charcot the opposing actions of women whom he described as hysterics. Freud and Janet were each the originators of a grand psychological theory which started from this observation. Beginning this chapter with a motivational conflict and a predicament is to follow in their footsteps. However, each explained this conflict slightly differently. Janet supposed that there was a failure of the mind to synthesize different tendencies, Freud that there was a conflict between different tendencies. This conflict was the dynamic: 'We do not derive the psychical splitting from an innate incapacity for synthesis on the part of the mental apparatus; we explain it dynamically, from the conflict of opposing mental forces, and recognize it as the outcome of an active struggling on the part of the two psychical groupings against each other' (Freud, 1910).

The two psychical groupings are the unconscious or the 'id' and 'super-ego', and the conscious or 'ego' (or almost all of it). The term 'psychodynamic' therefore implies an acceptance of these different 'groupings', of the existence of constant mental conflict, and of the existence of mental forces. Although it is not mentioned in the quotation, it is well known that one of the most important forces which Freud claimed to have re-discovered was 'lust'.

In addition to being a metapsychologist – a speculative theoretician – Freud was the originator of the 'psycho-analysis' technique. There are many psychotherapists whose practice has been greatly influenced by the techniques of free association and interpretation introduced by Freud but who would take exception to some aspects of the theory. Some of them might prefer the term 'interpersonal' to the term 'psycho-dynamic' because it does not have these theoretical connotations. But what about the term, 'psycho-analytic'? Surely this would be even more preferred, as it is the term used by Freud for his new technique for treating neurotic disorders. The answer to this question lies in the reasons that Freud gives for choosing the term 'analysis': '. . . we trace the symptoms back to the instinctual impulses which motivate them; we point out to the client these instinctual motives, which are present in his symptoms and of which he has hitherto been unaware – just as a chemist isolates the fundamental substance, the chemical "element", out of the salt in which it has been combined with other elements in which it was unrecognisable' (Freud, 1919).

This passage illustrates one of the strongest claims of psycho-analysis, and the reason why it has created such enmity. Freud believed that he was speaking with the authority of the scientist – that he knew, incontrovertibly, about the mind. Even though the analogy with science has been repeatedly rejected since Freud, and indeed science itself no longer seems so secure a source of authority about the world, this air of incontrovertible, superior knowledge flavours psycho-analytic writing and attitudes.

A psychotherapist who wanted to draw on psycho-analysis selectively, but eschew its authoritarian stance, might therefore much prefer to use the term 'interpersonal' to describe his or her work to the term, 'psycho-analytic'. But what would such a psychotherapist have taken from psycho-analysis? What has psycho-analysis contributed to interpersonal therapy?

Freud's single most important contribution is to have campaigned so effectively for the 'unconscious', or rather, for the recognition that we have motives, such as desires and inhibitions, which another person can see, and we cannot. There is no doubt that there are mental processes which lie outside awareness, but which influence our actions. No psychologist would deny this. What many psychologists would still deny, but what Freud asserted, is that there was unconscious agency. For example, I forget a lecture. I feel mortified, and I think of all the reasons: something distracted me from looking at my diary, or the lecture date had been changed at the last minute. But my analyst tells me that I had an unconscious wish not to give the lecture, and that's why I forgot it. My unconscious took control of my actions, and made me forget to go. Or, to take another example, I make a slip of the tongue or a slip of the pen because my unconscious has taken over my tongue or my hand for a moment to express its desires.

Freud's image of this is clearly based on a reality of the Austro-Hungarian empire, the censor. He supposed that 'an agency of the mind', the 'conscious', or, as it was later termed, the 'ego', acts as a censor to unconscious ideas and impulses, repressing those that offend its conception of the good. These ideas originate in another agency, the 'unconscious' or the 'id', and are able to find expression, sometimes, by tricking the censor. This notion that a person is not the master or mistress of their own mind has caused outrage since it was first propounded. Hull described the theory as a depiction of the mind as a bank manager watching his maiden aunt fight to the death with a sex-crazed gorilla. Freud dismissed such critics by interpreting their criticisms as defensive. He said that he wrote what others were trying to repress, and so he, too, was censored. However, whether or not psycho-analysis is true is not the point for us here. It will have already become clear that there is no exhaustive theory of psychotherapy. It may be that there never can be, because to believe a theory is to change one's self-perception and therefore to change oneself (Harre, 1983). It is a joke among psycho-analytic candidates that trainees whose psycho-analyst is Freudian dream about the Oedipus complex and those whose psycho-analyst is Kleinian dream about the breast. Readers who are interested in plumbing the rich and often intellectually fascinating history of the debates over psycho-analysis during the last century may wish to consult Erwin (1996) for a philosopher's view.

What is of more importance is the extent to which psycho-analysis has provided explanations of emotional and relationship difficulties which have endured.

Case example

Mr Foot had been severely beaten by his father as a baby, and had several bones broken in his leg. He was also neglected. He was taken into care at the age of 3 months, and subsequently adopted. He grew up to be an angry, quick-tempered man with an energy and an intellectual ability that enabled him to rise in business. However, he had a good relationship with his adoptive parents, called them 'mother' and 'father', and never felt that he wanted to trace his biological parents.

He never met a woman with whom he felt that he could have a long-term relationship until, as the managing director of a medium-sized company, he got involved in a takeover bid for another company – L. King of Droitwich – a family firm in the same line of business as Mr Foot. He became quite emotionally involved in the takeover. He disliked Mr King, the man who ran the other business, but felt an attraction towards his wife, also a partner in the business, even though she was much older than himself. The family firm was ailing financially and could not resist the takeover. The terms were that Mrs King would join Mr Foot's company as a director and that Mr King would get a share option but no job. Mr King became depressed, and in the course of time, Mrs King divorced him and married Mr Foot. They had two daughters.

Mr Foot knew that he should be happy, but he wasn't.

Why was Mr King unhappy, and what does psycho-analysis have to say about it? One possible interpretation is that Mr Foot did wish to harm Mr King, but Mr Foot had always been told by his parents that such wishes are destructive. Mr Foot therefore did not allow himself to see that this is what he wanted. Or, to rephrase this interpretation in more psycho-analytic terms, Mr Foot repressed his wish to harm Mr King, keeping it unconscious, under the influence of his super-ego, the internalized representation of his father. When the harm came about, his super-ego – his 'conscience' to use an older term – punished him because in the world of childhood, when the super-ego is formed, to have a wish to do something and doing it are equally culpable.

As it turns out, there are lots of problems with Freud's formulation of the super-ego. It is inextricably entangled with male rather than female development, it assumes that civilization consists of reigning in the primitive destructiveness of unfettered human nature, it reifies processes, making them the activities of mental structures, and it emphasizes too strongly a single moment in childhood development. Some, but not all, of these points have been successfully addressed in later revisions by Klein (1948), Lacan (1977), and others. However, no psychotherapist has questioned the formative role that censure plays in society, or the fact that feeling good is strongly associated with having the approval of others, and with being popular. Indeed, there would be as much support for these ideas among neurobiologists as among psychotherapists. Attachment theory, with its emphasis on security from anxiety, brings together experts on the amygdala and on animal behaviour, and psychotherapists, each of them stressing the importance for defence against anxiety of being able to be close to protective others.

We are strongly influenced by our actual relations with others, as has been stressed in some of the non-psycho-analytic relationship theories considered below, but we also perpetuate our relations with remembered or imagined others. It does not seem necessary to suppose that we can only do this by 'internalizing' these others i.e. making a part of our minds over to them. We can perfectly well continue a relationship in thought, in imagery, or in enactments, like visiting graves or wearing clothing that was given to us by the other. Mental conflict or mental turmoil does provide an explanation of anguish or mental suffering which many people accept. And many people will also accept that we can sometimes blind ourselves to the consequences of our actions until afterwards, when we realize what we have done and may feel regret or remorse for it. For many psychotherapists, mental conflict does not need to be between internalized mental objects, and not being aware of all the implications of what we are doing does not imply an animalistic unconscious at war with a socialized conscious. We can deceive ourselves (Mele, 1997) and we can deny things to ourselves without needing to suppose an unconscious.

One account of how we can deceive ourselves, which seems an impossible task at first, is that we can do it through conversations. We can tell comforting stories about our motives, and can allow ourselves more latitude than we allow other people in judging their purity. We can simply skirt around issues, which therefore remain unassimilated (Stiles, 1999). We can do this in conversation with others, but also in conversation with ourselves.

Internal conversations linked to predicaments very often take the form of a debate: should I, or shouldn't I? This debate can also be carried on in a self-deceiving way or in a way that denies some of the reality of the situation. According to this narrative development of psycho-analytic theory, the role of the therapist is to participate in this debate, speaking the part of the chorus who will not go along with self-deception or denial. This process is very similar to debates among philosophers who seek to prune away error and faulty inference in each other's work, but retain a respect for the good intentions of their opponents. It is therefore not surprising that some of the newest arrivals to the group of people that can help one resolve a personal crisis are philosophical counsellors, applying Socratic dialogue or other philosophical methods of enquiry to psychotherapy.

Many psycho-analysts would say that such approaches are superficial: that they deal with what a person can be aware of, and chooses not to be aware of, rather than what is hidden from their awareness. The mind to them is like a landscape. A mound can be flattened by removing topsoil, but it needs deeper digging to discover that the soil has accumulated on the site of an old building, and even more digging to discover that the building was there because there was an outcrop of a different and harder rock at that point. Removing the soil may resolve an immediate problem, but when the same pattern recurs over and over, the underlying factors need to be dug out.

If the depth analogy is true, then it might explain why the psycho-analytic approach is still pre-eminent among psychotherapies which are not focussed on symptom relief. For if a person's deepest wishes and impulses are hidden in a special region of the mind, then perhaps only trained psycho-analysts have the knowledge and the experience to discover them. But are there impulses hidden in all of us?

Mr Foot, as it turned out, laughed off the possibility that he had become unhappy thinking of the consequences of his takeover of Mr King's company for Mr King himself. Mr Foot was of the school of macho businessmen who saw struggle as a sacred duty, and losing as a personal failing. The therapist asked him, 'If this was not the cause of his unhappiness, what was?'. Mr Foot seemed

unwilling to give his opinion about this at first but then said that he first felt that there was a cloud on his horizon when a business colleague said to him, on meeting Mrs Foot for the first time, 'She's very like you'. Mr Foot had glanced in the mirror, seeing himself and his wife together, and thought, 'We could be mother and son'. Mr Foot began, the following day, to try to trace his mother. He discovered that she had been a Mrs Jocasta King, wife of Mr L. King, of Droitwich . . .

Readers will probably have recognized Mr Foot to be a modernized incarnation of Oedipus, the emblematic figure of psycho-analytic theory. When Mr Foot, or Oedipus as we should now call him, traced his mother, Jocasta, he found that he had married her, after getting rid of her former husband, his father. In the original story (Sophocles, 1982), Oedipus had killed his father in an act of road rage, and had much later met and married his widowed mother . . . Sophocles makes clear that neither Oedipus nor his mother recognized each other. Nor did Oedipus know his father, since he was separated from him at birth and had been brought up to know another man and woman as father and mother.

It is well established that mothers and sons separated since early life have a strong and often sexual attraction to each other (Greenberg & Littlewood, 1995). There is likely to have been this special attraction between Oedipus and his mother, although they would not have known that it should be distrusted. It is commonly the rule in mammalian groups composed of one male and several females that male offspring are driven off when they reach puberty. This would seem to support the psycho-analytic theory that sons want to couple with their mothers, but are prevented from doing so by being driven out of their preoccupation with the family home and into the world by the threat of retribution from their fathers. Freud thought that human male children experience the same sequence of events. He gave this sequence, and its psychological consequences, the name 'Oedipus complex', because Oedipus succeeded in doing what Freud imagined all sons want to do. Oedipus challenged his father, overcame him, and subsequently married his mother.

Both parricide and incest are abhorred in every human culture. The only exceptions to this rule are made for religious or dynastic reasons, as in Pharaonic Egypt or in the Greek myths about the succession of the Gods. However, it seems unnecessarily convoluted to suppose that the abhorrence exists *because* every son has a wish to kill his father and mate with his mother. According to this form of argument, which has become widely diffused in psycho-analytically influenced psychotherapy, the reason that a person is violently or irrationally repressive of some idea or behaviour is that he or she is forcefully repressing the same belief or wish in themselves. It is all too easy for a self-opinionated therapist to use such an argument to stifle their client, for the more that the client objects that the therapist has misunderstood, the more the therapist can claim that the client is in denial.

Clearly, there must be some arrangements which ensure that incest, and parricide, are anomalous, but it may be that familiarity is normally enough to prevent the shock of excitement that normally leads to sexual attraction or murderous rage (Erickson, 1993). As has been pointed out by many commentators since Freud, the myth of Oedipus is not really relevant to Freud's theory because Oedipus's mother's name was not Jocasta, but Periboea, the woman to whom he had been given as an infant and who had brought him up as her own. Oedipus, when he met his mother, had last seen her when he was a newborn baby. It is inconceivable that he recognized her. The plays of Sophocles and Euripides are tragedies precisely because none of the protagonists intended to do what they did. In fact, Oedipus left Corinth and went to Thebes precisely because the oracle at Delphi had warned him that he would murder his father and lie with his mother. He was not to know that Corinth was only his adoptive city, and that Thebes was his native city, and the city where his parents lived.

Blows of fate like the kind that Oedipus suffered when he discovered the truth about his life place people in a different sort of predicament to the one that has been considered up to now. They are not concerned with choosing between several possible pathways, but with knowing how to go on when the paths cease. When the unthinkable happens, how can one think about it? This issue has been addressed most directly in the existential approach, which is considered in the next section.

Perhaps Oedipus was caused to do what he did by nothing more specific than a violent temperament and the genetic attraction that existed between his mother and himself. But for many people, this reduces life to a level of meaninglessness that is unacceptable. If we can be struck down by random misfortune, what is the point of our aspirations and our efforts to reach them? I have argued elsewhere that people are inclined to attribute reasons to the actors in events retrospectively to fill in gaps of this kind. These reasons make sense of what has happened because they provide plausible motives for the actions. Once the reasons have been accepted as real, they have consequences for how the actions are interpreted. But it is a fallacy to think that the actors had these reasons in mind, or any reasons for that matter, when they acted. This is particularly obvious in the case of Oedipus since he could not have known that he was killing his father, or marrying his mother.

The reason that Sophocles gave for the tragedy reflects ancient Greek values which are now hard for us to understand. They considered that whole families might set themselves against the Gods, and against custom. But the Gods arranged repayment, in the form of fate. Oedipus' fate was just one example of this. Oedipus' grandfather was Labdakos, 'the Lame'. He opposed the worship of Dionysus, and was then killed by Maenads, worshippers of

Dionysus. His son, Oedipus' father, was Laios, 'the Left-handed'. He lived in exile for a while, in the court of King Pelops. Whilst he was there, he became infatuated with one of Pelops' sons, and abducted him. Although he was eventually forgiven for this, he died at the hands of a son parted from his father.

Sophocles' Oedipus had failed to live harmoniously with his given fate, but had wanted more. His punishment was to bring shame on himself, his family and his city. Freud's Oedipus feels guilt. He has to make amends for an offence that he, unconsciously, intended to commit. One difference between the two accounts is that Freud's Oedipus is autonomous. He might make a mess of things, but it is himself doing it. No-one messes with him. Sophocles' Oedipus is but a link in a chain of fate that dates back to his grandfather.

Freud's theories fitted with prevailing values, and had a flavour of the tragic hero which also fitted with the times. However, his insistence that Oedipus intended to marry his mother – that the unconscious knows what it is doing – seems a fatal flaw. This becomes even more apparent in the work of Melanie Klein, who attributes to infants phantasies which are far beyond their cognitive power, and even extends these phantasies to infants before they are born. What Klein, and Freud, do well to remind us is that whatever causes us to act as we do, other people will take the attitude that we intended the consequences of our actions. Even if a baby bites its mother's nipple hard because of the shape of its mouth, or her breast, the mother will attribute anger or voraciousness to the baby that will influence her attitude to it. And perhaps Klein was right. Perhaps one long-term result of such an attribution might be that the baby grows up into an adult who perceives him- or herself as dangerously destructive.

Existential

Mrs Wilson was a god-fearing, upright woman who was making an excellent job of bringing up two children and supporting her husband. He was not a high-flyer but he was a kindly man, and she was very happy with him. There were few clouds on her horizon, and those were only little ones. Then a van backed into her in a parking area. She saw it coming, and assumed that the driver had seen her. When she realized he hadn't, it was too late to get out of the way. Her head was crushed under the wheels, and she was very lucky (or so they told her) to survive with the facial injuries that resulted. Following the accident she did not feel lucky, but bitter. She was frequently weepy and had some anxiety symptoms, so her family doctor referred her to a psychotherapist.

Mrs Wilson's predicament was coming to grips with the randomness, the arbitrariness, of her accident. She would say, 'Why was it me?', and then reproach herself saying, 'Well, I suppose if it wasn't me it would have been someone else', as if there was a certain quota of accidents that 'Fate' had to meet. Thinking that if it had not been her, it might not have been anybody, was just too upsetting.

Existential psychotherapy is derived from the philosophies of the existentialists who include Kierkegaard, Heidegger, Sartre, de Beauvoir, Merleau-Ponty, Jaspers, Buber, and others. Their philosophies have been applied to psychotherapy by Binswanger, Boss, May, Yalom, and van Deurzen (1997), whose work includes an overview of the history and key concepts of existential psychotherapy. These authors stressed the inescapability of anxiety in the face of death and other 'limit-situations', as Jaspers called them (1951). Most of the time, a person cannot stand this anxiety and falls away into some sort of comforting fiction. Sometimes, as in Mrs Wilson's case, the fiction is stripped away. At these times it is easy to fall into another kind of fiction – that one is the plaything of fate or that one has merited such treatment. Chronic anxiety or hopelessness can be the result.

Mrs Wilson's helplessness became focussed on the hospital. She had told the neurosurgeon that she had a persistently runny nose, and he had raised the possibility of a dura mater tear, leading to a leak of cerebro-spinal fluid. Mrs Wilson was told that she might need to have a further operation, and that she should be on the alert for signs of meningitis. A test was arranged, but no results came through. Mrs Wilson was sure that they were positive, but that no-one had bothered to tell her because they were fed up with her demands. 'What demands?', the therapist asked her. Mrs Wilson had, as it turned out, been a model client but there had been complications of her initial emergency surgery, and she had been in hospital for a long time. Sometimes it became too much, and she would cry. Mrs Wilson looked back on these occasions with shame. What would they have thought of her? Surely she should have been glad of all that had been done for her, not upset or angry.

Mrs Wilson did not recognize existential anxiety, and that it was normal to fear death and suffering. Her predicament was that she thought that she should just go back to living life as she had before, but she did not know how to do it. When the therapist went through with Mrs Wilson how she would have felt to be a nurse with her as a client, she was considerably more understanding. Of course a person in her situation would get upset. It would be unnatural not to. But she could not give herself the same leeway. A turning point came when she received a letter from the hospital but, instead of opening it, she became uncharacteristically irritable with her son. She was sure that her family would have condemned her. The therapist thought differently. He thought that everyone else in the family would understand how worried she was, and how appropriate that worry was. She decided to test out what the therapist had said. Was her husband critical of her? When she asked her husband that evening, he said that they all knew how anxious she was, indeed they all were. It had been a relief to see her get angry. Normally, she kept such control on her feelings that he and the children felt they could not show their feelings of worry either. Mrs Wilson improved quite rapidly after this.

Existential principles are also useful in longer-term therapy and are discussed further in the next chapter. Their particular relevance to the psychotherapy of predicaments is the reminder that the resolution of many predicaments involves facing up to the inevitability of anxiety or loss, and not trying to escape them.

Mrs Milton's mother had died a year before. After her death, Mrs Milton had done her mother's washing, ironed the clothes and put them away. Her family doctor was worried because Mrs Milton had continued to be paralysed by grief, showing little sign of coming to terms with her mother's death. The therapist asked her what she had done with her mother's things. Mrs Milton said that everything was as her mother would have wanted it, put away tidily just as it was when her mother was alive. The therapist asked whether Mrs Milton planned to dispose of the clothes in any way. Mrs Milton was shocked. Doing that would be like getting rid of her mother, Mrs Milton said.

Mrs Milton could not face letting go of her mother, and her grief was blocked.

Sometimes, paradoxically, anxiety about other things can be an escape from existential anxiety. This is related to the idea of existential guilt, the anxiety that results from falling short of one's potential.

Mrs De'ath was a single mother who was struggling to keep going. One source of comfort for her was her house, which was in a quiet street in a good part of the city. She felt safe there. One day, just after getting home, she heard a noise and looked out of her window to see the woman across the road beckoning frantically to her. Her normal instinct was to draw the curtains and keep herself to herself. On this occasion she went across the road to see what was wrong. Her neighbour speechlessly led her into the house and pointed to something in a dark corner of the kitchen. Mrs De'ath saw that it was the woman's husband curled up in a corner, bleeding from at least three stab wounds. She felt repulsed but knew that she could not just leave him to die. She tried to stop the bleeding, but the more that she pressed in one place, the more it seemed to bleed in another. It seemed an eternity until the ambulance arrived. She was covered in blood by then.

Mrs De'ath heard later that the man had died. His wife said that a stranger calling at the front door had stabbed him, but another story began to circulate in the street, that it was a drug-related killing. This all came out later. On the day, Mrs De'ath just wanted to get home, and lock her doors and windows. This did not keep out the fear, which grew over the next few days to the point where she could not sleep but constantly roamed the house in case there had been an intruder. She was frightened too about her daughter, and disturbed her sleep by going into her room throughout the night just to see if she was OK. After a few days she arranged for her daughter to go to stay with her grandmother, but if anything, Mrs De'ath's anxiety was even greater when she was on her own.

Mrs De'ath was anxious about many things: that another murder might take place in the street, that the security of her home had been violated, that she should have checked earlier that an ambulance had been called, that she should have stayed at home and not answered her neighbour's signals . . . and so on.

Mrs De'ath needed to talk about all these fears to the therapist at first, but after the first session, one main fear began to predominate: that she might have saved her neighbour if she had tried hard enough. She explained the circumstances. It was dark in the kitchen, there was little room to move, the body was too heavy even to roll over, and blood seemed to be pouring out of him. The horror of the experience was still strong enough to communicate itself to the therapist in the safety of the consulting room. What Mrs De'ath found so terrible was the inexorability of death and her helplessness in the face of it. This existential anxiety could only be resolved when Mrs De'ath asked to talk to the pathologist, who was able to explain that the probable cause of death was a laceration of the abdominal aorta, which would have caused internal bleeding and would have been impossible to staunch. This acceptance by a professional with constant experience of mortality that death was sometimes inevitable enabled Mrs De'ath to face her own anxiety.

Supportive, expressive, person-centered problem solving

The example of Mrs De'ath could have been given as an example of supportive, expressive or person-centered therapies. These assume that a person in a predicament could work it out for themselves if they had a sufficiently supportive environment in which to do it. This simple principle was most clearly enunciated by Carl Rogers, who wrote:

. . . that the individual has within himself vast resources for self-understanding, for altering his self concept, his attitudes, and his self-directed behaviour – and that these resources can be tapped if only a definable climate of facilitative psychological attitudes can be provided. (1974, p. 116)

The facilitative environment was the subject of research by Rogers and his colleagues. Its essence was that the therapist or counsellor should remove all obstacles of understanding between her- or himself and the client. These obstacles include critical rejection or judgement of the client, a lack of understanding of the client's experience, that is a lack of empathy, and an inability to transcend any barriers of cultural, gender or social difference.

The emphasis of person-centered training is on helping the therapist to be more aware of these barriers in themselves. There is a de-emphasis on any barriers within the client. Those barriers that exist are assumed to be due to a failure on the part of the therapist to be able to make a therapeutic bond with the client rather than the client's failure to get on terms with the therapist or the therapeutic method.

For many therapists there is both considerable wisdom and considerable ingenuousness in the client-centered approach. Its emphasis on the influence of the therapist has itself been influential, even spreading back into psycho-analysis through communicative psychotherapy, which puts failures in understanding by the psycho-analyst centre stage in the therapist dialogue. It has strongly influenced counselling training in North America and the UK. Its emphasis on self-reflection is a valuable one for all health professionals.

The premise that people can work out their problems if given the right sort of listening ear is an empowering one which fits well with the values of practical psychotherapy. It also turns out in practice that many people *are* denied a listening ear. However, it is much less often true of those people who are referred on from first-line helpers. A person's ability to overcome ob-stacles is sometimes exceeded, as we have seen in some of the examples already mentioned.

Problem-solving therapy is included in this section because its efficacy, which has been proven in general practice (Mynors-Wallis et al., 1997), probably stems more from its common features with client-centered therapy. The addition of cognitive techniques of problem-solving – widening the option fan, questioning statements with 'should' in them, brainstorming possible solutions – are extensions of empathic understanding. It is not a lack of understanding that prevents people from considering all their options, but a lack of opportunity to rehearse them.

Personal constructivist, cognitive-analytic, applied relationship theory

There are approaches which seek to retain the collaborative flavour of the humanistically orientated approaches in the previous section, but which recognize that there are persistent styles in relatedness which affect a person's ability to resolve predicaments. The personal constructivists base this on Kelly's personal construct theory, a theory that people are influenced by 'constructs', that is concepts about others, their roles, and their likely emo-tional responses. Kelly's first fundamental postulate was that: 'A person's processes are psychologically channelized by the ways in which he anticipates events' (Kelly, 1953, p. 46). This postulate is, as written, entirely compatible

with the cognitive-appraisal theories of emotion which have strongly influenced the symptomatic treatments considered in Chapter 5. However,
Kelly's use of the word 'channels' points to a rather different emphasis, which
becomes clearer later in the chapter when he writes, 'Channels . . . are laid
down by the devices which a person invents in order to achieve a purpose. A
person's processes, psychologically speaking, slip into the grooves which are
cut out by the mechanisms he adopts for realizing his devices' (ibid., p. 49).

The concrete and somewhat mechanical flavour of this passage, due to the
use of words like channels, grooves, devices and mechanisms, is striking. We
shall see that this concrete flavour pervades all the approaches grouped in this
section. It attracts practitioners, and clients, who are seeking a science of
psychotherapy but it may also give a spurious appearance of knowledge to
what is, after all, only metaphor. The mind does not have channels or grooves
in it, any more than it has internalized objects. However, any carpenter will
recognize the metaphor. Just go wrong on a saw cut, and the saw imperceptibly drifts back into that groove and increases it. Unless the sawyer concen-
trates hard on putting a contrary tendency on her or his stroke, the saw will of
itself increase the groove and its divergence away from the desired line. So,
according to Kelly's metaphor, is it with people. Once a tendency to react in
certain ways has been established, once there is a groove, then this tends to
deepen the more it is used.

The extent to which a particular groove is used is determined by groupings
of similarity and difference. If I tend to react to my son in a particular way,
along a particular groove, I am likely to react to anyone that I consider to be
similar to my son along the same lines (to extend the metaphor further).
However, the category 'my son' may not be unitary. I may have one groove
for one son, and not the other. Or two grooves for one son, depending on
when he is being kind, or when he is being angry. Therefore, how many
grooves I have, and what they are for, is to some extent determined by how
many things I think fit together in one groove, or are differentiated into
several grooves. Kelly called the maps of similarities and differences personal
constructs. Pursuing this line of similarities and differences, Kelly assumed
that most constructs were also dichotomous and gained their meaning from
contrast, for example black and white, man and animal, scientist and artist.

Case example
John Rogers was referred because of his uncontrollable temper. He felt that it
was imperilling his job and his marriage. In the past, he had always thought
approvingly of himself as someone who could stand up to anybody. Now he
began to see that he had a problem. He had hit a friend with whom he was
playing golf because he thought that the friend had moved his ball, he had
assaulted his neighbour who had criticized the fact that John's garden was
messy, and he had punched a car-driver through the open window of his car

because the driver had cut him up. John described his father as a completely selfish despot whose success outside in the world only mirrored his callous coercion of his children. John's construct of his father included all other men. Until proven otherwise, they too were out to tyrannize John and would do so unless John was even stronger than them. This construct of man was the polar opposite of woman, and also the construct of self. John saw women as non-aggressive, understanding and supportive, and himself as much exercised but basically kindly.

Emotional reactions reflect the failure of constructs to provide adequate guides to action. So anxiety is the 'awareness that the events with which one is confronted lie mostly outside the range of convenience of one's construct system' (Bannister & Fransella, 1986, p. 21). Hostility is 'the continued effort to extort validational evidence in favour of a type of social prediction which has already been recognized as a failure' (ibid., p. 22). John's hostility would, according to this way of looking at things, be driven by his wish not to differentiate his concepts of men and women. Interestingly, a psycho-analytically orientated psychotherapist might arrive at a similar conclusion, although couching it in other terms. One interpretation might be that John splits all the badness of people, and his disappointment with them, into one object – his father specifically, and men in general – and all the goodness, and his hopes of care, into another object – his mother specifically.

Kelly, and personal construct therapists since him, have developed various techniques for helping people to develop new grooves. Some of these techniques involve helping a person to become aware of the grooves themselves, for example by writing an account of themselves in the third person, a process which Kelly called 'self-characterization'. Other methods that Kelly used included role playing someone who is psychologically at '90 degrees', as Kelly put it, in their self-characterization to that of the client. He stressed that not only should the person undertaking this exercise react in a new way, but that they should dress the part, and adopt tastes and habits fitting the new character.

Kelly invented a diagrammatic method, the repertory grid, to elicit and display personal constructs. It has been used widely as a means of characterizing personality and has the advantage that it combines emotional tendencies and beliefs in a richer way than trait theory or the schemata of cognitive therapy.

Repertory grids were used not just for assessment, but as a tool to help clients understand their difficulties, by Anthony Ryle, then a psychiatrist working with university students. A workshop on short-term psycho-dynamic psychotherapy given by Davanloo (see below) inspired him to attempt a synthesis of short-term psychodynamic and Kellyan principles. The result is strongly reminiscent of personal construct therapy, although the grooves are now termed 'reciprocal role procedures'. A procedure is a mental process, followed by an action, followed by consequences. Most procedures are modified by experience, but some remain resistant to modification even though they lead to distress and to problems in relationships with others. These resistant procedures are termed 'snags', 'traps' and 'dilemmas' according to the factors that make them resistant to change.

Both personal construct therapy and cognitive-analytic therapy (CAT) are didactic. In the case of cognitive-analytic theroy, clients are given a formulation letter, which may be followed by a reformulation letter. This sets out the various snags, traps and dilemmas that prevent the client from reaching their desired goal. The letter may be supplemented or replaced by a diagram giving the same information. The use of these tools is similar to the use of Kellyan self-characterizations, or repertory grids. They are designed to make a person stop and think, and look around for new ways of acting and reacting.

There is quite a ritual in the formulation letter or diagram. It needs to be agreed with the client since both Kelly's and Ryle's approaches place strong emphasis on collaboration. Many clients carry the letters around with them, and may look at them in moments of crisis or difficulty. They are a good way of helping clients feel that they have the goodwill and support of the therapist with them at all times. Whether or not people do actually behave as they do because they experience snags, traps and dilemmas in the world is less clear. As is the case for many psychotherapies, the theory outruns the evidence. Perhaps we have to accept that there is something inalienably unreachable about a theory of psychotherapy. As Bannister put it:

. . . we have almost totally loose circumspective psychologies such as Freudian or Existential psychology. This is the kind of speculative vague psychologizing which leads to papers of the *Unconscious aggression and overt sexual fantasies as quasi-religious substrata for international conflicts* type. At the other end of the spectrum we have the tight world of the pure learning theorist dealing in the highly defined and fragmentary and providing us with the *Short-term memory for T mazes under electrically induced stress conditions in the decorticate woodlouse* type of paper. (1970, p. 70)

Bannister concluded that it was necessary for science to move constantly between tighter and looser hypotheses, and that personal construct theory was a means of characterizing this movement. However, it does not seem to me that personal construct theory is any more able to avoid the limitations of other theories. Indeed, the reader might conclude, rightly in my opinion, that no single theory of psychotherapy will ever suffice. Facts or trends or probabilities can be established more or less incontrovertibly. The theories that link them together into a meaningful whole will still vary. Elsewhere I have argued that there are two distinct kinds of account of why a person does things. One account is about the causes of a person's actions. The second account is about the meaning which is placed on those actions retrospective-ly. Much of psychotherapy is concerned with the second, meaningful, kind of account, even when it purports to be of the former type.

Psychotherapy theories are narratives: stories, perhaps even songs, about the world. Some of them have the grandeur of national anthems, others have the evanescent popularity of chart-toppers. Some convey truths about the human condition which are timeless and which cannot be captured in any other way. Many need to be performed correctly by people skilled in the art for their qualities and their effects to be apparent. But none of them exhausts all that might be said on the subject.

Family, systems, networks

What if a person's predicament is not a result of their own conflicts or inability to see ahead in their lives, but a consequence of someone else's actions, or of their interaction with someone else? This might be someone at work who is bullying them, or a parent, friend or neighbour, but it is most likely to be a partner, at least in adult life. Various therapeutic approaches to help people with relationship problems are applicable to predicaments. They are best classified according to the frame of the intervention, that is, the characteristics of the people who are included, and excluded, in the therapy. The choice of the frame is determined by who is considered to be responsible for the predicament. If the predicament is thought not to be resoluble unless others change, then the frame of the therapy is drawn around these others. The frame may include a whole community, as in the network therapy based on Navajo healing rituals (Speck & Attneave, 1973), a family with or without children or grandparents, a couple, or, as we have seen, individuals.

Family therapy has introduced many theoretical ideas which have per-meated all types of short-term therapy. Not the least of these is the 'strategic' approach (Haley, 1963). This has some similarities to Foulkes's concept of dynamic administration (Foulkes, 1964) since it stresses the impact of the organization of the therapy on the progress of the therapy itself. Administra-tion is dynamic, Foulkes considered, when the way that it is conducted, and the concern and understanding of others that is apparent in that way, provide a model of good relating for other family or group members.

Strategic therapy is influenced by systemic theories such as general systems theory (von Bertalanffy, 1974) and catastrophe theory (Carver & Scheier, 1999), theories which allow for large events having little effect and small events having substantial and lasting effects. Strategic therapy sets out to identify where effort can be applied which will produce change most effi-ciently. Framing a problem is one strategy that almost always has a substantial effect.

Case example

Mrs Johnson had serious mental health problems. She suffered from regular bouts of low mood, and frequently took overdoses. She drank heavily, cut herself, and could be violent towards her partner. She was referred for psychotherapy and attended the assessment session with her partner. She asked whether he could be involved in the therapy. It was agreed that a further assessment visit should be arranged, but with both Mr and Mrs Johnson attending together. In the meanwhile, Mrs Johnson was referred to an individual psychotherapist.

At the joint assessment, Mr Johnson began by telling the story of how his wife had stormed out of the house the previous week and ended up being sexually assaulted by a taxi driver. The therapist knew enough to know that Mr Johnson was unlikely to be blameless in all of this, but it was difficult not to side with Mr Johnson in thinking that the problem that needed to be addressed was his wife's mental health problem. Indeed, Mrs Johnson herself thought this. It was only at the end of the session that it emerged, almost by chance, that Mr Johnson was regularly in contact with his ex-wife. In fact, the starting point of the row which led to his wife leaving was that he had spent the day at his ex-wife's house, mending her washing machine. Subsequent sessions focussed on Mr Johnson's difficulty in separating from his ex-wife, and the reactions of Mrs Johnson to this, rather than on Mrs Johnson's personality difficulties.

In fact, the individual therapist that Mrs Johnson was seeing reported a substantial improvement in her mood, suggesting that her predicament was not, on this occasion, best understood as a consequence of her difficulties in making relationships but as a response to her husband's ambivalence.

It was important in helping Mrs Johnson to resolve her predicament to frame it as a marital problem since, otherwise, her husband would have considered her objections to his continuing contact with his ex-wife to be a result of her unreasononableness.

Similar strategic judgements have to be made about whether to include the children when seeing a couple who have been referred because their children are out of control, or whether to include management as well as clinical staff when convening a staff group in a unit in crisis. There are no hard and fast rules, because the position of the frame will alter the salience of different preoccupying concerns. Seeing Mrs Johnson on her own brought her own concerns about her mental health and her own emotional reactions into salience. Seeing her with her husband put these into the background and brought the marital problems into the foreground.

Framing a predicament is an important step in resolving it. Which frame is the 'best' depends partly on the flavour and values attached to each frame, and partly on where a simple intervention can be most effective. Mrs Johnson had previously had therapy for her personality difficulties, and was constantly having them discussed by her husband. She was therefore somewhat refractory to more of the same kind. However, the idea that her husband should share some responsibility for causing her outbursts was a novel one in their marriage. An intervention along these lines was therefore likely to have a large effect.

The flavour of marital therapy is hard to describe but instantly recognizable to anyone who has experienced it. Family and marital therapists are more concerned with the actualities of relationships than many other therapists. Sex is often on their minds, but not the cerebral sex of the psychoanalyst. Family therapists are interested in how couples actually have sex, how often, and who initiates it. Crowe and Ridley (1990) advocate partners using sexual concessions as a reward for desired behaviour by the other partner.

Family therapists have been quick to embrace new theories, such as narrative theory, and seem to enjoy experimenting with new apparatus. The two-way screen, supervisors who can ring up the therapist during the course of the session, and video-taping sessions for future discussion with the family, are all innovations which first appeared in family therapy.

This zest for the playful, the unexpected and the charismatic has led therapists to be attracted to strategies which undermine or disrupt family expectations and therefore, it is hoped, family patterns of interaction that cause distress. The paradoxical injunction, or prescribing the symptom, is one example. A family member may be told to carry on with whatever they are doing which upsets other family members. Indeed they may be told to do it even more. The reason given for this intervention is that this behaviour prevents something even worse happening. The girl who diets to the point of anorexia nervosa may, for example, be ensuring that her parents have to stay together to look after her. If she resumed her normal weight, they might split up and so she is told to keep dieting. Either way, after the intervention, dieting cannot be the same. Either the daughter continues to diet, but is now carrying out the wishes of the therapist rather than striking a blow for her own independence, or she stops dieting to show the therapist how independent she is, but she now has to face up to her parents' marital problems (Shoham-Salomon, Avner & Neeman, 1989).

Paradoxical injunctions have appealed to many psychotherapists because they seem so powerful. However, they gain what power they have from a kind of coerciveness that raises ethical problems (Foreman, 1990). Not stigmatizing or blaming one particular person in the family is one of the key values of family therapy, as is openness and preparedness to change. Siding with the unpopular member, or making oneself a scapegoat, are positions which family therapists often adopt and can convey positive values of acceptance without recrimination. However, sometimes there is a degree of insincerity in a very powerful charismatic therapist taking a one-down position which may connote the negative value that underhand means are justified by their results.

Much of family therapy's history has been bedevilled by the value that 'it's all the fault of the parents'. The early history of autism which suggested that it was caused by 'refrigerator parents', Laing and Esterson's (1964) family research in schizophrenia which suggested that people with schizophrenia were sane and it was their parents who were mad, and more recent work which has attributed relapse in schizophrenia to parental expressed emotion: all of these trends have left some parents feeling betrayed.

This is just one aspect of a problem facing all psychotherapists and their clients: who is responsible for placing them in the predicament in the first place? Laing and others helped people with schizophrenia to feel better about themselves by insisting it was not they who were at fault, but their parents. But, not only were many parents demoralized and distressed by these accusations, but the person with schizophrenia found themselves in a new predicament. Either he or she had to cut off contact with their parents, a course of action sometimes insisted upon by psychiatrists in the 1960s, or carry on being ill. Providing an easy answer solves one predicament but only at the expense of creating another.

But avoiding conflict by taking all responsibility on oneself is not a psychologically satisfactory solution, either. Resolving predicaments requires something more than blaming someone else, or accepting the total responsibility for a situation oneself. Blaming other people is a potent cause of conflicts failing to be resolved. It is time to look at short-term psychotherapy approaches that have been especially designed to help people through predicaments by trying to find a middle way which avoids these two extremes.

Conflict resolution

Conflict resolution is a procedure that has been developed in mediation between two or more parties. Surprisingly, mediation is often used in individual therapy, too, despite only one of the parties to the conflict being present. In practice, the same principle applies in both situations. Conflicts fail to be resolved when people stop listening to each other. Conflict resolution is about making the parties to the conflict more receptive to listening and less ready to attack or defend. Conflict resolution does not aim at reconciliation, but at settlement. The principles of mediation are shown in the Table 7.1.

The difference between psychotherapy and non-therapeutic counselling, including mediation, is that psychotherapists, as I have already quoted one of my clients as saying, 'interfere'. Psychotherapists deal with situations in which it is not enough just to change a person's situation. The person themself has to change.

Sometimes conflicts do not resolve despite providing the right situation

Table 7.1. Steps in resolving conflicts in the workplace

---

1. Identify the parties involved in the conflict and obtain their consent to the resolution process.
2. Meet each party separately.
3. Consider whether the conflict is about issues or identity.
4. (Work to establish identity independent of the conflict.)
5. Identify the issues and present them to the parties.
6. Listen to the interests of each of the parties and the resolution each party wants.
7. List possible options for resolving the conflict.
8. Evaluate the options.
9. Select an option or options: give a date for a decision if necessary.
10. Document the agreement(s).
11. Agree on contingencies, monitoring and evaluation.

Modified from Hicks (1996–2000).

for them to do so. The parties still do not listen to each other. This is because what the other person is saying has become unpalatable, and is not taken in. Or, to use the militaristic metaphor that many psychotherapists use, it is as if each of the parties has insulated themself against the other person behind fortifications of justification for the status quo. These fortifications – called defences by many psychotherapists – are so thick that the other person cannot be heard any more.

The psychotherapeutic approach to conflict resolution therefore involves providing the right situation, but also interfering with the defences of at least one of the parties, to make them more open to listening. Obviously this carries with it an increased vulnerability to hurt, and so the psychotherapist needs to be sure that this is done carefully. Various techniques can be used.

Metaphor

Roger is an industrial chemist with long-term problems about his own feelings for other people. In one session, he reports that he is fighting constantly with his daughter. 'We're like oil and water', he says. 'What you need is a detergent', comments the therapist. Roger retorts, 'Oh, that soft soap stuff'. 'No', says the therapist, 'detergent. An astringent cleanser, not to be used without dilution and, if necessary, gloves. Each of you has probably developed a bit of a crust, as a result of all your other bumps and scrapes with each other. And I know you, Roger. You tend to hide your real feelings under a lot of camouflage. What you both need is a detergent that will wash off the camouflage and let you both see each other for what you are. I know, from what you have said about your daughter before, that she is very worried that you will judge her negatively. And I know that you are very inclined to think that people are rejecting you. If you could both show your vulnerability to each other, and not your hard shell, I think that you would find that you would mix'.

After this session, whenever Roger reported that he had been in an emotional situation with someone, but had focussed on incidentals and not on what really mattered, he said, 'I needed more detergent'. And, as the therapy progressed, Roger said that his detergent supply was increasing.

Confrontation

Hannah said that her husband was impossible. He was only concerned for himself. She had been desperate to get out of the house, almost anywhere, after a week stuck at home. It was alright for him, he was at work every day. She had said, 'Let's go to town. You could do with some new shirts. Let's see what's in the sales', but he had said that there was a good football match on the television. She had replied, with some asperity, 'I'm only thinking of you. I just want you to look smart at work', and they had not spoken for the rest of the day.

The therapist said, 'I know it's difficult for you to ask for something directly for yourself. But you did make this trip to town look as though it was for your husband. And he, not unreasonably, told you that it was better for him to watch television. What would have happened if you had said, "I'm going stir-crazy in this house. I have to get out. Will you come with me? We could go to the sales"'. Hannah thought for a while, and then said, rather grudgingly, 'I suppose he might have come . . . But if he really thought about me, he would have known that I needed to get out'. The therapist said, 'Is that true? Did you know how he was feeling? Did you know why he didn't want to go out? I know that you look after him very well on the material level. After all, you did want to get him new shirts. But are you as in touch with his feelings as he would like you to be? Is the problem not so much that he is insensitive, but that you have each lost the ability to know what the other is longing for?'.

Interpretation

Amanda and Luke were both successful career people. They were tackling their relationship problems as if they were business setbacks, and had been doing so well with this – with the help of a counsellor – that they had recently committed themselves to buying a house together. However, each time that they found somewhere that was suitable, something went wrong. They had become, to use their own words, quite 'dysfunctional' about it. After some reassuring discussion, Luke told the counsellor that the problem was that Amanda wasn't very realistic about the property situation. Amanda, looking angry and hurt, said that that wasn't the problem at all. Luke was just dragging his feet. In fact, she wondered if he really wanted to move at all. Perhaps they had made a mistake thinking that they loved each other, and that they were ready to commit themselves.

They talked further about the places that they had seen. The counsellor thought that there was a strange lack of enthusiasm about the way that they both talked about all of them, even those for which they had made an offer. She said, 'What is it you are looking for?'. Luke gave a succinct description of the area and the price range, and Amanda of the number and layout of the rooms. 'No', said the counsellor, 'What do you really want from your home together. What are you looking for, really?'. Luke looked at Amanda, who looked at Luke. Amanda said, 'Somewhere that we can be alone together' and Luke said, 'Somewhere that no-one can get at us'. The counsellor noted how similar the answers were, and asked if the places that they had so far tried to buy met these criteria. 'Not really', both Luke and Amanda admitted. 'Perhaps', interpreted the counsellor, 'You really knew that each of you wanted this degree of closeness. Perhaps you didn't pursue the offers that you made because you knew that the houses weren't really right for you. You want to be so business-like about everything, and yet there is a deeper, emotional level to things. And the interesting thing is that you both understand this and work with it. The problem is that you can't respect that side of yourselves. I have the feeling that if you just trusted to each other, and to your being tuned in to each other, and to your love for each other, you'll come up with a place that will suit you much better in the long run'.

Relationship or couple therapy

Conflict resolution techniques like the above may be less effective when the parties to the conflict are listening, but they are listening to a voice from the past: when, that is, the conflict has a history. This is often the case in relationship or couple therapy, when the history may go back to previous generations.

John and Mary are arguing about the children. They have become noisy romping with John, then Mary comes in, ignores John, and tells the children that they should know better than to behave in such a stupid way. John shouts at Mary that she is undermining his authority as a parent, and how dare she? Mary, who dares most things with John, tells him that if he can't set them a good example, is it her fault? The row lasts for some time and only looks like dying because both parties are becoming exhausted, but just as their voices drop, Mary says: 'If you knew what you looked like when you came home last Thursday you wouldn't wonder why I don't respect you'. This is a reference to John coming home drunk and incapable. He feels that the introduction of this new issue is quite unfair, especially as he does feel ashamed of this incident. But he says, 'The trouble with you is that you're such a control freak that you can't stand anyone having a bit of a drink'. The episode of John being drunk never got properly resolved, and bringing it in adds fresh fuel to the present row, which promptly bursts into flame again.

Bringing in past conflicts is a common feature of marital conflicts and family conflicts. Therapists often deal with it by setting a 'one thing at a time rule': that one conflict has to be resolved before another one can be tackled. Another way of dealing with it is by asking the parties what the two conflicts have in common. Is there an issue which is common to them both? Mary might say, for example, that she had in each case hoped that she would come home to find that John had tackled some of the outstanding jobs around the house, but instead of that he'd either been fooling around with the children or had gone to the pub. John might say that there was a common issue for him, too. They had got the balance in their life wrong. Too much time was spent in drudgery, and not enough time enjoying oneself. Life was short, and not to be wasted just being dutiful.

Finding the issue which underlies several different rows is useful. In John and Mary's case it might help them to see that the other person was doing more than just thwarting them. They could recognize that each of them was acting more or less appropriately, but according to different values. Depending on whether or not the conflicting values could be resolved, John and Mary might find themselves either getting closer together or feeling more distant, but less angry.

The common issue might not be a matter of content, but of emotional meaning. John might say that Mary picks on him when he knows that he looks a bit foolish, and that is because Mary wants to humiliate him. Mary might say that, far from wanting to humiliate John, she feels completely blanked by him. When he knows that she is really het up, he behaves in a completely selfish and frivolous way. It is as if he wants to show her how stupid he thinks her worries are, and how little he cares about them.

This way of looking at things might be quite new to John, as his way of looking at things was new to Mary. Again, if they could stop and listen to each other at this moment, it would be possible to move the conflict to a new level. It might be possible to look at what emotional meaning each of them gave to what the other said and how, given that meaning, each of them was not being quite as unpleasant or malicious as the other one thought.

Each of these stratagems is designed to allow John and Mary to stand back from their conflict, to invite them to work together on finding a common account of their difficulties. But this is to assume that they have an identity of purpose.

Time-limited therapy

Almost all psychotherapies have started out to be brief interventions. Many of the analyses that Freud reported were short term, for example. However there is, in psychotherapy, an almost irresistible drift towards longer and longer treatment. Cognitive-analytic therapy (CAT), to cite another example, was originally developed to provide effective treatment with eight sessions, but is currently being described as requiring 16–24 sessions to be effective, and trainees in CAT are advised to have 'long-term' cognitive-analytic therapy.

There may be several reasons for this drift. One is that the attitudes of psychotherapists, like those of other health care professionals, are influenced most strongly by the clients that are most often seen. Many clients are seen once by psychotherapists and not offered treatment. Many more drop out of psychotherapy in the first six sessions (Piper et al., 1990). The impression of clients' neediness is therefore created by the minority of clients who continue to persist with their attendance. These tend to be people with the most difficulties in forming relationships with other people (ibid., 1990).

If it can be assumed that people drop out because they are improved, then, arguably, this shows that the system is working. However, a principal reason for people dropping out of therapy in one study was that people did not feel that their symptoms were being addressed (Last et al., 1985). In one naturalistic study of outcome and length of treatment, it was estimated that 50% of clients were 'measurably improved' after eight sessions (Howard et al., 1986). However, a later study, using the same methods of probit analysis, showed that acute distress responds most quickly to treatment, followed by chronic distress, followed by 'characterological symptoms' (Kopta et al., 1994). These findings strongly support the tenor of previous chapters that matching the treatment with the preoccupying concern (and, of course, with the emotional meaning of the problem and the values of the client) is important. They are also consistent with the presupposition that termination by agreement is better than clients dropping out, or being discharged.

Time-limited psychotherapies presume that the agreement about the length of the treatment is the fundamental place to start. Setting this time-limit determines which preoccupying concerns can be addressed effectively. If the time-limit is set at four sessions, it is likely that a person's current predicament, or the distress that it is causing, can be addressed. If there is a time-limit of 12 sessions, then it is realistic to address not only the current predicament but any false beliefs or wrong sentiments that have led to a person becoming stuck in the first place.

Setting a time-limit is sometimes portrayed as an uncaring intervention. After all, if someone had cancer it would be quite wrong for the oncologist to tell them that they could only have 12 sessions of treatment and, after that, they were on their own. It is true that setting a time-limit *is* often a reflection of the exigencies imposed on the therapist rather than being in the service of the client. And, of course, such exigencies exist, particularly in care that is paid by the state or by third-party payers like insurance companies. Counsellors working in primary care in the UK are sometimes given such time-limits. They may be told, for example, that they can only undertake six sessions of counselling and that they then need to discuss the case with the family doctor.

But, if we return to the example of the oncologist, he or she would be remiss if they did not tell their clients how many treatments they were likely to receive. A client having chemotherapy wants to know how many injections, and how many periods of nausea, diarrhoea and hair loss, to expect. What the oncologist would not say is that the number of expected injections is the limit. At the end of this treatment, clients not in remission would be considered for other procedures.

Time-limited psychotherapy is not, in practice, about limits at all, but about time-*frames*. It is about negotiating what can be done in a particular time boundary, and how this matches with what concerns the client. It also includes a statement detailing the options if, at the end of the agreed number of sessions, the desired result has not been obtained. The intention of time-limited therapy is to empower the client, not to deprive him or her.

If there is a theme to the wide range of different time-limited psychotherapy approaches, it is the concept of negotiation, seen as a process in which what a person wants and what is available are brought together. It is therapeutic because the psychotherapist deals with the emotional obstacles that prevent a person either admitting to what they want, or accepting what is available. The emotions that time-limited approaches confront are social ones, often arising from the wish to be approved or accepted by others. Many time-limited psychotherapists deal with these by confrontation, modelling a more open, and less conforming, social persona. One of the major exponents of this approach, Davanloo (1978, 1980), has been termed a 'relentless healer' in a review of his work (Molnos, 1998).

was, but that it was no thanks to Sydenham. Sydenham said, on the contrary, he had set his Lordship the task of finding a mythical physician because it was the cure for his ailment. (Hunter & Macalpine, 1982)

Generally speaking, psychotherapists do not prescribe actions although there may be some exceptions, for example if a person is at risk of serious physical harm or sexual abuse. There are grey areas, of course. Some counsellors or psychotherapists may consider it appropriate to indicate to a woman who is in an aggressive relationship with her husband that it is not her fault, and that she would be better off leaving him. Prescribing actions may, however, be ill-advised or even unethical. In reality, the consequences of actions may be indeterminate and recommending a particular course of action, even if it seems obviously in the client's interests ahead of time, may lead to an unforeseen, adverse outcome. It is also inadvisable for a psychotherapist to rely on being uninvolved emotionally with his or her client's problems. And, if the psychotherapist is involved, it is likely that any action that he or she recommends will be influenced by what would be good for the psycho-therapist if he or she were in the same predicament as the client. This may be quite different from what is good for the client. A final ethical consideration applies particularly to western cultural values. In the West, autonomy is the dominant principle in medical ethics (Gillon, 1994). Prescribing action almost always runs counter to this. However, in non-western cultures, where interdependence may be more important than independence (Neki, 1976), prescribing a psychologically meaningful action may be ethical.

A Yoruba man consulted a traditional healer because he had been having such bad stomach pains after his father died that he was unable to work, or to satisfy his wives. The healer told him that he had not taken sufficient trouble to appease his ancestors, and that they were angry with him. He was told to visit several sacred sites, and to make a sacrifice at each of them.

Within this particular Nigerian healing culture, the traditional healer was expected to know what was wrong with the client without having to ask the client much about his symptoms. In this case, the healer recognized a link between bereavement and the symptoms, but instead of exploring the feelings that the client had about his father's death, he prescribed an action which would expiate them.

In practice, a client does not expect that a psychotherapist will prescribe an action. That is still the role of the priest, the physician or the traditional healer. People consult psychotherapists if they experience themselves as having an emotional life, an inner world, which is in disarray. Malan is therefore right in concluding that addressing what is missing in this inner world is a universal technique of psychotherapy, although we should not extend this to assume that it is a universal technique of resolving predicaments. Nor should we assume that it is always a problem in a person's inner world that creates their predicament. In fact, it would be quite hard to find any criterion that would allow us to distinguish an inner from an outer world.

What can be concluded is that there is a technique of predicament resolution which is universally practised by psychotherapists which takes as its focus the emotions of a person who experiences themselves in that predicament. Furthermore, this universal technique is based on the assumption that when a feeling or an impulse is hidden there is a corresponding action which is ruled out, and vice versa. So the universal psychotherapy technique of predicament resolution is, as Malan states, to reveal such hidden feelings or impulses and so enable new actions to be made possible in the expectation that one of these new actions will be the way out of the predicament.

Attentive readers will note that there is an elision here between feelings (the word used by Malan), impulse (Whitaker's word) and emotions. There is, I believe, little practical difference in using one or the other, but some theoretical difference. A psycho-analytic psychotherapist might say that a person has wishes or impulses to act in certain ways, and that some of these actions are prevented because the wish to undertake them is repressed. Enabling them to act in new ways means de-repressing the wish.

I have various objections to the notions of the unconscious and repression. One of these is the one put by Sartre, that it involves a paradox: either the unconscious cannot foresee, in which case it cannot wish for some desired event, or the unconscious can foresee consequences, in which case it is unlikely to wish for something that will have destructive consequences. Another is the practical objection which is discussed later in this section. A third is that invoking wishes as an intermediary cause of actions falls foul of Wittgenstein's strictures: 'When I raise my arm "voluntarily" I do not use any instrument to bring the movement about. My wish is not such an instrument either' (1958, para 614).

Contemporary definitions of emotion have been extended to include intention. For example, Oatley's definition is that an emotion is a 'mental state of readiness for action . . . normally based on an evaluation of something happening that affects important concerns' (1992, p. 20). This definition makes it possible to say very simply that the psychotherapist is concerned to bring to light hidden emotions and that this is the same as bringing to light new dispositions to act.

Revealing what is hidden

For Malan, as for other psycho-analytically orientated psychotherapists, revealing what is hidden involves a special process called 'interpretation'.

Interpretations are a form of divination. They reveal the hidden meaning of something, as the diviner sees the future in a dream, and they show how that hidden meaning is encoded in the surface meaning.

36. And two youths entered the prison with him [Jusuf]. One of them said: I saw myself pressing wine. And the other said: I saw myself carrying bread on my head, of which birds ate. Inform us of its interpretation; surely we see you to be of the doers of good.
37. He said: There shall not come to you the food with which you are fed, but I will inform you both of its interpretation before it comes to you; this is of what my Lord has taught me; surely I have forsaken the religion of a people who do not believe in Allah, and they are deniers of the hereafter . . .
41. O my two mates of the prison! as for one of you, he shall give his lord to drink wine; and as for the other, he shall be crucified, so that the birds shall eat from his head, the matter is decreed concerning which you inquired.
(Koran)

Dreams are here described as having a single hidden meaning, which they were intended to convey by God, who sent them. A person who knows the mind of God, as Joseph does, can read that meaning. It is as if a dream is an inscription over which moss has grown. Joseph reads the meaning of the dream as unequivocally as someone who rubs off the moss can read the inscription.

Semiologists have gone further than most in considering how signs may apparently mean one thing, but also convey a hidden meaning. Barthes was a leading exponent of this approach, which he presented in several books, including one entitled *Mythologies*, in which can be found the following:

I am at the barber's and a copy of *Paris-Match* is offered to me. On the cover, a young Negro in a French uniform is saluting, with his eyes uplifted, probably fixed on a fold of the tricolour. All this is the *meaning* of the picture. But, whether naively or not, I see very well what it signifies to me: that France is a great Empire, that all her sons, without any colour discrimination, faithfully serve under her flag, and there is no better answer to the detractors of an alleged colonialism than the zeal shown by this Negro in serving his so-called oppressors. (1973, p. 116)

Barthes interpreted the hidden meaning of the *Paris-Match* picture as a negation of French colonialism. Like Joseph, he lays claim to a special ability to divine what is present underneath the surface of another's experience. No doubt he was a doer of good, as the youths recognized Joseph to be. No doubt, too, he was a man who was not afraid to tell the truth, even if it was not in his apparent interests, as Joseph's story shows that Joseph was. Both Roland Barthes and Joseph bar-Jacob could be described as prophets.

The question is, is uncovering hidden feelings really like this? Do clients resolve their predicaments because they meet a psychotherapist with prophetic ability who can see into their souls and find there a meaning which the client him- or herself has buried? I used to think so (Tantam, 1984). Readers must make up their own minds. Any who would like to have another view might want to consider the alternative possibility that interpretations are rationalizations after the fact (Tantam, 1999a) rather than secret messages.

Some readers might consider that this is all 'splitting hairs', but I am not so sure. The act of interpreting is a claim to a special, and perhaps higher, authority. Making this claim may be legitimate or it may be a disguised attempt to dominate the client. Certainly, in Joseph's case, his eventual rise to be Pharaoh's right-hand man seems to have been based entirely on his apparent ability as a diviner. It might not always be to a client's advantage to have a therapist who claims special knowledge. In fact, the evidence seems to be that the frequency of interpretations made by a therapist is *inversely* proportional to the outcome of therapy, not directly proportional to it (Piper et al., 1991).

A further problem with the divination model of interpretation is that once an interpretation is accepted as correct, it shuts off the possibility of other interpretations. If we accept Barthes's view of the image from *Paris-Match*, we do not search for another interpretation. But there is another interpretation, in fact one which is in direct opposition to that of Barthes. The image can be taken as a reminder that people from ethnic minorities are over-represented in the French armed forces because other, less dangerous, work is closed off to them. The picture would then be a confirmation of racism, not a rebuttal of it.

Speaking, or thinking, aloud

Let us for the moment put to one side what is meant by revealing a hidden emotion, and consider the other aspect of interpretation which Malan mentions. He writes that a fundamental rule of interpretation is to interpret the defence before the impulse. He gives the following case example: (Malan, 1979, p. 75–9)

Malan's case example: the interior decorator

The client, an interior decorator aged 26, was unable to consummate his marriage. His wife had made hurtful allusions to his lack of manhood. The client told the therapist that he was aware that he had hurt her in the past by telling lies to make himself look big. This seems to have been a test of how the therapist would respond to a secret because in later session, the client said, 'Yes, that's the heart of the whole thing. There's something I'd like to ask you. If my wife is wearing a mackintosh, I could kiss her and never stop. I know this kind of thing does happen to people, and it's called a fetish. Is it very abnormal?'

The therapist does not answer this question, and notes that the client is completely 'taken aback' and says, 'Can you give me a lead about what I should talk about?' The therapist then says, 'I think the reason why you can't go on and want a lead is because you are angry with me. You asked me to reassure you about something, and I wouldn't do it'. The client flatly denied any anger, and there was an impasse [*this is what Malan calls 'interpreting the impulse'*].

In the next session, the therapist refers to this moment and says that when the client gets angry, he doesn't show it but goes the other way, and submits himself completely [*this is what Malan calls 'interpreting the defence'*]. This linked various things up for the client, for example the fact that when he is angry with his wife, he tends to do the housework for her, and a rapport is re-established between the client and the therapist.

The client then went on to admit that this pattern of submitting was characteristic of him, and that it stemmed from his fear of losing his temper. He had never shown his temper to anyone other than his mother. Certainly not his father who had a temper himself, and would certainly have exploded at any sign of his son's aggression. Shortly after this there is a discussion about the relationship of the therapist and the client, and the client says, 'I think you would give it to me straight', indicating that this permits openness on both sides.

There are several noteworthy features of this vignette:
(1) There is a consistent emotional meaning throughout it. There is a flavour of shame or humiliation in each of the important episodes. The decorator feels ashamed of his past boasting and also of his fetish, and asks the therapist whether the latter is shameful. When the therapist does not answer, the client humiliates himself by requesting guidance. The client sees anger, too, as something to be ashamed of, perhaps because of the embarrassing nature of his father's outbursts, and denies being angry himself as if he has been accused of something shameful. He can only show anger with his mother who, it seems, does not shame him. In circumstances when others might be angry, he humiliates himself. He is probably ashamed of this, too. Certainly, his presenting complaint is that he is not a manly man, often a source of shame in itself.
(2) The level of rapport between the client and the therapist seems to be proportional to the extent to which the client is speaking aloud about shame or humiliation.
(3) The therapist knows, or learns, that he, too, needs to be speaking about shame or humiliation, and not about anger or anxiety.
(4) The therapist's ability to speak aloud about shame or humiliation facilitates the client's ability to speak about it. As the client says, '. . . I like your face. I like the way you look me in the eyes and give it to me straight. I want you to give it to me straight'.

I think that there is no need for the therapist to have made any interpretations to the interior decorator at all, except perhaps when it was necessary to refocus the topic back onto humiliation (the moment termed 'interpreting the defence' in the vignette). There was certainly no need to reveal any hidden meanings to the client.

Stiles (1999) suggests that the core of psychotherapy is 'assimilation' of warded-off experiences, or 'voices'. Using this metaphor, we could say that it was the voice of shame that was heard in the therapy of the interior decorator and that the therapy was successful inasmuch as this voice could speak, and be heard. Stiles has developed a scale, the Assimilation of Problematic Experiences Scale (Stiles et al., 1991), for assessing the progress of assimilation. This has three implicit dimensions: the clarity with which the client talks about (1) the experience, (2) emotions and (3) feelings, and bridges between the client's understanding of the meaning of the problematic experience and the meaning of other experiences.

Stiles et al. describe a characteristic trajectory of feeling as a person begins to speak about a previously warded-off experience. First, there is little feeling. Then, as the person speaks more about it, there are bursts of intense but unfocussed feeling, which make the person 'panicky'. Finally, the feelings become more composed, and then dwindle. The story of a patient of a traditional healer whose treatment the author observed in Zanzibar provides an example.

Case history

The woman had run away from her family after a quarrel with her husband. She was in an acute anxiety state, not surprisingly given that in Zanzibar, deserting your husband ran the risk of becoming an outcast. The healer told her that she was possessed by a djinni, and an exorcism was arranged. She was seated, with a cloth over her head, in amongst a band and a group of singers. To a background of intrusive rhythmic chanting, she was repeatedly asked to say the name of the Devil possessing her. A rather menacing pair of scissors was constantly clacked near her face. The healer gradually came closer and closer to her, eventually whispering in her ear. This lack of interpersonal distance between a woman and a strange man was rare in Zanzibar, and must have caused the client great anxiety. The fact that her head was covered and that she had absolutely no control over her situation must also have been very frightening. The client was clearly becoming increasing distressed until a moment when the djinni left her body and passed into that of the healer. The cloth was whipped off the woman's head, and she was quickly removed from the room. The cloth contained the djinni, momentarily, but the djinni took the opportunity to pass into the person holding the cloth, who happened to be the healer. The healer fortunately had an assistant who then conducted a second exorcism, but this time of the healer himself. The client was reported to have made a good recovery and to have returned to her husband (Tantam, 1993).

This account of an exorcism in Zanzibar demonstrates a similar trajectory of feeling to that described by Stiles et al. The client's feelings were first aroused to a point where, one supposes, her distress must have been almost unsupportable, but then there is a moment of crisis, after which the client seems much more in control of her feelings which, over the course of a few days, abate completely.

If there is really a universal technique of psychotherapy, then we should be able to find it not only in the Malan's triangular formulation of psychoanalytic psychotherapy, but also in the exorcism in Zanzibar and in the observations made about the case of the interior decorator.

I hope that the reader will share my intuition that there *are* discernible universal principles. A possible list might be:

- A procedure for shaping feelings and accommodating to the natural trajectory of strong feeling to a point of crisis, and then dissolution
- A container for the feelings, which makes them safe (the djinni in the head cloth in the exorcism, the interpretation of the defence in Malan)
- A procedure for facilitating acceptance rather than rejection of the feelings expressed by the client (the interpretation of the anxiety in Malan, the community in the exorcism, the therapist's ability to 'talk straight' about shame in the case of the interior decorator)
- A special relationship with the therapist

Perhaps not unsurprisingly, these four factors are comparable to the universal principles of remoralization described by Frank (1984): a ritual, a rationale conceptual scheme or myth; a healing setting; and an emotionally charged confiding relationship with a helpful person.

A therapist wanting to carry out therapy according to the universal technique might still find a lack of specificity in the list given above. What, for example, constitutes a procedure for facilitating acceptance of feelings? And what constitutes the special relationship with the therapist which enables confiding to take place?

The eyes of the therapist

The existential psychotherapists, Freud, Janet and many others, have placed anxiety in the forefront of the therapeutic process. But what is anxiety? For Freud, whose view has been very influential, it was the signal that the mind's integrity is under threat, rather as pain is the signal of a threat to bodily integrity. For Kierkegaard (1960), anxiety was 'the dizziness of freedom', the experience that we have when we look into what *The Hitchhikers' Guide to the Galaxy* calls 'the vortex', in which we see ourselves measured against universal values.

Consider the young primate who ranges further and further away from her mother. At a distance, she will be startled and will experience an urge to flee back to her mother. She will experience separation anxiety. Perhaps she looks back at her mother and, reassured, continues her exploration. Or perhaps she just turns and runs back. In both cases anxiety is signalling being alone, but in the first scenario the young primate tolerates it and ultimately is able to extend her range further, while in the second, the anxiety cannot be tolerated, and the youngster learns to limit her explorations.

Take this thought experiment a bit further. Consider what would happen if, when the young primate glances back, her mother deliberately moves away from her, or snarls, or turns her back. The separation anxiety that erupts at that moment would not be due to an outward contemplation of the world outside the primate domestic circle, but to the collapse of security from within. The emotional meaning of exploration would not be given by the pure and high-minded anxiety of a person confronting the infinite, but by the rejection of the carer. It would not be an experience of danger to be mastered, but inadequacy to be hidden.

There are probably many moments in all of our lives when we, metaphorically speaking, look to someone important and find rejection written on their faces and in their eyes. It is a consequence of the tension between being ourselves, and being socialized. Those people who cannot be immobilized by being shamed or by experiencing others' disgust are dangerous within society. We are inclined to call them names like 'psychopath', and to want to sequester them away from society.

What clients ask for in a therapist is that the therapist does not re-enact that experience of social rejection. It is not enough that the therapist does not do this in response to specific emotions. The therapist also needs to convey his or her commitment not to reject the client's feelings, whatever they are. This, I take it, is another way of formulating the 'unconditional positive regard' which has already been discussed as a therapeutic factor in client-centered therapy.

A professional man was having a terrible row with his equally accomplished wife. It was about him having interrupted her when she was having a telephone conversation with someone else. His wife was making some arrangements about furniture that had belonged to her family, and the husband wanted to discuss these arrangements with her before she committed herself. Eventually, she finished her phone call and accused him of wanting to humiliate her in front of her friend. 'She would have heard you bossing me about', she said, 'You never let me make decisions for myself. You just want to weaken me until I am no longer a threat to you.' The husband felt rejected by this comment. He was a man who always tried to do the right thing, although he often lacked the instinct of doing so and ended up being seen by others as being selfish and in the wrong. His wife's rejection re-evoked a long-held shame about being called a bully as a child. He became enraged and, quite unreasonably, attacking of his

wife. However, this was not solely about trying to cover up his shame. There was also a disappointment in him that his wife had not seen how inadequate he felt when faced with her attachment to her past. 'If only', he thought, 'she could see how excluded I feel'.

Not rejecting the client, or having unconditional positive regard for them, is therefore not only about accepting manifest feelings, but also about seeing and accepting the feelings that they conceal.

- The therapist must be able to continue to look the client in the face, and not flinch, nor harden his or her gaze. Actually, being unmoved or indifferent is not enough. It is not enough that the eyes of the therapist do not harden, they must actually soften, showing that the therapist is open to some part of the client's distress or pain.

The response to the client's feelings cannot be a purely intellectual one if it is to be meaningful to the client. Meaning is conveyed by the change in the emotional world of the therapist in response to the feelings of the client. This openness to the client's feelings is what Rogers meant by facilitation and what humanistic psychotherapists term 'being authentic'. The exchange of emotional meaning at these moments is what Malan terms 'rapport', and what gestalt psychologists have called the '*erlebnis*' experience. Heidegger describes a similar experience, which he calls '*die augenblick*' ('moment of vision'), in the following way:

In resoluteness, the Present is not only brought back from distraction with the objects of one's closest concern, but it gets held in the future and in having been. That *Present* which is held in authentic temporality and which thus is *authentic* itself, we call the '*moment of vision* . . . This term must be understood in the active sense as an ecstasis. It means the resolute rapture with which Dasein is carried away to whatever possibilities and circumstances are encountered in the Situation as possible objects of concern, but a rapture which is *held* in resoluteness. (1927, section 338)

The arms of other people

Resolving a predicament always means finding a way to act in relation to other people. As we have seen, it often means starting to speak or think aloud about a hidden feeling or experience, but that usually means acting in new, and previously avoided, ways towards other people. Contrary to many psycho-analytic psychotherapists, I think that the emphasis should be placed on what has never been acted upon, not what has never been thought. One might say that the unconscious is not a region of the mind that contains unthought impulses, but a pile of dramatic scripts that have never been performed. The barrier that keeps feelings hidden is not an intrapsychic zone patrolled by a part of the ego called the 'internal censor', but the real censorship of social opinion. There are enough secrets to explain people's predicaments without needing to invoke unconscious impulses.

Nayer had an English mother and a Kuwaiti father. She was about 14 years old and living in Kuwait city when it was invaded by the Iraqis. Her father told her to stay in the house, but she felt too confined and one day felt that she could not stand being cooped up any longer and went for a walk. She thought that she would be safe if she stayed within one street of her house, but she was mistaken. She was spotted by two Iraqi soldiers and raped. She was left lying in the street, otherwise uninjured, and she managed to get home, somehow. She knew that her family would be ashamed of her if they knew what had happened, even if it was not her fault, and so she concealed what had happened. Fortunately, her mother decided that it was best for Nayer to go to an English school, and Nayer and her mother moved to the UK shortly after. Nayer did well, but when she was 16 years old her father wanted her and her mother to return to Kuwait. Nayer felt that she had no way out. Either she went back and faced certain shame when the truth came out, as it would, or she stayed in the UK, but against her father's wishes, which would mean being ostracized by her family. Nayer took an overdose, thinking that there was no way out, except to die.

Nayer's terrible secret cut her off from her family. When her mother held her in her arms, Nayer did not feel that her mother was really holding her, but that it was a sham. When she thought of how her father would react if he knew, she thought of his arms being crossed, excluding her from his affection. She felt ashamed of what had happened and would have liked to unburden herself, but thought that if she did she would be shunned. When she found herself in a situation in which concealing her shame was no longer possible either, she felt paralysed. She was not paralysed because of something she had repressed into her unconsciousness. Nor was she paralysed by anxiety. She was paralysed by an overpowering shame of something that was all too present to her, and all she could think of doing was to hide from it in unconsciousness.

Nayer's therapist was a woman with considerable intuitive therapeutic skill, and personal experience of living in two cultures. She was moved by Nayer's predicament. She thought it entirely understandable that Nayer had not wanted to stay at home during the invasion. She was a bright girl, brought up by her English mother to be curious, and this was a historic moment. Nor was the therapist fazed by rape, or by the shame that attaches to it. She had counselled women before who had been raped, and knew the way that families could turn on the victim when the perpetrator was unknown. Nayer did not have to hide her experiences from the psychotherapist therefore, but talking about the experience was a different matter to resolving the predicament. In fact, it was after she talked about what had happened that Nayer took the overdose.

Fortunately, Nayer's family doctor was a motherly woman who reminded Nayer of her own mother. The therapist obtained Nayer's permission to discuss Nayer's experiences with this doctor, and Nayer went to see her subsequently. She arranged various checks to ensure that Nayer had not caught any disease, and confirmed to Nayer that she was not pregnant. This activity seemed to give Nayer a sense that there were things to do, even when faced with such a horrible predicament. However, it was clear that the only way to deal effectively with her father's insistence that she should return to Kuwait was to tell him why she would not feel safe there. Both the family doctor and the therapist suggested that Nayer should talk to her mother and ask her advice. Nayer asked that the therapist should be present at this discussion. Nayer's mother was at first shocked, and then angry with Nayer that Nayer had kept her in the dark. However, the therapist acted as Nayer's advocate, explaining that Nayer had been afraid of forcing her mother to choose between supporting Nayer or going along with what was likely to be the prevailing view – that she had brought dishonour on the house.

Nayer's mother looked at her daughter with tears in her eyes at this point, and opened her arms to her.

Nayer seemed deeply reassured by being held by her mother, and was willing to accept her mother's suggestion that she, the mother, would talk things over with Nayer's father. Nayer's mother felt sure that if she approached the father in the right way, he would sympathize with Nayer, rather than reject her.

Nayer left for Kuwait shortly afterwards.

- Nayer's case shows that getting in touch with hidden feelings makes new courses of action possible. But this is not enough. It is still necessary to choose between different courses of action. It is also necessary to pursue the chosen course of action in a way that is most likely to be accepted with open arms by others.

Conclusions

Bullet points have been placed alongside passages throughout this chapter to indicate what I think have been the enduring contributions of each of the theories under consideration to a theory of how predicaments can be resolved. It is important to stress again, as has been done at frequent intervals, that there is unlikely to be a single theory which will work in every situation and with every therapist. The effectiveness of an intervention depends on the values with which it is associated, and the emotional meaning which it conveys. These will be different for different people, and in different cultures.

Readers are therefore encouraged to arrive at their own synthesis of the various approaches considered which fits best with their values and which conveys an emotional meaning that is most palatable to them.

My own synthesis can be derived from bringing together each of the bulleted paragraphs, in the following way:

- A predicament is a situation in which certain actions or conversations are required to move the situation on. But the emotions which tend to these actions or conversations are hidden, and so the actions or conversations are precluded. This lack of freedom in conversation is concealed from ourselves and others by various means (considered later, in Chapter 10). Sometimes this lack of freedom is apparent in an abnormal absence of anxiety, sometimes by gaps or unexplained associations, and sometimes by traces of the hidden feeling. However, therapists who believe that they know what is hidden may be deceiving themselves. What therapists can do is to create circumstances for relevant conversations. In particular, therapists can clarify what the focus of the conversations should be, that is, they should agree with the client that the client is in a predicament and on the nature of the predicament. Therapists should aim to have conversations with their clients in which the client can speak about their hidden feelings without feeling ashamed or fearful about the therapist's view of them. Translating these conversations into action outside the therapy may be something that the client does without consultation with the therapist, or may be explicitly discussed in the therapy. One issue will be the frame in which the action is carried out, i.e. the social setting, and the participants in that setting.

The deftness, sensitivity and poetry required of a psychotherapist in this type of therapeutic conversation is evocatively conveyed by Hobson (1985).

9

Relinquishment and releasement: changing something about me

This chapter is about addiction: why it is difficult to give up a way of life that has become destructive or to relinquish certain ways of reacting, including symptoms, which have gained a hold despite being unwanted. It is also about how people give up their addictions, and therefore about what therapists can do to help them. It will turn out that overcoming an addiction is rarely a matter of vanquishing it but more often a matter of giving in to a realization of the need for something bigger and more powerful than oneself, a process that Heidegger terms 'releasement' (von Deurzen, 1997). The word 'addiction' is used advisedly here, even though it is no longer fashionable. It has generally been replaced by the words 'dependency', as in chemical dependency, or by the term 'misuse', as in substance misuse. Dependency connotes a particular image of someone who is needy and dependent on other people. There is no evidence that these personality traits are particularly linked to becoming addicted, however. Misuse does not capture the imperative nature of the problem. Heroin, as an illicit substance, is misused every time that it is used. Yet there are people who manage to confine their heroin use to a level which they would not consider to be problematic. The 'demandingness' of heroin addiction – its admixture of pleasure and self-destruction – is not really conveyed by the much more neutral term, 'misuse', which could apply equally well to the recreational user. The mix of pleasure and risk, the compelling quality of the behaviour, and its social condemnation also apply to some sexual deviations, to eating disorders, and to some other habit disorders. These, too, may have an addictive quality (Szmukler & Tantam, 1984).

It was a very unusual family session. The previous week, mother had been working, so father and son had come alone. Father had talked of his failure to set his son adequate limits or to support his wife. For once, he had not been derailed by his son's disparagement. This session, mother was present but said that she was taking a back seat. The session was not just unusual for this reason. Father said that there had been a reduction of family tension. He reported that, despite being suspended from college, his son had tried hard to overcome the problems that he had had in the past, and he complimented his son. The son said that he felt that he had been supported by his parents, and particularly by his mother, during this difficult time. The therapist was so surprised that he checked out whether this was intended to be a compliment. It was. The therapist then commented, truthfully, that this was the first time that he could remember in about 10 sessions that the son had said anything positive about his mother. There was a long, tense silence and then mother started criticizing both father and son. The atmosphere lightened considerably. The son began to slag off his mother, and father became increasingly detached.

In this family, it was hard to move away from a long-established pattern of hostile and intimate interaction between mother and son, with father being a detached observer. This session began in a new way, but the old pattern reasserted itself. It would be wrong to say that the family was addicted or dependent on this way of behaving, or that they got a perverse satisfaction from it. But they did find it difficult to change their interaction despite knowing that it led to mother getting depressed, and to the parents feeling increasingly distant from each other.

This difficulty in relinquishing a behaviour despite knowing that it is self-destructive is a characteristic of what many psychiatrists call a 'habit disorder'.

Sarah gets a bit red-faced being unable to engage reverse in her new car. Her husband smirks in a superior way, and she exculpates herself by saying that she has got into a habit of pushing the gear-stick to the left, where reverse was on the old car, and not to the right, where it is on this new one. 'But', she says, 'I'll soon change my habits'.

Sarah has an unwanted habit which is the product of memory traces that have not yet been extinguished. However, it differs from a habit disorder because pushing the gear-stick the wrong way is inadvertent, and because it quickly stops as a person gets used to a new car. Habit disorders involve voluntary actions, however apparently meaningless, and they are maintained, even strengthened, by repetition.

This chapter will treat all addictions and perversions as if they have common properties, and it will be these that will be the subject of the chapter. Whilst there is some empirical evidence for this (McLellan et al., 1994), it *is* a generalization and should be treated with appropriate circumspectness. However, it also has some advantages, at least in the practice of psychotherapy, since it uncovers common difficulties and common remedies which can guide psychotherapists who are working with any kind of addiction.

The general scheme of the chapter will be to use examples from people with different kinds of addiction to illustrate the different stages of treatment as, in fact, the choice of a particular addiction is less important than the fact of the addiction.

In practice, addictions (or a misuse or dependency problem) and perversions (or sexual deviations) are actions that are hard to stop. It is this which makes them habit disorders, although unlike simple habits, they are also compulsive. There are two elements to this compulsiveness (Leshner, 1999). One is that the substance that is misused or the deviant sexual gratification that is achieved is an antidote to shame or self-disgust, the other is that it satiates a craving.

Riccardo was an only child. His father died when he was young, and he was brought up by his mother in a small town in Tuscany. The family was very poor, but his mother doted on Riccardo and they were happy. However, his mother was also very strict. If she thought that Riccardo was misbehaving at school, or he was cheeky at home, she would first tell him off and, if that did not work, would become ill. One day, the teacher found a window broken in the school room. 'Who had done it?', he demanded. No-one would own up, and the teacher threatened to punish the whole class. Riccardo felt that he had to do something, so he said that he had done it, even though he had not. He was put in detention and so was late home. When he arrived, his mother was already in an advanced state of anxiety. When she found out that he had broken a window (Riccardo could not explain that he had lied), she became carried away with grief and tried to throw herself through the window, saying that she could never hold up her head again.

Riccardo married a local girl, and moved to the UK to work for his brother-in-law. His mother came with him. Riccardo prided himself on his virtue. Never a day went past when he did not do someone a favour, or buy his daughter a present, or sort out a row at work. When he was passed over for promotion, which he invariably was, he told himself that it was because he was always willing to humble himself so that others might benefit.

Riccardo had experienced great love from his mother, but it was conditional. At any moment, a slip on his part would change it. It was not that his mother would become angry. Then, he could have fought back. It was that a slip made her ashamed of him, and she would become physically unwell. When this happened, Riccardo would become filled with shame himself. He would just wish that the earth would swallow him up. He dealt with this successfully for many years by never doing anything that would push him ahead of anyone else or make him stand out in any way.

His wife wanted to move up in the world, but Riccardo was not interested in that. His main interest was in getting on with everyone, and in being above reproach. However, he was not insensible to his wife's feelings and so he talked to a local builder about having an extension built onto the house. This was done to everyone's apparent satisfaction. However, the neighbour claimed that it was longer that it should be. The council was involved and confirmed that it was 6" (15 cm) too long. The builder said that Riccardo had approved all the plans, and that he could not take any responsibility. The neighbour told Riccardo that he was trying to 'pull a fast one', and wanted it pulled down. The builder became abusive because Riccardo did not pay the bill while the argument was ongoing. His wife became tearful and said that she had really wished that Riccardo would stand up for her interests a bit more.

Riccardo became depressed, but more than that, he became preoccupied with his loss of irreproachability. He had never wanted to be a saint, or someone special, but he had always wanted to think of himself as beyond criticism. Now that had gone, and he craved it back.

Riccardo had an extreme sensitivity to shame. He had effectively protected himself over many years by avoiding any possibility of reproach. Now, despite his best efforts, he was plunged back into the shame and ignominy of a wrangle with his neighbour over the extension.

Riccardo's colleague at work said that he had to ought to go out and get drunk. It was the only cure for this kind of trouble. Riccardo never drank normally, and refused his colleague's offer on several occasions. Eventually, the colleague implied that Riccardo was refusing because he felt too superior to drink with his friends, so Riccardo went. He quickly became quite drunk, and behaved in a quite uninhibited way. Instead of feeling embarrassed by him, his friends laughed and egged him on. Riccardo felt humiliated, but also felt that it didn't matter – that he had risen above it. He enjoyed himself more than he had done for years. When he got home, his wife was understanding, but his mother berated him. However, instead of being mortified, he must have still been a little drunk because he laughed in her face.

Riccardo was very sick the next day, and vowed never to drink again. But he found himself proposing a drink to his colleague a few days later, and it became a regular habit to go out, firstly once a week and then almost every day. He would drink a bit more if he had had a bad day at work, and it would always make him feel better. On a day like that, if he could not go out, Riccardo was moody and irritable. This created a barrier between himself and his family, and they started to want him to go out, rather than coming home and bringing his moroseness with him. The pub became Riccardo's real home.

Drink became a strong emotor (see Chapter 3) for Riccardo, i.e. it made him silly, and open to reproach, but it also made this no longer matter because it was blended with a feeling of male companionship and of euphoria. It insinuated itself into the life of Riccardo and his family, becoming for Riccardo an increasingly effective antidote to his shame-proneness and his inhibition (see Toneatto (1999) for a similar account of the effects of addiction). Every time he got drunk, the shame would be dissolved into the previous blend of shame and euphoria and would be made harmless.

At this stage, Riccardo was compelled to drink by his wish to get rid of feeling ashamed, but he had no craving for drink itself. When something went wrong for Riccardo, he imagined having a drink and dissolving the anxiety that he was to blame that filled him. If he saw a comedy on the television, in which someone was making a fool of themselves, he felt like having a drink, but not when he watched a drink advertisement. On a good day, Riccardo had no interest in drinking. In fact, he would often say, in answer to his family's criticism, that he could take or leave alcohol.

Whatever Riccardo said to his family, he began to go to the pub more and more. If he did not go out to the pub, he felt hard done by. He imagined how much better he would feel in the warmth of the pub, with his friends, and how different that was to the oppressive atmosphere at home. He could imagine the glow as his first drink of the day went down. He felt an almost irresistible craving to have that first drink. Now almost anything difficult or upsetting made him feel like having a drink. If his wife wanted him to go shopping, an activity that he disliked, he felt like having a drink. If he had a difficult drive, he felt like having a drink to steady his nerves. He liked to see bottles, and he developed a special fondness for Campari. It reminded him of home. He would also start an evening's drinking with a glass of Campari and lemon. Seeing an advert for Campari on the television gave him an almost irresistible desire to have a glass of it himself. Riccardo could feel it in his mouth, and if he didn't have any available, he felt an emptiness inside him which was the most unpleasant feeling that he could remember having – worse even than feeling ashamed.

Craving

Riccardo developed a craving for drink through repeated exposure. This is not to say that he was physically dependent. He was compelled to drink to get rid of symptoms, true, but these symptoms were those of any craving, however caused. A feeling of emptiness associated with a constant preoccupation with drinking was what took him back to the pub, not tremor or anxiety.

Although cravings for particular satisfactions have specific names – hunger, thirst, love-sickness, cold turkey – there are many similarities between them. In fact, it seems likely that craving of whatever origin is associated with a particular brain state – specifically increased neural activity in the anterior cingulate gyrus (Childress et al., 1999) and frontal cortex (Maas et al., 1998) involving increased dopaminergic activity (Volkow et al., 1999).

The psychotherapeutic treatment of addiction therefore involves taking account not only of the complex emotional factors that maintain it, but the neurochemical changes that it induces. These are not changes induced by chemical effects of the addictive substance. The recent studies just cited show that cocaine craving can be induced by watching a film about cocaine, not only by withdrawal from cocaine. Addiction is an area in which psychotherapy and neuropharmacology are converging, but it is probably only the first of such areas of overlap.

Changing values through addiction

Many people in the world experience hunger and thirst on a regular basis. They are a part of life. However, in the developed world, it has become possible to lead one's life so that one is never hungry, or never thirsty. Having once experienced freedom from hunger and thirst, though, it is difficult to return to a life where these are routine afflictions. It is as if one's sights have been lifted to a new, higher kind of life where more important goals than feeding one's body hold sway.

A woman starving in the desert can feel better once she and her family move to a feeding station. But the very experience of having regular meals may create a wish never to hunger again, and exacerbate the fear that she will do so when the charitable flow of food ceases. Giving her lots of food in the short term will not satisfy her wish never to have to worry about food again. Telling her that she never wished for freedom from hunger before, so she should not wish for it now, will not work either. The only way to relieve her of her fear for the future is for her economic relations to be permanently changed.

Addictions also create new expectations. In fact, it has been argued that the addictive potency of psycho-stimulants is due to their ability to increase new associative learning because they release dopamine in the striatum and elsewhere which increases synaptic plasticity (Berke & Hyman, 2000). Addictions open vistas beyond the everyday which the addict is unwilling to give up, however scary or unpleasant. An addiction creates a new expectation, as well as a craving. This expectation can be stilled in the short term by the provision of positive esteem and acceptance. This may be the reason for the success of community-orientated approaches like Alcoholics Anonymous or concept houses. Strong religious convictions may also provide this positivism for the minority who are believers. However, satisfying the expectation does not change it. Only a change in the way of living, and of relating to others, can do that.

Treatment

Lucy was the ambitious and compliant daughter of two ambitious, but compliant, parents. Her father was a delivery man, but all of his spare time was taken up by competitive running. Her mother was a successful business woman. She was of a similar size to Lucy, and often used to wear her clothes. Her mother used to say that she had missed out on her teenage years, so she was having them again, through Lucy. She also used to say, thank God that Lucy wasn't selfish, like her sister. Diane, Lucy's sister, had a turbulent adolescence and had left home under a cloud. However, she was now studying occupational therapy, and doing well for herself. Lucy became very depressed about her GCSEs and was sure that she would fail. She began to withdraw from her friends at school. Then she began to diet. She became quite tyrannical at home about her parents' diet. She often cooked for them, and insisted that they never leave anything. She made her father stop running by having a tantrum every time he left the house in his running gear. However, she ate less and less herself. Within a very short time, she had lost a considerable amount of weight. Her periods stopped, and she started to faint. However, she told her parents that she had never been better. There were terrible rows about her weight but she was adamant about not eating in a way that her parents had never known her to be about anything before.

Eventually, Lucy was admitted to hospital, and given a combination of psychotherapy and a high-calorie diet. With enormous difficulty and distress she managed to get close to her target weight (set at her weight before she began dieting since this had been appropriate for her height and age), but never reached it. Once back home, she could not seem to increase her weight any more. Family sessions were begun, but Lucy seemed to get more distressed as a result of these and there was no increase in her weight. Then she started to see a young psychologist on an individual basis. He and Lucy hit it off immediately. They discussed what Lucy should say to her friends about her anorexia, what boys she liked, what she should say to her mother when her mother wanted to borrow her clothes, and how Lucy should deal with her parents' expectations. Lucy began to put on weight again, reaching her target weight and then stabilizing without further difficulty.

Lucy found that feeling empty actually reduced her depression. She experienced herself as never feeling better. It was a state to which she found that she needed to return more and more often, and with greater intensity. Szmukler and I have previously suggested (Szmukler & Tantam, 1984) that anorexia nervosa is a type of addiction. We suggested that starvation might induce euphoria, possibly through the production of endogenous opioids (Demitrack et al., 1993). One characteristic feature of anorexia, as with some other addictions at a particular phase, is that the affected person, usually a young woman, can contemplate her emaciated state with equanimity, even satisfaction. This has perplexed psychiatrists, and has motivated study after study to investigate whether it is a delusion.

How could someone who is not psychotic say that they are a bit fat when they are obviously dangerously emaciated? How could Lucy say this? One possible answer is that Lucy, like other people with an addiction, was able to compartmentalize her thinking. She could judge others by one standard, and herself by another, but could also keep these rigidly separated. From one perspective, this is sometimes seen as denial: the refusal to admit to something that is self-evidently true to others. From another perspective, it is a kind of dissociation – a split in the mind leaving some beliefs and feelings disconnected from others. This may be a common feature of addictions, and I shall return to it.

In practice, it is often best, when puzzled by something, to go back to what a person said and consider whether it is true. Perhaps Lucy was simply speaking the truth when she said that she was not abnormally thin. Perhaps what she was denying was not thinness, but abnormality. The reader will probably have guessed where this discussion is heading: to the proposal that her emaciated appearance had become a strong emotor.

The emotional meaning of Lucy's anorexia

Knowing *why* someone is addicted is probably less important than knowing that they *are* addicted. Or at least, it is not the first concern to address. But knowing why someone is addicted does tell the psychotherapist *how* it happened in the first place.

The prevailing explanation for how anorexia nervosa begins is that a certain proportion of the girls who diet (the theory largely applies to the teenage girls who make up the majority of anorectics) are anxious about their developing sexuality. These girls discover that dieting slows down the development of these characteristics and, if it is taken to an extreme, actually causes regression of secondary sexual characteristics. These girls become averse to gaining weight, weight phobic, and seek to lose more and more weight in the same way as agoraphobics avoid more and more any situation which is reminiscent of the crowded supermarket (Crisp et al., 1991).

This explanation does account for anorexia nervosa being particularly common around the time of puberty, although it does not fully explain why it should be commoner in girls than in boys. It also focusses strongly on anxiety about sexuality, although one of the commoner anxieties that precedes its onset is worry about examinations, as in Lucy's case.

Lucy did not think that she was weight phobic. She said that she did not have any worries about sexuality, and did not know why she became anorectic. There was no conscious process of avoidance, and no anxiety about sex to reduce. She also thought that there was nothing wrong with her. She felt better than she had felt for a long time. When she looked at her emaciated body, she saw health.

Far from having a happy childhood to which she was clinging, as the adult phobia theory might suggest, Lucy was an over-compliant child who felt little independence from her parents. In this she was typical of other people with anorexia (Troop & Treasure, 1997). Since she had become anorexic, she was back in a body reminiscent of that childhood state, but instead of feeling cowed, she was throwing her weight around. She had taken over the food shopping, and dictated what her parents ate, for example. She was having the battles over her weight that her sister had had over boyfriends and staying out late, but Lucy could not be accused of being bad because she was suffering, not having a good time, like Diane. Her child-like frame had been transformed into the vehicle of a powerful and autonomous social agent. The helplessness that she associated with herself, the weakness that she had always seen when she looked at her child's body, was now blended with the euphoria of the starvation into a triumphant overcoming of humiliation.

What is being described is not a conscious decision, or even a specific happening, but the modification of the continuous and constant emotional meaning of the body. By chance or random exposure, Lucy dieted, in the same way as some other girl might be given some heroin or another girl might cut herself experimentally. The feeling of being in control that dieting gave her had a particular meaning in her world. The minute changes in her body that she noticed were both a move back to childhood experience and a blending of the impotence of that experience with a new sense of being able to control her shape, for herself and without any interference. This combination, of helplessness and of control, produces the emotional meaning of helplessness overcome.

One could say to Lucy that the key to her preoccupations about herself, the examinations and her parents is the question, 'How is she to become a person with weight and value?'. But clinical experience suggests that there is little value in making interpretations like this. The emotional meaning of her disorder is determined through predominantly involuntary emotional processing, possibly involving the non-dominant hemisphere in particular. Lucy cannot introspect these processes. Her understanding of the emotional meaning of anorexia can only be determined by the same process, and with the same error, as that of the clinician. Making an interpretation is likely to have its principal effect through adding to the emotional meaning of the therapeutic relationship rather than in any other way.

In fact, as the case history showed, Lucy began to feel able to eat normally more as a result of being taken so seriously by the young psychologist than because she gained insight into her problems. One can see, in retrospect, how this came to be so. He treated her as an adult, and respected her views about her difficulties. He recognized that her struggle against her parents showed that she was a young woman of considerable determination. It was a very different relationship to the one that she had with her parents or, indeed, to the one that she had with her psychiatrist.

By the time that Lucy had started to see the psychologist, her weight had been fairly close to her target weight for about 3 months. She was nowhere near as desperate about putting on weight, or as elated if she lost weight, as she had been previously. Her craving for thinness had considerably diminished. However, there was still the unresolved issue of feeling powerless, for which starving had proved an antidote. The psychologist was not tainted by any sort of commitment to Lucy's parents. Nor had he had the experience of being confronted by Lucy when her weight was so low as to become a danger to health, as had the psychiatrist. The psychiatrist had become a parental figure, too, as a result of that experience. The psychologist was much more able to relate to Lucy as another young person and knew himself about the difficulties of creating a space for oneself in a family or, in his case, in an organization. Lucy and he shared many of the same values. Moreover, the emotional flavour of the therapeutic sessions with him was, for Lucy, much more like the flavour of a relationship with a friend than a relationship with a parent. Her concerns over her independence could be dealt with in a new and more effective way as a result, especially as her struggles for power in the family on behalf of her anorexia had irreversibly altered her family's perception of her from the baby of the family to seeing her changed her family position in thewere therefore very nor did he stand in a pseudo-parental relationship which is how the psychiatrist experienced his independence and mastery.

First steps in treating addiction: addressing the craving

The longer that a person has been addicted, the more that craving dictates their activity, and the more important that the first step in therapy is to tackle the craving. Because being an addict threatens social and physical extinction (Winship, 1999), the addiction itself becomes a strong emotor which effaces the concerns that led to the addiction in the first place. When an addiction has become firmly established, then psychotherapy for other concerns is not appropriate. Even during the initial phase of enthusiastic abstinence, it is relapse prevention which usually dominates the agenda and not wider psychological difficulties.

Craving is associated with desire, but also affects attention, and executive functions, like goal setting. It is, as we all know, relieved by obtaining whatever it is that is craved. The relief may be physical, for example when someone eats when they are 'starving hungry', or psychological, for example when someone is reunited with someone for whom they have been pining. The distinction between physical and psychological relief is probably much less than would appear at first sight, however. Hunger can be reduced by fear, and increased by other psychological means, and as far as brain representation is concerned, the cingulate gyrus is equally activated whether someone craves for a lover or craves for cocaine.

The emotional concomitant of a craving – the desire which accompanies it – is very contagious. Relief of a craving is deeply satisfying. This satisfaction adds to the emotional meaning of whatever is craved. When a person longs for a drink and then has one, it is as if the glass, the bottle and the drink itself are friends. Sometimes they can become their closest friends. If so, they are jealous friends, who leach the emotional meaning out of family, friends, work and any other meaning not associated with the addiction.

There is a tendency for the emotional meaning of an addiction to spread, as well as to deepen. 'Cues' related to the addictive experience become imbued with emotional meaning because of their contiguity to it (Shiffman et al., 1996). In this chapter, I have discussed this in terms of the transmission of emotional meaning between associated emotors. In the animal literature, it is termed 'conditioned place preference' and is usually described in relation to psycho-stimulants. The place where cocaine, for example, is administered to a rat becomes a place in which the rat prefers to be even if no further injections are given (Tzschentke, 1998). Actions that the rat performed in relation to drug administration can also become involuntary routines which the rat will perform in that place even if no drug administration takes place (Ellinwood & Kilbey, 1975).

Cravings become a problem when what is craved becomes out of reach, for example when another, adored, person fails to reciprocate romantic feelings, or when the craving is for something that has become dangerous, expensive, or unhealthy.

Dealing with craving

Motivation for change

Prochaska and DiClimente (1982) described three stages (recently expanded to six by Prochaska & Velicer (1997)) that a person passes through *en route* to a confrontation with craving and a change in their behaviour. Most people who have not sought help, but been offered it by health professionals, are in the first stage, 'pre-contemplation'. They have never seriously considered change, or whether or not it would be in their interests. People in the second state of 'contemplation' have considered change, but are in two minds. Only when a person is in the third stage, 'action', is change likely.

Rollnick and Miller (1995) have developed what they describe as a directive client-centered counselling approach – motivational interviewing – to address these problems. They point out that scaring people as a motivator, far from decreasing addiction, tends to increase it. Telling someone that if they continue drinking, it will kill them, makes them drink more rather than less. The reason is apparent from the previous discussion about strong emotors. Attacking a person means that their identity is in question. People with an addiction are already vulnerable to extinction of their identity. That is why they have developed the addiction as an antidote. Their response to this kind of attack is therefore to need to make more antidote, i.e. to pursue their addiction more rather than less.

Miller (1994) contrasts motivational interviewing with other, more coercive, approaches. It builds on two important principles of change. One is to make values explicit and, in the process, become aware that the values associated with addiction are inconsistent with other values, which may be more dear and more important to the client – not to the therapist. The second is to create a safe therapeutic environment in which the client can own up to this inconsistency, and consider ways of resolving it.

Values, and the means by which a therapist might in practice elicit them, are discussed in Chapter 2. One of the important issues when it comes to their application in motivational interviewing, or in other brief interventions, is the therapist's values, and the values of the therapist's organization. If the value of either is that clients should be persuaded to stop drinking, put on weight, give up cocaine or otherwise stop their addictions, then it is unlikely that the client will be able to be open about their values. Therapists, and organizations, should have confidence that few people who are drinking excessively, or have any sort of 'habit' that they cannot change but which they have to conceal, will be content. Most people will be motivated to change if they just allowed themselves to think about the reality of their situation. It is, however, very easy to think of motivational interviewing as a form of subtle manipulation towards a goal set by the therapist. If it is used in this way, motivational interviewing is destructive rather than constructive. In a recent evaluation of motivational interviewing, the poor results of the study overall could be attributed to outstandingly bad results of a few therapists, and it seems likely that they were the therapists who believed that they had to manipulate their clients towards abstinence rather than work towards the goals set by the clients themselves (Project MATCH, research, et al., 1998).

Determination to change

Relinquishing an addiction means coping with the craving with which it is associated. If craving is severe, psychotherapy has little role to play, although practically orientated counselling may be useful (Crits-Christoph et al., 1999) and may be combined in specialist units with drug therapy, e.g. naltrexone (Jaffe et al., 1996) or acamprosate (Pelc et al., 1997), which may relieve its severity.

Craving is most severe when a person's life has become organized around their addiction. They are likely to have friends who share the addiction, and they are likely to experience many of the day-to-day details of their lives as associated with drinking, and therefore as potential cues to a craving for drink. Addiction may be inextricably enmeshed with loss of control so that the possibility of a controlled return to alcohol, dieting or having a flutter is unrealistic. This is particularly likely to be the case if the addiction has been long-standing or, in the case of alcohol addiction, if there is a family history or an early age of onset, suggesting a biological predisposition.

Follow-up studies indicate that an important factor in the successful outcome of addiction treatment is 'self-efficacy' (Allsop, Saunders & Phillips, 2000). A person needs to feel that they are more than just a void which has to be filled. Only if someone has an identity independent of being an addict can they experience themselves as being able to set goals and achieve them. And only if a person can focus their determination on abstinence is this likely to be achieved.

Addicts may fill the void that is in them by belonging to a community or a religious group, and this may be enough to enable them to regain a sense of themselves. Sometimes such groups require abstinence first, which may be putting the cart before the horse.

Legal sanctions may enforce attendance in community treatment programmes and employers may increase abstinence in their employees by making it a condition of continued employment, but experience suggests coercion is not an effective treatment. Coercion may, however, force a re-evaluation of the situation.

Terence was an academic physicist who had been both an able and an extremely assiduous student, and had achieved considerable academic success. He was, however, never quite confident about his own abilities. He dealt with this partly by over-extending himself, and partly by being fiercely competitive. This did not help him when it came to writing papers. These were a too-naked expression of his ability for him not to fear that they would be condemned as drivel by his peers. He got into the habit of stopping off on his way home from work to have a drink in a country pub. He would not socialize, but would sit at a remote table over a pint or two, and write. It solved many problems. He was less anxious about the reviewer's reaction when he had had a pint or two, and he wrote well in this situation. He did not feel guilty about the drink because he was using it to help him work. And he enjoyed having a breathing space before facing the demands of family life.

As his reputation grew, Terence became a consultant on physics to several large companies. He found this even more difficult. Perhaps he would give advice that would be simply dismissed, or that would result in the firm losing a lot of money. He used alcohol to relax himself when he travelled, and again this helped with his lack of self-confidence too. He developed a liver problem, but his doctor put it down to some idiopathic hepatic disorder, and Terence dealt with it in his usual method, by out-competing it. He took up running, and soon was running further than anyone in the university. He told himself that there could not be much wrong with his liver if he could run as he did.

Then his wife made an appointment to see the doctor. Her husband had a drinking problem, she said. This came as a shock to the doctor and to Terence, but Terence took it in his stride. He would change his schedule and try to cut down, but he thought it was quite a minor problem. What was more important was his current book. The day came when Terence had to give a lecture to some distinguished visitors, and he had a drink or two to loosen his wits. His speech was obviously slurred in the lecture, and his thoughts were muddled. The visitors were dismayed and made their displeasure known to his head of department. He saw Terence the same day, suspended him with immediate effect, and banned him from the campus. Terence was admitted at his own request to a private alcohol treatment unit, where he did very well. He became even more proud, and preoccupied, with his fitness. He became militantly anti-alcohol. It became for him a test of his will-power to remain abstinent and he was determined not to fail. However, the defining moment for him was his realization that he and the head of department shared the same values. Both of them had a conception of the academic life which was almost religious. Terence realized that he had allowed other values – to make money, to feel easy in himself – to dominate what had been his ideal all his life, that of intellectual improvement. It was this realization, more than anything else, which fixed his determination on recovery and helped him to succeed.

Relapse prevention

Even if a person is determined to change, there will be moments when relapse is particularly likely. It is better to be honest about this from the beginning of the therapy. One way of doing this is to encourage the client to identify the circumstances in which relapse is most likely. It may be helpful to remind the client that what seems achievable as the client is sitting talking to you, the psychotherapist, in the relative security of your office, will be very different from what is achievable when faced with an ever-tightening spring of tension and a triggering event.

'Relapse prevention' is the name often given to this honest discussion. It usually involves four main elements (see Table 9.1): treating co-morbid psychiatric disorder, coping skills, avoiding high-risk situations, and coping with relapse.

Coping with craving

What seems a very good reason for giving up something when one is replete may seem very insubstantial when the satisfaction has worn off. This is one reason why the motivational interviewing approach, or some other clarification of what the client's preoccupying concerns are, is important. As noted in a previous section, a person needs to have convinced themselves that they want to change in order to be able to hold on to this motivation when the going gets rough. But they also need some means of dealing with craving.

Table 9.1. Relapse prevention

Element	Example
Treating co-morbid psychiatric disorder	Antidepressants for depression
Coping skills	One day at a time
	Distraction (but see Chapter 6)
	Re-focussing on reasons for abstinence
Avoiding high-risk situations	Cue
	Trigger
	Spring
Coping with relapse	Expecting relapse, and preparing for it

In a study of the reports of women who repeatedly harm themselves, Huband (personal communication) found that there were two pathways to self-wounding. The woman might experience a slow insidious development of tension associated with thoughts of self-harm (the 'spring'), or a sudden impulse (the 'trigger') to self-harm which might be immediately translated into self-cutting or which might increase the urge to self-harm to unbearable proportions. The emotional content of the descriptions of trigger events suggested that they had acted as triggers because they had led to the woman feeling shame, or that she was disgusting to others. These negative emotions may trigger action sequences which may have become involuntary, leading directly to relapse. Studies in other fields have confirmed that it is negative emotion that is most likely to trigger the addictive behaviour (Price, 1999).

Most models of dealing with craving consider only the 'spring' model of relapse or, as commonsense psychology terms it, the 'temptation' model. According to this approach, a person feels an increasing temptation to do or have whatever is craved. Temptation involves an increasing preoccupation with, and desire for, whatever is tempting. It is increased by exposure to cues that are associated with what is craved. Relapse prevention approaches have been developed which attempt to deal with this by de-sensitisation, by exposing people to addiction-related cues, but without satiation. For example, smokers may be encouraged to make a list of situations in which they would normally smoke – after a good meal, perhaps, or after making love – and then to imagine themselves in these situations, but not smoking. Exposure to cues with response prevention does reduce temptation to smoke in people giving up cigarettes, and may reduce temptation in other addictions, but it seems to have less impact on preventing relapse (Shiffman et al., 1996).

The reason for this may be that relapses are more likely to be 'triggered' than response to temptation.

Oliver was 25 years old. He had autism and, although not mentally handicapped, had attended schools for people with learning disabilities. When he reached puberty, his parents had sometimes heard him remark about girls' breasts to his brother and they were, on the whole, pleased that he was developing normally. He left school at 19 and started attending a day centre, but the atmosphere there was much more stressful. There were some other attenders with uninhibited or challenging behaviour, and Oliver began to copy them. His parents noted that Oliver began to rub himself through his trousers, and that his remarks about breasts became more outspoken. They discussed this with him, and tried to explain about sexual propriety, but Oliver got angry. Over a period of time, Oliver's preoccupation with breasts deepened, to the point where he would begin to rub himself even if he saw a brassiere hanging in a shop. He would be more likely to masturbate in public if he was tense, but he could be in an apparently calm mood and then pass a woman in the street who was wearing a low-cut dress, and begin to masturbate there and then.

Oliver's autism meant that he did not use language for communication very much. Nor did he have much sense of himself as an agent of communication. It was not therefore possible to develop a coping strategy with his collaboration. In fact, he did not understand why his parents and others were scandalized by his masturbation, and would become aggressive if they tried to stop him.

Rising sexual tension did not contribute to the likelihood that Oliver would masturbate; his parents had not observed any correlation between the likelihood of Oliver masturbating and the length of time since he had last done it. In fact, rising sexual tension seems to be a myth. Sexual activity is more likely, at least between couples, if there has been recent sex than if there has not. Masturbation did become more likely as Oliver became more anxious or tense. But this 'spring' explanation did not fit the many occasions when Oliver seemed calm but then caught sight of a woman's breasts.

The A–B–C of addiction

People in the learning disability field write about what they call habit problems, or challenging behaviours, quite differently from workers in the drug dependency field who write about addictions, and differently again from psychotherapists or counsellors working with sexual deviations or perversions. However, there are many similarities. Perhaps one of the most useful frameworks for understanding the similarities is the A–B–C model, which emanates from the learning disability field and which has begun to percolate into drug dependency services (Clark, Leukefeld & Godlaski, 1999). 'A' in A–B–C stands for antecedents, 'B' for behaviour, and 'C' for consequences. Confusingly, rational-emotive psychotherapists also have an A–B–C model (Kwee & Ellis, 1997) but, for them, 'B' stands for beliefs and the consequences of 'C' include the person's behaviour and not, as for the other A–B–C model, the consequential reactions of other people.

Some of the antecedents of addiction have already been discussed. They include the factors that contribute to the winding of the 'spring' of craving, and the cues that 'trigger' relapse. The 'B' of behaviour is important because it indicates that the addictive behaviour changes. People with alcohol problems become increasingly addicted to a particular drink, and not just alcohol in any form. People with a long-standing eating disorder or those who misuse drugs may go on to develop an alcohol problem that replaces the original addiction. In the learning disability field, attention is sometimes given to fading out one behaviour with another, more acceptable, one. This is one way of understanding the value of self-help groups: that they provide, for a while, a new kind of addiction which attenuates the former addiction and which makes it more possible to give it up.

Coping with relapse

Thinking about the 'C' of the A–B–C model – the consequences of the addictive behaviour are also important.

Choosing abstinence makes relapse almost inevitable. What matters, therefore, is to ensure that the relapse frequency is minimized and that relapse, when it does happen, does not mean the collapse of the determination to return to abstinence. When relapse does occur, it is important that it does not go so far that it rekindles the exultation of shame or disgust that fuelled the addiction originally. Rehearsal of what will happen when the person relapses may help a person to hoard up some measure of self-control for when the time comes, whilst denial of the likelihood of relapse increases shame or disgust. Other people's reactions to relapse are also important. Criticism, shaming or disgust have the effect of increasing the likelihood of relapse because they increase the need for an antidote to social extinction.

Harm reduction

So far in this chapter, the treatment issues have been predominantly those of treating craving and the void that is left when someone with a long-established addiction loses the social identity of being an addict, and the 'friendship' of the paraphernalia of addiction.

However, there are people who seek treatment when their addiction is not so well entrenched. Sometimes, too, a person might realize that there are more fundamental problems than the addiction and want help with those.

Practical experience suggests that symptomatic psychotherapy can be effective even in the context of an established addiction. But working on predicaments, or in longer-term therapy, may be impossible unless the addiction is first controlled. The reason is that self-disgust and shame are such pervasive emotions, and are so readily aroused in psychotherapy, that a person is increasingly tempted to deal with them in the same way as before – by an increase in the addictive behaviour.

Psychotherapy of a person who is addicted presents one further challenge that needs to be considered. A person who is ashamed or believes him- or herself to be an object of disgust or scorn learns to hide, to dissimulate. An addiction partakes of this flavour. It is something to be minimized or kept secret. Sometimes a person's values seem to uphold this. Their motto might be, 'What the eye does not know, the heart does not grieve over'. However, this motto only holds true if what the eye sees and the heart experiences are in two quite distinct compartments. Most spouses of a person who has been secretly carrying on an addiction, however, wonder whether there are other secrets – secrets of more direct concern to the spouse – that have been concealed. The addiction is experienced as a sort of unfaithfulness, or a lack of commitment. A spouse might wonder if their partner would give in to other kinds of temptations if they were already unable to control their temptation for drink, drugs or whatever else they are addicted to.

Psychotherapists, too, are likely to resent this type of concealment, but there is a more serious problem about it. It obfuscates the client's real concerns. The client lives in a magical world in which actual consequences are hidden by wished-for outcomes which are achieved through the liberal use of the addictive 'antidote'. The emotional difficulties of the client are evaded because in this magical world there is a kind of glamour over everything which seems to make everything rosy. At best, this means that any benefits of the therapy are likely to be achieved almost by chance. At worst, it means that the therapy is misdirected.

One way of dealing with this problem is by combining therapy with checking on abstinence: weighing the person with anorexia, checking the liver function tests in someone with an alcohol problem, or analysing the urine samples of a drug addict. This will irrevocably change the nature of the therapy, especially if it is the therapist him- or herself who is carrying out the investigations. The client who professes gratitude to the therapist for stiffening their resolve to quit their habit may seem like a success, but he or she is still depending on the psychotherapist, if not on the original addictive behaviour or substance.

Many clients who have been addicted will discover that they still need some antidote to shame or self-disgust. Their preoccupying concern is likely to become what makes them so prone to these emotions, and this may naturally lead on to the longer-term therapy discussed later in this chapter, and in Chapter 10.

Most psychotherapists would consider that their intervention has only been successful if it leaves the client more autonomous. These psychotherapists may consider that gratitude indicated a degree of dependency on them which betokened a continuing predisposition to addiction. A psychotherapist of this persuasion might conclude that only those clients who go into longer-term therapy are really dealing with the root of their problem.

However, some clients may not want to change themselves. They may view the addiction as something that they caught. This is a prevalent view among lawmakers. The rationale of preventing the ingress of heroin into the country is that anyone exposed to heroin is likely to become addicted, because heroin is so addictive. Similarly some pornography – the kind that can be seized on a magistrates' order in the UK – has the power to 'deprave and corrupt'.

Psychotherapists should not be prescriptive about the therapy that is right for their clients. Clients who think that they 'caught' an addiction have a similar view of their difficulties, and similar values, to clients whose preoccupying concern is a symptom. We have already noted that symptomatic psychotherapy rests on values which are much more like those of the medical model. Because the symptoms are like something a person has, rather than something that a person is, it is possible for the psychotherapist to be beneficent without weakening the autonomy of the client. And, in fact, sometimes people who have given up an addiction develop anxiety or depressive symptoms which – to use a common form of words – they have been self-treating with the addiction. If these symptoms become a preoccupying concern for the client, it may be appropriate to move on from the addiction-orientated approach described in this chapter to symptomatic psychotherapy, as described in Chapter 5.

Remedying symptoms of psychological disorder is one aspect of the harm reduction approach. Other aspects include reducing the addiction, and reducing the personal and social impact of the addiction. The approach is similar to the treatment of anxiety. A person works with the therapist to set targets, to identify alternative means of coping, to anticipate future situations which might be associated with an increase in addictive behaviour, and to plan ways of minimizing the harm to others.

Roger was into pornography, and had been all his sexual life. It had become more of a problem after his relationship with his wife had broken down. He had discovered the Internet and become compulsive about masturbating to pictures of women that he viewed on his computer. Whilst Roger was single, he had thought of his behaviour only as a way of solacing himself. However, he had begun a new relationship which was much deeper than the one that he had previously had with his wife. His new partner, Connie, felt excluded by Roger's pornography. She told him that she could never be sure that, when he was making love to her, he was not thinking of some other woman that he had masturbated over. It did not matter that they were strangers. Roger was

sensitive about the issue. He knew that his partner's attitude was, if anything, more moderate than many other women's might have been. After all, he was participating in a trade which certainly did degrade women. But he told himself that he was not making anybody do anything. He was just a passive observer. And, anyway, he felt enormous comfort in just downloading the pictures. He was not being unfaithful. It was more his way of keeping himself calm than anything really sexual.

Roger had become an internet addict (Putnam & Maheu, 2000) and Connie recognized this. She knew that if she criticized Roger, he would simply withdraw into the non-judgemental, dream world of virtual reality. So she decided to work out a harm reduction approach with Roger.

She decided that the most harmful aspect of his addiction was the fact that it excluded her. She therefore agreed to go with Roger to buy magazines and videos which they would look at together. However, it became clear to both of them that this would not work. Connie still felt that Roger was in his own private world but Roger felt that he could not really be himself sexually with Connie watching him. He still downloaded pictures whilst she was out. They therefore agreed that if he had to do that, he would always tell her when he had, and he would not masturbate. He agreed, and this worked for a few months. But it did not really make Connie feel more secure. Then Roger discovered sexually explicit cartoons. Connie found that she liked these too. The women in them were exaggerated, and she could not believe that Roger would ever meet another woman in reality who was remotely like these steatopygous figures.

Roger and Connie had succeeded in reducing the harm of his addiction to a substantial extent, and in fact, Roger gradually stopped looking at sexually explicit pictures. But Connie did not think that he was completely over it. He was still an addict, even if he was in remission. Somewhere, Connie thought, Roger still had a hidden pocket of sexuality that was closed to her, and she resented this. Moreover, whilst his addiction was still present, even if not indulged, she felt that Roger was continually being tempted to re-use it to deal with the various challenges in his life, including those in his relationship with Connie. She could never be sure whether or not one of these challenges would prove too strong and Roger would return to his pictures, blaming her for needing to do so.

Dissociation and deception

Certain secrets are fatal to a person's identity once discovered. Very often, these are secrets that would invite disgust or shame, as Connie feared she would feel if she knew about Roger's actual fantasies. A person who harbours a shameful secret may become mortified by it, so that their identity is gradually hollowed out and eventually collapses (Tantam, 1991). However, this would not happen with Roger. He did not feel shame or disgust at his own fantasies. He had long since turned his pornography into strong emotors by which his own self-disgust had been transformed into its antidote. However, his success in doing so created another danger. There is a metaphorical 'stop' button on most people marked 'disgust' and one marked 'shame'. These are important means of social influence and control. Freud was wrong in supposing that people feel anxiety over misdeeds as a form of expiation, or 'guilt'. The anxiety is created by the fear that a misdemeanour will cause others to push one of these safety override buttons and that this will lead to such a flood of shame or self-disgust that the miscreant will want to hide from others rather than interact with them.

Connie believed that if Roger did not feel any disgust at some of the sexually explicit material that he watched, or shame at his lack of sexual inhibition, his disgust and shame responses would be more generally warped. In this, she was expressing a common assumption: that no part of a person's emotional life can be sequestrated. Our emotions are entire. If, as many people think, we show cruelty to our pets, we express a general sentiment of cruelty and we will be cruel to children or defenceless people too.

Hidden emotions are considered further in a substantial section of the next chapter. Extreme sequestration of emotions may result in 'dissociation', i.e. the ability to have quite separate states of mind, each associated with a distinctive capacity to think, feel and act. Often, this will result in a person seeming quite normal, and having normal reactions, but being able to switch into an abnormal state of mind under certain conditions. However, it may be that a person who dissociates frequently comes to believe, sometimes under therapeutic influence, that they are 'really' two people and so constructs a separate narrative of their dissociative self, giving this self a different name. This process often rapidly accelerates if given credence and encouragement by others, creating what ICD-10 calls 'dissociative identity disorder', but what is more often called 'multiple personality'.

Dissociation is linked to addiction because it is often closely associated with the addictive act. Deliberate self-harm has been described as an attempt to terminate dissociation, but dissociation may also be induced to enable self-harm to take place, or it may be the consequence of deliberate self-harm (Huband, personal communication).

Dissociation has been described as a way of opening an escape hatch in the mind to escape from intolerable stress, for example in people in front-line battle situations (Shalev et al., 1996) or in the victims of abuse (Kolk et al., 1996).

There is evidence, at least in normal subjects, that deliberate attempts at forgetting increase the possibility of dissociation (Hout, Merckelbach & Pool,

1996) although once the faculty is established, which may only be possible in susceptible individuals, it may become involuntary.

Fred was a bit of a wimp. His father and elder brother were both strong individuals who worked hard, and yet never seemed tired. He worked in the family business, too, but he found it very hard going. He got completely hardened to his father's lectures about his weaknesses, especially as he could always rely on his mother to intercede on his behalf. If things were really bad, he would suddenly go off on holiday. Sometimes no-one would know that he had left until he rang home from Tenerife, or Corsica. He had married, but this relationship had broken down – unreasonably, Fred thought. His wife had made much of the fact that one afternoon, when both he and his mother-in-law had been drinking, they had a bit of a dalliance. Fred really didn't think much of it at the time, or later.

Despite his insouciance, Fred was often anxious. He had relied on drink for many years, and at the time of referral to a psychotherapist, he was drinking so heavily and so regularly that he had 'the shakes' on Monday mornings, and sometimes had to have an eye-opener. His income from the family business was also dropping as his brother, who was the foreman, began to dock his wages if he came in late. In order to make the money to buy drink, Fred began to deal in stolen goods. He would buy electronic goods from acquaintances in pubs at knock-down prices, and sell them on to friends and relatives.

Fred did not say that the goods were stolen. Once his father challenged him on it, and he loudly and long protested his innocence. Fred said later that he really felt outraged that his father would make this suggestion, 'to his own son' as Fred put it. In the less pressurized atmosphere of the therapy sessions, Fred was prepared to say that the goods were sold to him at unusually low prices, and that they were always unpacked. This did make him suspicious, but he was not one to look a gift-horse in the mouth. Once Fred came drunk to the session. He had been drinking with his mates, and was still in a boozy, expansive frame of mind. He boasted that he made a good killing on some radios that had 'fallen off the back of a lorry', but collected himself when he saw the therapist's face and said, 'They really had you know. This whole box was found on the A6. The driver must have forgotten to latch the tail-gate'.

Fred is an example of someone who, under pressure from his father, considered himself to be unfairly judged and in that mood was convinced himself that he had done nothing wrong. And since he had done nothing wrong, the goods were not stolen. When speaking to the therapist, he was disingenuous and self-deceptive, except on the last occasion when he was, frankly, lying.

Highly suggestible individuals like Fred may deliberately deceive someone else about something, then persuade themselves that the something has not happened (self-deception), then be unable to remember that the something has happened. Memory is not an engraving, but a dynamic record that is constantly being overwritten with the prevailing narrative about the past.

Therapists should be sceptical about the cognitive distinction between deception, self-deception and dissociation. Moralists and lawyers would like these to be distinguished, since it would be convenient if people could be condemned for falsehoods, exhorted to greater moral strength if they deceive themselves, and forgiven if they dissociate, since then their memory has become unconscious and therefore inaccessible.

It may be better to think of the line between deception and dissociation as a continuum of attentional restriction. Like the child who will not look at the cup that they have broken, and will say, 'I didn't do anything', a person may omit unpleasant or conflicting evidence from their consideration. Attentional restriction is a general problem for the psychotherapist since a person may have an emotion whether or not they attend to it. The emotions connected with addiction have many ramifications. If a person dissociates from them, or even deceives him- or herself about them, they will still have their effect.

Harvey was a successful businessman who was burning the candle at both ends. He went out to clubs and bars until the early hours, and he worked long hours during the day in stock-broking. He began to use amphetamines, and quickly became dependent on them. They made him feel fine. He had never felt much pleasure in anything before, just going through life as if it was a sort of purgatory, but now he felt contentment. He did not see that his amphetamine use bothered anyone, and he saw no reason to change it. He began to think that he was a sort of machine that just needed a particular kind of fuel. From this thought, he went on to thinking of other people as machines too: complex ones with complex needs for fuelling and tending to, of various kinds, but machines nonetheless. Then something went wrong at work. There was a complaint about his handling of a personnel matter. He realized that he had no support. People had picked up his mechanical approach to them, and resented it. Despite a continuing amphetamine supply, Harvey plunged into despair that was inexplicable to him. He could only think that he needed a better combination of drugs.

The longer-term psychotherapy of addiction is therefore likely to begin with a stage during which the therapist provides the safety for a person to enlarge their attention (Ross, 1989) and begin to consider what is problematic about the pseudo-safety which their addiction provides. The technique may not be any different for a person who dissociates as for a person who self-deceives or deceives. In each case, the client must have sufficient concern about changing his or her situation to build with the therapist an honest and open relationship, at least some of the time, that can be a basis for further enlargement of the therapeutic relationship.

Releasement

Case example

In February 2000, the *Honolulu Star Bulletin* contained the obituary of Vincent O. 'Vinny' Marino. 'He climbed from the degradation of addiction', his daughter said. 'He went through the system several times . . . it took him a long time to wake up. He was the example of turning the worst into the best. He had a hard head, a big ego, he was very controlling, but he had a big heart. Habilitat was his life . . . that is his legacy'. The obituary continues, 'He opened his facility in a two-bedroom Kailua house in 1970 and the community effort to evict him was just the beginning of numerous encounters with officialdom over licensing, financing and other issues . . . His office reflects Marino's success, memorialized in a row of framed congratulatory proclamations from government and private agencies, and his thirst for celebrity, in photographs of Marino with entertainers, framed covers from his autobiographical books and clippings of lifetime highlights'.

Undoubtedly, there are numerous routes to the overcoming of addiction. One is to live as an addict in remission, moderating or avoiding the craving as best one can. Another is to acknowledge that there can be a vision in addiction of wanting to go beyond the previous constraints of life. 'The idea that there is a goal that we can never quite reach can expand into a moral revulsion of the way that things are, and a yearning that they be put right', writes Roger Trigg, apropos of Nietzsche's philosophy (Trigg, 1988, p. 131). It is all too easy to fall back on the antidote for revulsion and yearning that addiction represents, and therefore all too easy to lose the vision of something more in the performance of something less. 'Vinny' Marino is reported, for example, to have relapsed four times before he managed to kick the habit.

Not enough is known of the factors that strengthen resolve. Psychotherapy theory has concentrated mainly on factors that restrict people. However, the 'Vinny' Marino example suggests that resilience involves acceptance of what one is – Vinny apparently was somewhat taken with himself – and finding a place in society in which that particular combination of characteristics is valued. Vinny's forcefulness may have been unacceptable when it was simply exercised in his interests, but when it was in the interests of other addicts, it became a virtue.

Acceptance as a means to transcendence is termed, by Heidegger, 'releasement' (Deurzen, 1997). It is one of the criteria of happiness that will be considered in the next chapter.

10

Re-narration: finding happiness

Sophie---Psychoanalyste
« Pour plus de jouissance »
Tel. 01 . . . .
Advertisement in *Psychologies* magazine 173, March 1999

What is Sophie offering? And is it anything to do with health? In an illness-led service such as the British NHS, happiness seems like an accidental consequence of lack of illness, rather than something for which the doctor could, or even should, aim. Happiness might be the stuff of escapism, of Mills and Boon fantasy, or of religious zealotry, but not of the clinic or everyday life. Or so it might seem. Argyle (1997) has argued that happiness is an important determinant of long-term health. Happiness is also the single most important determinant of quality of life according to a panel of UK residents brought together to develop the WHO International Quality of Life instrument (Skevington, Mac Arthur & Somerset, 1997).

How important happiness is, what constitutes happiness, and whether or not its absence should make us change our lives, are all questions that can only be answered in relation to our personal values. What to a psychotherapist might be hedonism might to his or her client be the activity that makes life worth living.

Stories of happiness

Long-term therapy requires some theory of what it takes to be a person – a theory of human nature (Trigg, 1999). Arguably, this should account, as a minimum, for the following: the givenness of circumstance and of temperament; the recognition that each of us experiences ourself as an agent seeking to further aims or reach goals; that each of us experiences ourself as having needs or desires which may sometimes be in opposition to our goals; that each of us experiences ourself in relation to others; that others experience us as having a particular identity; and that each of us believes that we are different from other animals because we seek moral goodness or spiritual salvation.

There is no single theory which can be said to be 'correct' when applied to human nature. As repeatedly noted in this book, the adoption of a particular theory is more likely to be determined by its emotional flavour and the values with which it is most attuned than by its theoretical content. The advantage of narrative theory is not that it is any more 'correct' than, say, cognitive-behavioural or psycho-analytic theory, although it may be richer than the former and less inconsistent than the latter. Its advantage is that it uses the language of commonsense psychology, albeit condensed by literary convention. It is a way of understanding life that comes naturally. As one sufferer from prostatic cancer wrote: 'My initial experience of illness [prostatic cancer] was a series of disconnected shocks, and my first instinct was to try to bring it under control by turning it into a narrative. Always in emergencies we invent stories. We describe what is happening, as if to confine the catastrophe. The client's narrative keeps him from falling out of his life into his illness. Like a novelist, he gives his anxiety a shape' (Broyard, 1990).

Psychotherapy is sometimes criticized for being too verbal a medium. Critics point out that thinking about themselves in the way that psychotherapists do may be foreign to many people of practical rather than propositional intelligence. Caleb Garth, in George Eliot's *Middlemarch*, is like this. '. . . his virtual divinities were good practical schemes, accurate work, and the faithful completion of undertakings: his prince of darkness was a slack workman. But there was no spirit of denial in Caleb, and the world seemed so wondrous to him that he was ready to accept any number of systems, like any number of firmaments, if they did not obviously interfere with the best land-drainage, solid building, correct measuring, and judicious boring (for coal). In fact, he had a reverential soul with a strong practical intelligence.'

Caleb's narrative about life was told not in words but in 'business', and particularly in the improvement of the land. Caleb says later to Mr Featherstone that: 'It's a most uncommonly cramping thing, as I've often told Susan, to sit on horseback and look over the hedges at the wrong thing, and not be able to put your hand to it to make it right'. Caleb never engaged, unlike some of the other characters in *Middlemarch*, in discussions about psychology, but he could respond to narrative in music: '. . . when he could afford it [Caleb] went to hear an oratorio that came within his reach, returning from it with a profound reverence for this mighty structure of tones, which made him sit meditatively, looking on the floor and throwing much unutterable language into his outstretched hands'.

Caleb Garth's biggest reverse in *Middlemarch* occurred because he lent money to Fred. Vincy and Fred bought a spavined horse with it, and so lost it. Caleb's business collapsed as a consequence of the resulting cash-flow problems, and the Garth family went through very hard times as a result. Caleb felt his own over-trusting nature was responsible. It is impossible to say whether or not Caleb would have benefitted from seeing a psychotherapist in this crisis. However, Caleb's regular discussions with his wife, Susan, are a feature of their relationship which is unique. No other couple in the book talks through the day as they do.

Narrative approaches are based not in psychologizing but in story-telling, something which everyone, from every culture, probably does. In fact, narrative approaches may be more applicable across cultures than other approaches (Bilu & Witztum, 1993; Howard, 1991). Narrative is not restricted to words: dance, music or graphic art may have a narrative and these may be more appropriate media for psychotherapy for some people.

Caleb Garth may have been someone who responded better to the impersonal narrative of music than to the analysis of character which he left to his wife and best-loved daughter, Mary. However, had he been prompted by one of them to seek psychotherapy – as he was prompted occasionally to talk to Mr Farebrother – he would have been unfortunate indeed to be assessed by a psychotherapist who mistook his lack of psychological mindedness for unsuitability for therapy. Despite his lack of articulacy, or rather his distrust of articulacy, Caleb has a strong narrative awareness that can be put into words. At one point he says to his wife, apropos of the inheritance that is one of the major sub-plots of the novel, 'The ins and outs of things are curious. Here is the land they've been all along expecting for Fred, which it seems the old man never meant to leave him a foot of, but left it to this side-slip of a son that he kept in the dark, and thought of his sticking there and vexing everybody as well as he could have vexed 'em himself if he could have kept alive . . . The soul of man, when it gets fairly rotten, will bear you all sorts of poisonous toad-stools, and no eye can see whence came the seed thereof'.

What George Eliot was observing through Caleb was that, as Caleb's story was consistent and unswerving, the same in the small details as in the big, so the story of Mr Featherstone was convoluted and its real meaning was hidden. Caleb's story is as coherent as Mr Featherstone's is incoherent.

Coherence and distress

One possible conception of long-term psychotherapy is that it is, like the *USS Endeavour*, only motivated by one mission: 'to boldly go where none has gone before'. Or rather, it is to increase the coherence of a person's life-story by bringing into it events and experiences which have remained unincorporated, or 'warded off' to use Stiles's term (1999). Sigmund Freud's famous dictum, 'Wo Es war soll Ich werden' ('Where It was I will become'), refers to something similar.

One of the strongest influences that prevents this happening is distress, as both clinical and empirical studies show. An example of the latter is a study of 90 children aged from 2 to13 years who were treated for injury in a casualty department (emergency room). The children who were more distressed produced less coherent accounts, and made fewer evaluations of the impact of the trauma (Peterson & Biggs, 1998). Another study, this time of 157 victims of violent assault, found that 19% of the victims had an acute stress disorder after 1 month and many of them had gone on to develop post-traumatic stress syndrome at 6 months. However, victims were more likely to develop long-term stress disorder if their level of anxiety remained high and, instead of being able to process their experience, they continued to relive it in its raw form, re-experiencing it as if it was happening again rather than remembering it (Brewin et al., 1999).

Narrating events coherently may be essential for us to make sense of them, but it involves re-experiencing some of the distress of the events themselves. It can only be done if we are prepared to tolerate rather than avoid the distress, and if we are secure enough not to be overwhelmed by it. The therapist can help the client to be able to do this by providing a secure setting and a secure relationship.

Some of the important ways that the therapist can accomplish this security are shown in Table 10.1. Many of them will vary between cultures. For example, being alone with the therapist is important for many westerners who experience other people as potentially threatening. People from other cultures might experience being alone with just one other person as more threatening than being with more than one other person even if these are people who drop in and out of the therapeutic setting.

The unspoken and the unspeakable

Long-term person-centered counselling or psychotherapy, mediation, and some types of group therapy, are therapeutic mainly because they provide a therapeutic situation in which distress can be contained and so enable matters to be spoken about which would otherwise remain unspoken. It is assumed that this will result in their incorporation into the narrative of the counselling or psychotherapy session, and therefore into the client's life-story.

Case example (from Taylor, 1999)
Laura and Tim both worked in the editorial team of a journal. Shortly after Laura started with them, the team went for an after-work drink and Laura and Tim shared a taxi on the way home. Tim made a pass, which Laura rebuffed. The following day, Tim apologized, and the day after that, and the day after that. Laura felt that Tim's apologies were worse than the original pass. She became increasingly anxious around Tim, and the atmosphere in the office deteriorated. Eventually Laura decided to move to another team in the same firm. However,

Table 10.1. Factors to maintain the security of the client within a therapeutic relationship

Giving the client either autonomy (especially important in western world) or trust in beneficence	A therapeutic culture in which the client's concerns are never dismissed
	Confidentiality
	Negotiating significant changes in the relationship
	Collaborative style
	Warnings of changes
Maintaining stability within the relationship	Minimizing therapist absence
	In group psychotherapy, ensuring slow and predictable turnover of group members
Maintaining the setting	Invariant setting
	Comfortable, non-threatening
	Suitable for its purpose
	Minimizing intrusion or threat
Ensuring that the client does not have to protect themselves against exploitation or social sanction as a result of therapy	No outside relationships between the client and the therapist or, in the case of group therapy, between other group members outside the group
	No financial dependence of the client on the therapist or of the therapist on the client
	No sexual relations between the client and the therapist
	The therapist makes arrangements to ensure that he or she does not become emotionally over-involved with the client
Keeping time boundaries	Meeting for a specified time, and sticking to it (neither too short, nor too long)

The therapist's ability to function	Therapist maintains, in the face of anxiety or other negative emotional atmosphere:
	    interest
	    positive attitude
	    creativity

she was unhappy there and she began to feel aggrieved by Tim's behaviour, which now seemed to her like harassment. She went to see the firm's ombudsman.

The ombudsman thought that 'The first step toward finding a resolution of the conflict is to discover what Laura truly wants'. Laura said that she wanted to be able to cross Tim's path without feeling distress. The ombudsman thought that Laura was not the only one who was distressed, but that Tim was too, and so were the other members of staff whom Laura had invited to take sides against Tim. In fact, the ombudsman concluded that 'The common thread running through everyone's interests is the alleviation of anxiety'. The ombudsman proposed a 'facilitated discussion' between Tim and Laura, and they met in the ombudsman's office.

Tim and Laura were each given the opportunity to give their version of events, without interruption. Laura told Tim how helpless he made her feel. Tim told Laura that she was making him out to be a sociopath, and asked why she hated him so. The atmosphere in the meeting became very tense.

The ombudsman felt this, and took some time to collect her thoughts. She then said that she recognized that both Tim and Laura felt shame and guilt, and that both, too, had tried to be as open as they could towards each other. She asked them what they wanted from each other, trying to sound as calm and at ease as she could. Tim wanted to hear Laura say that she had fully accepted his apology. Laura conceded that she had not been as unequivocal about her acceptance of Tim's apology as she might have been, but now she could say that she had fully accepted it. However, Laura wanted Tim to acknowledge that his repeated apologies, far from helping her, had constantly reminded her of the tension between them. Tim half accepted this. Both agreed that they could now work with each other again without too much difficulty. A week later, Laura rang the ombudsman to say that she was leaving the company because she had now realized that she did not really want to work on technical journals. She would prefer to be an editor in a mainstream book publisher.

This is an example of the creation of a containing situation in which both Tim and Laura can express what they had not been able to before. As they did so, their own narratives of the events causing their conflict became more coherent. Laura recognized that she had been equivocal, and Tim that he had been more concerned with his peace of mind than with Laura's.

Long-term psychotherapy often consists of a series of re-narrations of episodes like these, each narration, although only a paragraph or a page of the person's life-story, subtly increasing the coherence of that story. Each time that a comparable episode is narrated, it has been changed by the previous telling, and the reception that telling got. Each of these small increments of change adds up to an eventual substantial narrative shift.

It was the first session of a group-analytic group. There was a heavy silence in the beginning, and then Charles said, 'I wonder how many of us are here because of our mothers'. Arlene looked angry, and then tearful although it would be several weeks before the group discovered that she had experienced this comment of Charles as an attack on her. Bill said, 'God, yes. My mother always wanted rid of me. She would beat me as easily as she would feed me'. The group were duly horrified, and expressed sympathy and concern.

In the eighth week of the group, Arlene spoke about her regret that she once lost control with her youngest child, and hit him 'harder than I care to admit'. Bill said, 'I remember an occasion when my mother hit me. I suppose she was under a lot of stress at the time. My father was in hospital, and she had three of us to take care of. On this one day, she just seemed to snap. She rounded on me, and hit me as hard as she could with a brush that she was carrying. It knocked me over, and then she hit me again'.

Between sessions 10 and 20, Bill was quite often taken to task for not listening to other group members, especially the female members of the group. 'It's as if you don't think we are worth as much consideration as you', one of them said. Arlene said, 'You don't seem to have any depth to you. You're just like a two-dimensional man'. Bill said, 'I think that people should be true to themselves, and not get so influenced by other people's opinions. I've never bothered much with what other people think of me, so long as I know that I'm doing the right thing'.

In session 28, Bill again remembered the beating by his mother. He said to Yvette, 'Something about what you just said, about being the death of your mother, made me think about this time when my mother beat me. She was very tired, I remember, and I hated her for it. I felt that she was only tired because she was worrying so much about my father, and not enough about me. I can't exactly remember what happened, but something triggered her off. Oh yes, I do remember. I did something that I knew would upset her. I got my father's clothes out of the wardrobe – I suppose that I was trying them on – but I got angry that they didn't fit and I threw them around a bit. Well, quite a lot actually. One of his shirts got torn. Then she came in, and instead of apologizing, I started to laugh. I suppose she couldn't stand that, so she lashed out at me. I laughed even more. I thought, ''Now I've got a reaction out of you'''.

In Bill's last session in the group, he said that he had visited his mother, whom the group knew was in an old people's home. They had started to talk about his childhood, and had reminisced about various good, and bad, times. She had talked about the time that she had hit him with a brush. 'I wanted to be able to share my distress with you so much, Bill', she had said, 'but you had gone all cold and unkind. I knew I had to get through to you or we would both go mad. I hit you as hard as I could and I wanted you to cry because then I could hold you. You just laughed, and I hit you again. I felt terrible, and I started crying myself. And then you cried, too. We clung to each other. I don't know what you felt, but I felt the strength to carry on creeping back into me. You have meant so much to me.' Bill became increasingly tearful during this recital. Then he said to the group, 'You've had to beat me, too, sometimes. But I hope that's because I've meant something to you'.

As Bill becomes more secure and accepted in the group, so his narrative about his past becomes more coherent. As his narration and re-narration of the paradigmatic episode of his mother's violence towards him shows, the character of his mother becomes more and more clearly delineated, and his own character is described in an increasingly complex way.

In the process, previously hidden sources of distress become revealed. Bill was obviously rivalrous with his father, and distressed that he could not carry off wearing his clothes. Bill had declared himself unconcerned about how other people regarded him in the middle phase of the group, but his worry about this had become clear by the time he felt ready to leave. The increasing security that Bill felt in the group not only enabled him to say things that he would normally have kept to himself, but it allowed him to speak about himself in a new way, to say what had previously been unspeakable.

Why is some therapy long-term?

Bill did not remember more and more details of his beating by his mother just because he was feeling less anxious. It was also possible for him to accept his own jealousy of his father, his angry rejection of his mother, and his reckless destruction of his father's shirt. All of these memories were so unpalatable to him previously that he had simply left them out of his life-story. The result was that Bill had seemed a very shallow character. As one of the group members had put it, in an early group session, Bill had been 'the original two-dimensional man'.

When someone has a problem like Bill's it affects all their relationships, including those with a therapist. Bill may have sought therapy originally for a number of reasons, but whatever they were, Bill would have also been unhappy with his life – hence the title of this chapter. However, Bill and other people who enter long-term therapy have a particular kind of unhappiness. They are not unhappy because others are oppressing them, but because they are unable to make and keep close personal relationships which give them satisfaction. When so much of what other people say and do seems unpalatable, then a person is unable to have a close relationship with anyone.

Many surveys of the public have shown that, at least in the West, the quality of relationships (Reis & Franks, 1994), especially love relationships at least for young people (Campbell, Sedikides & Bosson, 1994), is one of the most important determinants of quality of life.

This chapter is therefore also about gaining and maintaining intimacy with others – usually, but not always, other people.

The reader will have spotted that there is a particular difficulty about this. Up to now it has been possible to assume, with a little latitude, that the client considers the therapist to be their ally. Collaboration has been one of the major themes of previous chapters, and many of the approaches that have been described have relied on it. We cannot do this in this chapter. Whilst the therapist will still aim for collaboration with a client like Bill, he or she should not expect it. Bill or his counterpart is likely to find the therapist to be just as unpalatable as any other person. Indeed, there will be times when the client may regard the therapist as an enemy. There may also be times when the client seems to the therapist to be inappropriately attracted to the therapist.

By far the most influential approach to understanding this situation has been that promoted by psycho-analysis, and derived from Freud and Breuer's confrontation with a client who changed their lives, Bertha Pappenheimer (referred to as 'Anna O.' in the published case histories).

There is no doubt in my mind that irrational affection, hatred or other very intimate emotions develop between clients and therapists, particularly in longer-term psychotherapy. However, as the reader will discover later, I share, with other psychotherapists who are sceptical about psycho-analytic theory (Deurzen, 1997), doubts about the explanations that are routinely given for these phenomena.

The two concepts which Freud developed to understand Anna O., and subsequent clients, were termed by him, 'resistance' and 'transference'. These concepts have become so entrenched in psychotherapy, counselling and mental health that they are taken as incontrovertible by many. Questions about them feature, for example, in an examination set by the Royal College of Psychiatrists. I do not think that this book would be complete if the psycho-analytic account of these irrational phenomena was omitted, but it would also be incomplete if alternative explanations were not considered.

I shall try to summarize 'resistance' and 'transference' as fairly as possible in the next sections, and this will mean withholding critical comment for the time being. The reader should remember, however, that summarizing the theory is not the same as agreeing with it, and I shall propose an alternative approach later in this chapter.

Resistance

One of the important discoveries made by the nineteenth century hypnotists was that some people seemed to resist being put into a hypnoid state. In fact, it appears that an inability to be hypnotized is a more common cause of the failure of hypnosis than is resistance (Spinhoven et al., 1993). However, Breuer and Freud (1950) took over the term 'resistance' to apply to the resistance to change that they noted in the clients with psychological problems that they were treating, firstly with hypnosis and later with Freud's emerging technique of free-association. The striking way in which resistance seemed to present itself to Freud was one of the factors that led him to develop a theory of intrapsychic conflict, and repression of unconscious impulses.

It has since been pointed out that resistance to change in beliefs is a general reaction to new beliefs rather than a reflection of specific beliefs having a specially strong anchorage in the unconscious. It has the valuable side-effect that a person can hold stable beliefs. Resistance can also be attributed to social influence. However, what Freud was struck by was the extreme nature of resistance, for example the flat denial of what should have been manifestly true. Freud noted that resistance tended to increase as therapy progressed. Indeed, the true work of psycho-analysis seemed to be to overcome this resistance.

Resistance is a military metaphor which accords well with the territorial metaphor of the boundary around the self. It summons up a picture of a beleaguered city, its boundary walls thronged with defenders staving off scaling ladders. Why don't the defenders give up? Some may fight to follow orders, to defend their women and children from a fate worse than the death of the male member of the family. Some may even fight for honour or glory or habit. But more often than not, cities have fought to retain their identity. And, as already noted, this identity is strongly linked with the retention of the existing boundary. Being besieged, having one's identity threatened, and resistance, are strongly linked for the individual too.

The city metaphor appealed to Freud. He imagined psychological mechanisms inside all of us which corresponded to the different bureaux of government. He served as a doctor in the Austrian army and so it was natural to imagine a mental censor which corresponded to the army officer who read and censored his mail.

Freud initially speculated that people could not benefit from the therapist's interventions because they were unable to follow the therapist's instructions to play the word association game without censoring some of the words that came to them. Later, Freud speculated that resistance had stronger origins than this. One of these, Freud thought, was transference.

Transference

Transference is Freud's term for the situation that he thought typically develops in therapy ('the transference neurosis'). The client begins to behave in ways which are characteristic of him or her, rather than in ways which are appropriate to the current situation. As the standard dictionary of psycho-analytic terms has it (Laplanche & Pontalis, 1973), there is a 'process of actualization of unconscious wishes. Transference uses specific objects and operates in the framework of a specific relationship with those objects' (1973, p. 455).

Wilhelmina was a middle-aged woman who was often cross and put out. She could never say, 'no', and could never tell anyone that they were being unreasonable or asking too much. She was rarely late for her therapy sessions, so when she was very late one day, the therapist brought it up. Wilhelmina said that she knew that the therapist would tell her off, but she just couldn't help it. She'd had such a terrible headache, she didn't know how she had come at all. The therapist said that he wasn't cross, just curious. Wilhelmina said that she appreciated the efforts that the therapist was taking not to be critical, but that she, Wilhelmina, knew that the therapist was angry and indeed she knew that she was entitled to be. Wilhelmina went on to explain, 'I haven't been a good client. I told my friend that you were . . . you were . . . having trouble with me. My friend said, that's unusual. I've never known you to criticize anyone. I felt so guilty afterwards. I know you try your best. It's just that I was feeling a bit down that day. Don't get angry with me. I didn't mean to hurt your feelings'. The therapist said, 'It's only too true. I don't think that I have helped you very much', but Wilhelmina wasn't listening.

Wilhelmina was very used to being criticized, particularly for getting angry. Perhaps she had parents who couldn't stand her anger. Perhaps she had experienced this intolerance of anger in later life. Whatever the reason, Wilhelmina had become increasingly inexperienced in feeling angry, and was inclined to think that any assertion would be interpreted as unacceptable aggression. It seemed, too, that Wilhelmina made little differentiation between people when it came to being critical of her. She seemed to assume, for example, that the therapist would be critical even when he was not feeling that way at all. The therapist assumed that Wilhelmina's reactions to him were typical of her reactions to everyone, and that her experiences of an earlier critical figure were transferred onto any person with whom she was currently dealing, and whom she would assume was criticizing her even when this was not the intention. The therapist, who had read the definition of transference by Laplanche and Pontalis given above, thought that Wilhelmina had an unconscious wish to be angry, and this became the focal point of many of her relationships as a result. Moreover, the therapist also had an interest in the revisions of Freudian theory produced by Melanie Klein and other object-relations theorists. He therefore thought that Wilhelmina created a critical attitude in others in order to make a specific kind of relationship with them. This relationship was one in which the other person made more and more demands on Wilhelmina which she felt forced to meet, in order to avoid being criticized.

The therapist termed this relationship a 'projective identification'. He thought that it was the basis of the relationship between himself and Wilhelmina, which he called a 'transference relationship' or, when he wanted to hark back to Freud, a 'transference neurosis'. He thought of Wilhelmina relieving her own feelings of anger, by getting herself into a position where she could say to herself that other people were unreasonable or bad, and that she was good. Other people took, and she gave, the therapist imagined her thinking. When he had his more radical Kleinian hat on, the therapist imagined Wilhelmina having a sort of swamp of angry feelings somewhere inside her, in her unconscious he would say. This swamp festered inside Wilhelmina but, so the therapist imagined, she could at least partially drain it by projecting its 'primitive contents' into his mind. This made sense to him because he often came home with a headache after seeing Wilhelmina, and quite often got irrationally angry with someone on the way.

The therapist's understanding of Wilhelmina is consistent with psychoanalytic theory. Psycho-analysts think of the transference as the client perceiving the therapist in the light of what Laplanche and Pontalis term 'infantile prototypes', which emerge with a 'strong sensation of immediacy' (1973, p. 455). It is supposed that these prototypes – which may be abnormally positive or idealizing, or abnormally negative or hostile – emerge in relation to other people, too, and when they do, they disrupt any close relationships that a person might be developing with them.

Transference is the most important analytic explanation of why a person's close relationships might go wrong. Wilhelmina (or some person like Wilhelmina) would, or so a psycho-analyst would say, be unable to react to other people as they really are, but would impose on them a template which was formed by Wilhelmina's early childhood experience. A similar conception has been introduced into cognitive therapy by one of its founding fathers, Tim Beck, himself once a psycho-analytic candidate. Cognitive therapists emphasize that this template is a cognitive one, a 'schema'. The psychoanalytic conception is that it is a disposition to re-enact a particular relationship, and so is more than having beliefs about another person, but also includes characteristic emotions and ways of communicating.

This template, Freud suggests, is formed by the actual relationships that a very young child has with his or her caregivers, particularly during the Oedipal period. This period, from about the age of 3 years to about the age of 5 years is a period of rapid social change for many western children, who generally start school at some time between these ages. If there is to be a younger sibling, its birth will most commonly also occur during this time. It is also a period of rapid cognitive development, with the child developing a sense of themselves as a distinct person. One consequence of the social changes during this period is that any exclusivity of the child's relationship with his or her mother becomes attenuated. Freud chose the term 'Oedipal period' for the reasons that have already been discussed in Chapter 7, which were, in brief, that he assumed that the exclusive relationship was an erotic one, that it was attenuated by the father demanding his conjugal rights, and that the child wanted to kill his (and perhaps her) father in retaliation.

Klein and the object-relations theorists (Greenberg & Mitchell, 1983) put the crisis back by several years, suggesting that it dated from a much earlier period in the child's life, when he or she began to realize that the mother, or the carer, was not perfect. This, Klein supposed, began to be a problem when the child was about 3 months old, when the child did not just cry with the pangs of hunger or the discomfort of an irritated perineum, but cried to get the carer to come and deal with him. The child was then able to know when the carer did not come, even though called. This was a moment of crisis in parent–child relations that Klein thought was even more important than a third person interposing themselves between the child and his or her carer during the Oedipal period. As in the Oedipal period, the child experienced rage.

Klein (1946) speculated that, at this stage, the rage was not with the carer because the child did not yet have knowledge of the carer as a complete person. It was therefore with 'the breast', this term to be taken rather broadly to mean the comforter that the child wanted. Sometimes, Klein thought, the breast would be good and deserving of love, and sometimes it would be absent, or 'bad' and deserving of attack. Normally, Klein speculated, the child would come to realize that there was one breast and one carer, and that a breast just needed to be 'good enough', to use a memorable phrase coined by Winnicott (1965), one of Klein's analysands.

Transference, to a therapist of a Freudian persuasion, means that the client assumes a relationship with the therapist that is more in keeping with the client's previous experience than with the actuality of the therapist. However, it is still a relationship that the client has. A therapist of an object-relations persuasion considers transference to apply to a situation in which the client does not have a rounded relationship with the therapist at all, but sometimes treats the therapist like a 'bad breast' and sometimes like a good one. There is, to use another term introduced by Klein, 'splitting' of the therapist into two part-people, one hostile and one seductive.

The relationship with these part-people is described by Klein as 'projective identification'. Laplanche and Pontalis define projection as 'an operation whereby qualities, feelings, wishes or even "objects" . . . are expelled from the self and located in another person or thing' (1973, p. 349). What Klein speculated was that the child relates to the breast, and the Kleinian patient relates to the 'bad therapist' or the 'good therapist' not as an autonomous person, but as a receptacle. The baby, or the client, it is supposed, projects either good or bad feelings into this receptacle depending on whether the baby, or the client, feels satisfied or frustrated. But if enough feeling is projected, the baby, or the client, considers that the receptacle is an extension of themself. The baby, or the client, identifies the receptacle as part of him- or herself. This kind of transference relationship is not a relationship at all, but a sort of ownership. The client owns the therapist, as Klein imagines the baby owns the carer, because the baby, or the baby-like client, does not recognize that another person owns themself. If he or she has 'projected' something of themself into another person, and that other person has no owner, well he or she has squatter's rights.

Erica was seen by many as rather bossy, although there were many other endearing traits in her character that made her friends overlook this. She had a very bossy father, and it seems likely that she acquired her bossiness from him, although Erica would have said that she had spent her life trying to be the exact opposite of her father. Erica was happy that she had achieved this. She had harmonious relationships with her colleagues at work, until a new boss was appointed. This was a highly ambitious woman, who had a brief to introduce various new methods of record-keeping and time management in the department where Erica worked.

As soon as Erica met her, the chemistry seemed wrong. The new boss, whose name was Celia, had not worked at this level of authority previously. She was determined to be fair and respectful, but she was also determined – indeed, perhaps rather over-determined – not to allow herself to be pushed around by any of the previous staff. Senior management had given Celia to understand that they thought that this department had become a little set in its ways, and Celia thought of herself as giving it a bit of a shake up.

Erica wanted to argue, to say that the department was already very efficient. Celia would have none of it, and Erica began to feel very primitive. Her fingers itched and she felt that she would like to slap Celia, and tell her that she was a spoilt child who had been given too much authority. That evening, Erica could not stop thinking about Celia and about how impotent Celia made her feel. Celia became a sort of obsession. When Erica met Celia, or as soon as she got a message from her, Erica would shake and get palpitations. Celia had become an emotor of impotence and frustration. Erica's view of this was that Celia was a natural bully, that her character contained more than its right share of authoritarianism. Erica forgot that it was she that wanted to attack Celia when they first met. By the time that Erica discussed all of this with her therapist, Celia had become an almost inhuman figure, part-bully, part-idiot.

The Kleinian way of looking at this situation is that Erica had projected her own aggression onto Celia. It was a kind of projective identification because Erica credited Celia not just with feelings but with a character trait – dominance.

Issues raised by transference

Most psychotherapists who work long-term with clients will have experienced episodes when they believe that the client is no longer reacting to them in a 'real' way. It is as if the client was with someone else, in another situation, and in another time. These 'catastrophic reactions' were first mentioned in Chapter 5. The reader will have been left in no doubt in that chapter that I, like many of my colleagues, are convinced by my own experience that catastrophic reactions do occur and that Freud and Breuer made a significant contribution to psychology when they described them.

Some research evidence also exists to demonstrate that particular people have characteristic catastrophic reactions. Luborsky and his research group have developed measures of the 'core conflictual relationship theme', and have shown that recurrent themes can be found in both children and adults. Resolving them is linked to a good outcome of psycho-analytic psychotherapy (Luborsky & Crits-Christoph, 1998).

However, Freud's assumption that catastrophic transference reactions are due to fixed schemata of interpersonal reactions which are the result of childhood experience has had many critics. Its assumption that there is a stable self has already been questioned in Chapter 4. The assumption that childhood events have a disproportionately large effect on adult relationships does not seem consistent with research that shows that more recent events have more impact than more remote ones (Blanz et al., 1990; Rutter, 1980).

An early criticism of transference was that catastrophic reactions are the product of the abnormal situation of psycho-analysis itself (Macalpine, 1950). This would not be a bad thing if what the analytic situation did was to uncover existing, but hidden, infantile relationship tendencies, which is what practising psycho-analysts would argue that it does. It would, however, undermine the psycho-analytic position if the analytic situation created these tendencies, rather than uncovered them.

Whether catastrophic reactions are caused by a person's inability to face reality or by an unbearable interpersonal situation in which they find themself in is not merely a matter of theoretical interest.

Herman and Sid have been living together for a long time. Recently, there has been a coldness between them. Matters come to a head one Friday evening. Sid says, 'Herman, I don't want to have a row but, let's face it, you're hardly at home in the evenings any more. You seem to have more and more reasons to stay at the office and work. As I say, I don't want to row, or be critical or anything, but you're obviously angry with me about something. What is it?'. Despite Sid's protestations, Herman does feel that he is being accused. His strategies might include: suggesting that they should just be good friends and that the problem will sort itself out; denying that he has been coming home from work any later; appeasing Sid by offering to cook his favourite supper; or holding his chest and asking Sid to stop because he (Herman) has chest pain and thinks that he may be having a heart attack.

Sid, if he were sufficiently riled, might brand the first strategy as avoidance and the second as denial. The third strategy might strike Sid as a deeper kind of duplicity, and he might be inclined to tell Herman that he always covers up his anger by a show of kindness. In the case of the chest pain, Sid might be diverted from his path but, if he was really angry and had already been exposed to Herman's chest pain before, Sid might say that the pain was due to anxiety and was not physical, but psychological, in origin.

Herman might challenge Sid on all of these points, perhaps by asserting that Sid could always see other people's faults, but not his own . . . but let's draw a veil over the further progress of what promises to be a childish and somehow embarrassing squabble. Such squabbles are common between intimate partners. *Ad hominem* criticisms like 'avoidance' or 'denial' are typical of them. They serve the purpose of either vitiating or confirming one or other partner's account of the difficulty. They are not intended to teach the other person about themself, although they may infrequently have that effect. They are intended to position one or other partner as the aggrieved party.

As noted in Chapters 3 and 5, conflicts about identity are much more intractable than conflicts about issues. Sid chooses to deal with his loneliness not by attributing it to Herman's situation – that he has to work long hours – but by supposing that Herman has chosen to work so late. And from having taken this tack, it is a short step to both Herman and Sid discussing each other's psychological identity, i.e. their characters.

Professional etiquette normally restrains mental health professionals from voicing their attributions of bad character to clients, even when they covertly make them. Psychotherapists do not have such scruples. If Glenys says that she is late for the session because her car broke down, her psycho-analytically orientated psychotherapist may challenge her and ask if there is perhaps another reason, for example that Glenys wanted to avoid voicing the frustration that she was feeling about her lack of improvement. In fact, psycho-analytic psychotherapists have compiled lists of 'defences' which people might use to disguise their real motives. So well established are these lists that they are often taught to psychotherapy trainees as 'mental mechanisms'.

Making an attribution to character and not situation positions the person so impugned into the role of accused: not only are they supposed to be using defences, they are put on the defensive. The person who makes the attribution is safe, at least if they succeed in imposing their view of the matter, because the problem is now entirely attributed to the other person's shortcomings. However, their safety is at the cost of a substantial increase in the insecurity of the accused.

Clearly, an unscrupulous bully could use these tactics to maintain his dominance over someone else who was less psychologically minded than himself. Most mental health professionals assume that they are not motivated by a need to dominate their clients, although this view is not held by all commentators (Szasz, 1988). But psychotherapists can be bullies, just like everyone else who is in a position of power over others. The only protection for us and our clients is to face up to any tendencies that we may have to authoritarianism. How this difficult task might be managed is discussed in the next chapter.

Attributing an interpersonal difficulty to a person's character has another effect on the relationship with that other person. It makes the difficulty into an identity issue. This may make the conflict harder to manage. Even more seriously, it runs the risk of provoking a catastrophic reaction (see Chapter 5). But, as Sid might have said of Herman, if it is an identity issue, then this has to be faced. If Herman does have a problem about avoiding conflict, and consistently does this, then Sid and Herman might be able to work out a more enduring solution to their difficulties if they look at this.

Which justifications are justified?

There is no objective reality to which either Herman or Sid can appeal in order to show which of them is right. Nor can the psychotherapist appeal to an objective authority. Contrary to what Freud claimed, psycho-analysis is not an empirical science. It cannot rightfully claim that psychotherapists observe psychic realities (Grunbaum, 1986). Nor is prior experience an incontrovertible claim. The philosopher of science, Popper, demonstrates this in a vignette illustrating the fallacies of arguments by induction (Popper, 1963).

The vignette is drawn from Popper's own experience of doing voluntary counselling under the supervision of Freud's pupil, Adler. One day, Popper went to Adler with a particularly troublesome case. Popper asked Adler what he should do. Adler said that it was straightforward. He knew a thousand cases like it. Popper should do . . . and here Adler made specific recommendations. According to Popper, Adler did not ask him how these recommendations had turned out but, observes Popper wryly, he supposed that at some future time, Adler might say to another supervisee: 'That's easy. I've known 1001 cases. This is what you should do . . .'.

What Sid was doing when he told Herman that he was avoiding showing anger, and what the psychotherapist is doing when he or she makes a transference interpretation, is supplying a reason for a person's action. The difference between reasons, and their contribution to a humanistic science, and causes, and their relationship to empirical evidence in the material sciences, was extensively discussed in Chapter 1. It was indicated there that reasons have to be justified rather than proven.

Another term for the kind of reasons under discussion is 'attribution' (Heider). An attribution is an effort to 'predict and control the world by assigning transient behavior to relatively unchanging dispositions'

(Heider, 1963, p. 79). People can, and do, make external attributions, to situations rather than personal dispositions, but are less likely to do so. External dispositions are more likely to be made about oneself, and about other people, only if they seem constrained by circumstances.

Attribution theory suggests that people are more ready to make internal attributions, to a person's character, when something has gone wrong. The theory also suggests that people are more likely to be assumed not to have tried hard enough (rather than been unable), and that they have been trying to get something for themselves (rather than trying to avoid loss). Finally, people are blamed more if something has happened to them that we fear could happen to ourselves.

What should we make of resistance and transference?

The concepts of resistance and transference are so important to many approaches to long-term therapy that it is worth restating some of the conclusions in the previous section.

Almost all practising therapists in my experience recognize that their clients are not like the clients of accountants or bank managers. They do not just come for guidance, accept it if it seems good, and make the necessary changes. Their clients resist change even as they say how much they want it. There is an inherent resistance to change in all of us that can partly be explained by the normal tenacity of convictions and the ingrained nature of habits. However, there are times, especially times when therapists feel frustrated, when clients seem to oppose change out of self-destructiveness.

Freud and other psycho-analysts have explained this on the basis of opposing instincts: a rational one of self-preservation, and an irrational one of desire. Sometimes desire goes against self-preservation. In addition, Klein introduced the notion that a person may be more strongly motivated by anger with someone else, anger which might be communicated by withholding or by self-destructiveness, than by a wish to preserve themselves. There are good reasons for being suspicious of these explanations. They posit a split mind, they equate conscious decision-making with the good and the emotions with danger, and they assume that speculation about infant behaviour can explain adults' behaviour. Even more importantly, they make it likely that the frustrations of a client are going to be attributed to the client's own personal history, rather than to the here-and-now situation.

However, Freud, Klein and others have discovered characteristics of catastrophic reactions which had not been previously noted. People do seem to behave towards others as if they own the other person sometimes. People do split, one day being kind and another day being critical for no apparent reason. And, a person may be more inclined to see the shortcoming in someone else that everyone else sees in him or her.

- Freud's basic intuitions – that there is a resistance to change, and that something strange often happens in long-term therapy which results in the client seeming to enter a disturbing unreal world – would be upheld by many therapists.
- Resistance reflects the dual basis of change. Change happens because a person changes how he/she think about the world, and also because the emotional meaning of the world changes. Changing emotional meaning requires new emotional experience to transform the old. In longer-term therapy especially, and when a person wants to make more fulfilling relationships and to be happier, changing emotional meaning is what therapy is mainly about.
- Unreality in therapy, which I am calling a 'catastrophic reaction', is brought about when the client's identity is being threatened. When this happens, a person can no longer make sense of the world, because their narrative capacity is called into question.
- Since a change in identity may be what the client wants, many therapists would also believe that such catastrophic relationship shifts are opportunities for change as well as being potentially destructive to the therapy itself.
- Transference affects therapists as well as clients.
- Transference is associated with great insecurity, and people who are in the grip of it are very vulnerable. There is a risk that they can be exploited. Attribution theory indicates how easy it is to blame people rather than see people as labouring under various limitations. It is easy to overlook the contribution of the therapeutic situation to transference. It also easy to distance oneself from the person in the grip of transference by attributing self-seeking motives to him or her, when the person is actually trying to defend him- or herself against catastrophe.
- It seems unlikely that there are pockets of childish reaction patterns that are untouched by subsequent experience until they are evoked during transference. Transference reactions are probably determined most often by recent experience, although that will have been affected by earlier experience, and that by earlier experience, and so on, back to childhood.
- There are patterns in catastrophic reactions and these can sometimes be attributed to the client's self narrative. A split narrative is likely to lead to 'splitting' and 'projective identification' in relating to others, for example.
- People may be unaware of their contribution to relationship problems. This is particularly important when close relationships go wrong, and in understanding the difficulties that sometimes arise in longer-term therapy. But it does not mean that there is a hidden chamber of the mind in which our animal nature is kept safely contained. We do not need to posit an unconscious to explain unawareness.

An alternative account of resistance and transference

In the remainder of this chapter, I shall consider an alternative account of the phenomena discussed in the previous section. This account will consider catastrophic reactions not as the activation of infantile prototypes, as Laplanche and Pontalis described transference reactions in a previously quoted passage, but as responses to a challenge to the 'me' and to the 'I' of the client. I will argue that resistance in its milder forms is a response to a challenge to a person's self narrative, to their 'me'. But transference reactions are a response to a challenge to a person's 'I'. I shall assume that these challenges are associated with characteristic emotions: anxiety, in the case of a challenge to 'me', and shame or self-disgust, in the case of a challenge to 'I'. Finally, I shall argue that the coherence of a person's narrative will determine his or her response. What Freud called 'Oedipal' transference reactions, in which a person continues to make a relationship even if it is strained, are descriptions of how a person who has a coherent self narrative responds to shame. What Kleinians attribute to 'part-person' transference reactions are how I suppose someone will react if an already incoherent account of themself is vitiated by shame and the capacity to relate breaks down altogether.

This story suggests that working with shame is a much more important part of long-term psychotherapy than is commonly thought to be the case. Perhaps because psychotherapists have not been prepared to address shame directly, they have often omitted another element in human relationships, often very much tied in with shame. I am referring to deception. Psychotherapists will often assume that a person cannot help acting as they do, and the capacity to relate breaks down altogether because they are under the influence of an unconscious motive, but they are very reluctant to address the possibility that a person acts as they do with the intention to deceive. Self-deception is a special case of deception. It, too, may be shameful because it may indicate that a person is not putting sufficient effort into reviewing their reasons for acting, or is too self-indulgent in how they conduct this review.

Interpreting the unconscious: trumping the ace

Attributing motives to peoples' actions or feelings is what therapists do when they make interpretations. In Chapter 8, I cited the story of Jusuf and the youth who dreamt that he was carrying bread on his head, and birds swooping down and flying off with it. Jusuf interpreted the dream at the youth's request. Unhappily, Jusuf divined that it predicted the youth's beheading.

Jusuf was credited with having the divine power to see revealed what was hidden by others, and this was the power that Freud was claiming for psycho-analytic adherents. It continues to be the account that many psycho-therapists give of interpretation to this day. They feel the force come on them and they see revealed the hidden meaning of their clients' actions. In some ways, this account is more attractive than the alternative, painting-by-numbers, version. According to this, the therapist has a kind of cerebral code-book from which to read off the meanings of what he or she has been told.

The reader may remember that many objections to the validity, and to the value, of interpretations were considered in Chapter 8. One virtue remained – that interpretations are an effective means of dealing with anxiety. But, is this an unduly negative account? It does seem that many of the examples given in this chapter are of people who are unaware of the motives for their actions until other people point them out. Surely, this justifies the therapist interpreting motives for their client's actions, if the client seems not to be aware of them. The therapist who has been convinced by the arguments in Chapter 8 would not assert that these were the only reasons, or that they knew the truth about why the client acted in that way, or that there could be no other account of the client's actions. However, given these various caveats, surely it is justified to provide the client with feedback about what other people can see, even if the client cannot.

Jusuf certainly does not seem to be a good role model in this post-modern age. He thought that he knew the only truth worth having about his client's dream. But a less assertive therapist, one who is ready to co-construct an account with the client, is providing a very different kind of intervention. Or is he?

As a result of the constant bickering between himself and Herman, Sid went into psycho-analysis. 'After all', he thought, 'perhaps it is me'. The only effect that Herman noticed straight away was that Sid was now inclined to make interpretations. He would now say to Herman, 'I know that you think that you're working hard to get promotion, and that would be better for both of us, but unconsciously you're working so hard to please your father. I'm not criticizing you. I'm sure you're trying to do the right thing. But your boss isn't your father. I don't suppose he'll promote you just because you work long hours'. Herman found this sort of interpretation infuriating. It didn't matter that Sid was obviously trying to be kind and to avoid being critical. It was the superiority that it assumed that made him mad. Although he did have to admit that Sid had a point. When he thought about it, there was nowhere to promote him to. All the more senior management jobs were filled with young go-ahead men with whom he could not compete. He had been deceiving himself as well as Sid when he said that he was working to get promoted. The real reason was that he just didn't look forward to coming home any more.

I have cited this further episode in the story of Sid and Herman to illustrate what is, I think, a common reaction to an interpretation: that the interpreter has a superior view of the world that enables them to see what is hidden. Interpretation has, unconsciously I am tempted to say, become central to how many psychotherapists work in longer-term therapy. I think that this is unfortunate because it is almost inevitable that clients feel put down by them. They have much the same reaction as a bridge player whose carefully cherished ace is trumped unexpectedly.

Some experienced psychotherapists who consider that they use interpretations have actually found a different and much more helpful intervention. They join with the concern that is apparent in what the patient has said. Jusuf might have said, for example, 'the birds in your dream seemed to be undoing all the good work that you had done, almost as if they were consuming you as well as the bread'. This would be what Foulkes called a 'clarification'. The content of the dream was repeated back but in a more personal and more alarming context. It may well have enabled the baker to say to Jusuf, 'you say that I am being consumed. That's just it. Am I for the chop? Do I have to pay with my life for this mistake I've made?'.

Clarification of this kind is also more effective against self-deception, of the kind that Herman was practising, than interpretation. It can also take account of the fact that people very often act in response to the emotional meaning of their circumstances. They do not know why they have acted as they did, because they did not rehearse the action beforehand. They responded, as we all do, without thinking. There is a great temptation, if one is in the interpreting mode, to see this as just another example of unconscious motive and to imagine that one can reveal this. Confining oneself to clarification makes it easier to say, 'So you don't know why you acted like that', and make this the starting point for exploring the emotional meaning of the situation.

Changing identity

Foulkes, the group psychotherapist, described a kind of catastrophic reaction to a 'plunging interpretation' (Foulkes, 1975), of the kind that Jusuf made. He visualized this reaction as plunging so far through the boundary of the client that it threatened the core of the client's identity. Whitaker (1985) writes of the frontier of clients and says that some have their frontier very near the core of their identity, whereas it is further out for others. Whitaker was not the first to use this term in this way. As noted earlier, Kant also used it.

Both Foulkes and Whitaker are using these metaphors to illustrate how catastrophic reactions can be avoided in therapy. Another way of looking at the same issues is to consider the 'me' and the 'I' of a person. Attacking someone's values, degrading them in some way, undermines the person's 'me'. To put it in Goffman's terms (1956), it invalidates their self-presentation. What happens to the 'I' in this situation? We all of us have experience of it. If the 'me' that is being invalidated has little of the values which I hold dear and if it has little emotional meaning to me, my 'I' is unscathed. But if the 'me' carries the values and the emotional meanings that I hold dear, then shame or self-disgust result.

One might say that Whitaker is suggesting that it is always a good thing to present a 'me' to the world that is remote from the 'I', but the effect of this is to diminish a person's sense of personal engagement in the world.

Rowena was at that period of adolescence when peer relationships were particularly important and, potentially, particularly hurtful. Her parents had recently separated, and she had moved city and, of course, school. It was a considerable challenge, and she met it by creating a persona for herself as slightly zany and a joker. This worked well in the sense that she was readily accepted, but there were times when she felt that no-one really knew her and that no-one really cared. She cried sometimes when she was alone, thinking that she felt much more hurt than anyone could ever see, and there was no way to show this without betraying the persona that all of her friends expected of her.

Consistent with my general view that the therapist should seek to make the minimal effective intervention, it is my practice to minimize creating transference reactions.

How this can be achieved is implicit in the previous sections which described the situational determinants of catastrophic, transference-type reactions. Practical steps include:
- reducing the power imbalance
- focussing on the here and now rather than the past
- portraying the other person as an agent rather than as a victim of mysterious forces
- treating a person in a couple, family or group
- avoiding mystification

A person may be in therapy for a long time without developing significant transference. Bill, whose case was described previously, is an example. Receiving transference interpretations is certainly not the only way in which a person benefits from long-term therapy, contrary to claims made by some psychotherapists in the euphoric days of psycho-analytic expansion. Indeed, the more frequently a therapist makes transference interpretations, the poorer can be the outcome (Piper et al., 1991).

Other important therapeutic factors in long-term group therapy have been reviewed by Yalom (1985), whose work is strongly influenced by the interpersonal school founded by Sullivan (1953). Yalom concluded that there are nine primary factors in the therapeutic experience, of which interpersonal learning and group cohesiveness are the most important.

What is long-term therapy again?

Long-term therapy could be considered as the application of the techniques described in all of the preceding chapters in the context of a closer and more enduring therapeutic relationship. Much of long-term therapy is about dealing with a memory or an interpersonal difficulty, with each episode receiving some short-term therapeutic attention. As in the case of Bill, described above, the long-term perspective means that some of these memories and episodes can return as preoccupations. Each time that they do return, more work is done on them, so that the cumulative effect is more thorough.

What is happening during this process is what happened for Bill. The client's narrative becomes enriched bit by bit. In the process, the client's values change. A dogmatic person might become more open. A person who believes himself to be inferior to others might develop more confidence. Not only do values change, but so do emotional meanings. Getting close to another person may become more palatable as positive reactions from other people begin to outweigh negative reactions.

What is being described can only happen if there is, to use Winnicott's term, a 'good-enough relationship' between the client and the therapist, or the client and the group. One requirement for this is, to use Whitaker's metaphor, that the client's frontier is sufficiently far out to enable it to be moved without threatening the security of the self too much. No therapist can ensure that everything that they say is right, or that nothing that they say has unexpectedly unpleasant connotations. Some degree of tolerance of the unpleasant emotional meaning and acceptance of different values is necessary for long-term psychotherapy to take place with a minimum of catastrophic transference reactions occurring.

Note that transference reactions are not just a reflection of a client's intolerance. Therapists may also behave in ways that most people, and not just people with particular sensitivities, would tell themselves was hostile or uncaring. Circumstances which are out of the control of either the therapist or the client may also create sufficient distress to affect the client's ability to provide a coherent account of the therapy. Illness or pregnancy of the therapist are two examples of unexpected therapist absence which can have this effect.

Identity and value in long-term therapy

Hannah had been in therapy for 6 months. Her therapist, Dr Strong, was much older than her, and she had rather looked up to him throughout most of the therapy. However, the day before her next regular session, she received a phone call from his secretary to say that Dr Strong, unexpectedly, had to be out of the country on the following day. Hannah was upset as she had something important to talk about, but she told herself that Dr Strong was a busy man. Dr Strong was back the following week, and Hannah asked him if he had had a good time. Dr Strong was rather waspish in his reply, saying that he would hardly call a professional trip 'a good time'. Hannah started to be a bit put out. It happened that she used to chat with Dr Strong's secretary on her way in and out of her sessions and so, as she left this particular session, she casually asked his secretary whether Dr Strong had had a successful trip. 'Well, I don't know', said the secretary, 'It was just some kind of jamboree paid for by a drug company. I suppose he must have enjoyed it. He was very keen to go'.

Hannah described her reaction to a friend later as feeling crushed. She felt that she was a person of no importance. Her friend said that Dr Strong was a creep, and why didn't she feel angry? Hannah could not respond to this. She felt that she had plunged into a deep well of black despair. She was of no account even to someone who was paid to see her. What point was there to her, if even he found any excuse to avoid meeting her? Later that day, she rang the secretary to say that she would not be coming back to see Dr Strong again and that she did not want Dr Strong to try to get in touch with her, or for him to write to her family doctor. In fact, she wanted nothing to do with him ever again.

Hannah's reaction might be considered extreme. Dr Strong would certainly think that she had taken his absence too personally. The fact is that Hannah's account of the therapy had assumed that Dr Strong found her a worthwhile person who could do something with her life. That belief had been vitiated, not so much by Dr Strong's absence as by his evasiveness. She would never trust him again. Hannah's account of the therapy was now very different. She felt that she had been duped. This account was only one chapter in a longer narrative about herself as weak and of no account.

Reactions like this can be triggered even in short-term therapy. Malan's extended case example of the 'interior decorator', which has already been discussed in Chapter 8, provides an example.

The interior decorator had been talking about his fetishistic interest in his wife wearing PVC. He became anxious about the therapist's reaction to this and asked him for reassurance by saying, 'Is it very abnormal?'. The therapist had refused to answer. This led to a withdrawal by the client, who said, 'Can you give me a lead about what I should talk about?'. The therapist said, 'I think that the reason why you can't go on and want a lead is because you are angry with me. You asked me to reassure you about something, and I wouldn't do it'. This comment, as it usually does, made things worse. The therapist then thought some more about the situation and commented on the decorator's tendency, which had emerged in earlier sessions, to submit whenever he had a quarrel with someone. Perhaps, the therapist commented, this was happening now. He and the client had a disagreement, and the client was dealing with it by submitting himself.

The interior decorator confirmed that this had happened, and that this is what he did. He believed that getting angry was wrong. He had seen his father have too many tantrums to want to be like that himself.

Malan uses this example, and a subsequent fictional example, to make the case that every predicament brought to therapy has an underlying transference component. Consequently, Malan asserts that no predicament can be resolved in therapy without there being work on the transference through what he calls the 'triangle of insight'. Interestingly, the fictional example given by Malan also includes a therapeutic error which leads into the transference problem.

Malan and I do seem to be in agreement that transference reactions occur when the client cannot 'write' new happenings into their life-story without undermining the narrative coherence of that story. In both the cases mentioned by Malan, the discrepancy is that the therapist does not seem to value being helpful to the client.

Fortunately, in both of the Malan cases, the therapists (both real and imaginary) reflected on what had happened and were prepared to open up the issue. Both of them took the client's view seriously. They both modelled two even more important and helpful values than being right: the ability to accept that one has been mistaken and the concern to try to improve understanding. These values were consistent with a narrative by the client of the therapy as being hopeful and helpful.

There are people who value themselves so little, and consequently have such a skimpy self-narrative, that they find it difficult to maintain an account of therapy as being helpful even when the therapeutic situation is as good as can be expected. These are often people who have experienced crushing adversity or chronic isolation and rejection. They are quite often categorized as being borderline by psychiatrists.

Angelica had taken numerous overdoses. She was chronically dysthymic. Angelica constantly complained that the therapist could not help her, but she never missed her therapy sessions. The therapist felt exhausted after every session and wondered each time whether Angelica got any benefit from the sessions and whether to go on. Came the approach of the summer break and the therapist told Angelica when he would be away, and then said, 'But you so often say that I'm not helping that it will probably be a relief not to have to come'.

During the subsequent week, Angelica took a large overdose of tablets, and cut herself on numerous occasions. She was not able to explain why this had happened, but in retrospect the therapist came to the conclusion that Angelica had interpreted his remark as mocking. She was probably reminded, the therapist thought, of her father, who went out of his way to ridicule her in every way. Angelica was preoccupied with being safe from her father, and seemed to feel that she could be safe in the therapy. The therapist's remark had, it seemed to the therapist, robbed her of this safety and provoked this catastrophic reaction.

Kernberg, perhaps one of the leading contributors to the literature on the psychotherapy of so-called 'borderline clients', recommends that constant attention needs to be paid to the transference if clients with these problems are to be helped. This is sometimes interpreted as needing to make many transference interpretations, particularly focussing on anger, as did the therapist of the interior decorator.

My experience is that it usually makes matters worse to talk about someone being angry because most people are taught to value being in control of one's temper, not losing it. Telling someone they are angry just seems like a further dismissal.

However, what does work is for the therapist to be ready to move the focus of the therapy on to the issue of the client's identity, on to the client's struggle to keep hold of their 'I', whenever transference seems to be a problem. A way needs to be found, a narrative form needs to be created, for the client to be able to recover their own account of the treatment. And the therapist needs to be willing to reconsider his or her actions from the client's perspective. This means that the therapist needs to value understanding more highly than being right. Not so easy for many professionals to do!

When transference reactions are most intense, it is not just the client but the therapist who is fighting for the supremacy of their account of the therapy. The therapist, as well as the client, may feel threatened emotionally. As we shall see in the next section, both may feel that there is a risk of being shamed or rejected. The therapist's task is to be able to work whilst flooded with the anxiety associated with this danger.

Something similar may happen to groups which are paralysed by their fear of annihilation. They, too, need to reaffirm their identity. Helping the group to tell its experience in a way that others can hear is important. But it may also be important to discover who the narrators of the story should be.

One of the first tasks of a mediator faced with an intractable conflict, or a family therapist faced with a family at war, is to decide where to draw the boundary, and which are the relevant parties to include. But this will depend on whose identity is at issue. Consider the conflict in Northern Ireland. Whose were the identities at issue there? If they were 'Republicans' and 'Unionists', the boundary ran through every community in Northern Ireland, with Britain on one side, and the Irish Republic on the other. If the identity was Ulster, then the boundary was between the whole of Northern

Ireland on one side, and on the other, the Irish Republic, Britain, and Irish communities in the United States. Some mediators have recently argued that the breakthrough in resolving the conflict was to include the Irish American community in the process, a move reinforced by appointing someone from North America as the mediator.

Identity issues have been discussed previously, in Chapter 5. It was suggested there that the most intractable issues, the ones that involve a person's 'I', involve shame or disgust. It is to these emotions that we now need to turn.

Shame and disgust: the other story

Sooner or later, however much a person's 'me' has been attuned both to their 'I' and to the expectations of the society in which they live, there will come a moment when their self-narrative, their story about their 'me', fails. At that moment, it can be not only the narrative that fails, but the story-teller who seems to have lost his or her voice. A person feels that their very identity, their 'I', has failed. At that moment, a person faces the shame or self-disgust that attends the breakage of the bonds that link us to others.

Janoff-Bulman (1992) describes this as the shattering of the assumptions that the world is benevolent and meaningful and that the self is worthy. She considers that people's 'seemingly paradoxical and maladaptive responses like self-blame are in fact strategies to restore the illusions of comprehensibility and control, and the psychological equilibrium these illusions maintain'. Shattering of identity can be brought about by bereavement, by being sacked, by ill-health, by mental illness, by rape . . . and by psychotherapy.

All of us are, in fact, conscious in some way of this danger. Some, like the shame-prone people that have been described elsewhere in this book, feel that every day they walk a knife-edge of possible humiliation or rejection. As always, there are stories to help us come to terms with this.

In the short story, 'The ones who walk away from Omelas', Ursula le Guin describes a blissful city state in which the citizens live an unregulated life which also succeeds in being satisfying and mutually respectful. However, somewhere in the city is a child who lives on two bowls of gruel and grease a day, locked in a cellar with two mops and a bucket. The child is afraid of the mops.

Every other child in the city visits this child once. All these children are disturbed by the visit but they know that: 'If the child were brought up into the sunlight out of the vile place, if it were cleaned and fed and comforted, that would be a good thing, indeed; but if it were done, in that day and hour all the prosperity and beauty and delight of Omelas would wither and be destroyed' (Le Guin, 1976).

Le Guin's account is very sympathetic to Freud. Consider that Omelas is not a city but a person – Salome in fact. She thrives and is happy as long as she can confine everything bad and everything cruel in herself into one hidden chamber, which we might call 'the unconscious'. Le Guin goes further than Freud by considering that doing this is a kind of choice which everyone faces in childhood. They visit the child, and know that by confining it in this way they are complicit with the repression. A very few leave the city – we do not know where they go, just as we do not know what will happen if we do not try to suppress aspects of ourselves which are unpalatable to us.

The Bluebeard legend was created by Perrault and anthologized in Andrew Lang's *Blue Fairy* Book. Bluebeard, according to Perrault, was a serial murderer who married and then murdered women for gain. The legend describes the last wife's escape and Bluebeard's demise at the hands of her brothers. What makes the story memorable is that Bluebeard has a locked chamber in which he keeps the remains of his former wives. What makes the Bluebeard legend particularly disturbing is that he gives his wife the key to the chamber, but forbids her to enter. It has provided inspiration not only to some famous serial murderers, but to many artists, including Angela Carter, in whose short story, 'The Bloody Chamber', Judith is saved by her mother, and Bela Balazs, who wrote the libretto of Bartok's opera, 'Duke Bluebeard's Castle'.

Blood is as much a motif in Balazs' libretto as it is in the other stories, but it is Bluebeard's blood, not that of his previous wives. They are alive, but locked away from him by their own wish to penetrate the last of his seven rooms. The prologue, which is not performed, begins with the lines: 'The tale is old that shall be told but where does it belong: Within? Without?' . . . and this is often taken to mean that the castle is in Bluebeard's mind.

The opera describes the early days of Bluebeard's marriage to Judith, his last wife. She takes Bluebeard and his castle as she finds it, but begs leave to open some of its windows and doors. At first this goes well. Sunlight enters the castle. A vista of Bluebeard's pastoral domain is revealed. But then Bluebeard wants her to love him, and to stop opening doors. Judith sings: 'Two more doors. Not one of your great doors must stay shut against me . . . Though I perish I fear nothing. Dearest Bluebeard'. Bluebeard capitulates and Judith opens the next door on to a lake of tears . . . Bluebeard's tears. Judith and Bluebeard make love, but she remains determined to open the last door, and Bluebeard tells her that she will extinguish all the sunshine that she has brought into the castle. Despite his admonition, he gives her the key and she opens the last door to reveal his three previous wives, arrayed in crowns and sumptuous jewels. Bluebeard does obeisance to them and, placing a heavy cloak over Judith's shoulders and a crown on her head, gazes after her as she and the other wives withdraw into the chamber. He sings, 'Thou art lovely, passing lovely, queen of all my women, my best and fairest . . . Henceforth all shall be darkness, darkness, darkness'.

Each of these legends refers to a truth about self-consciousness, described by many psychotherapists and also, perhaps, partly created by them: that the more clear and coherent a person's narrative about themselves, the more likely there is to be something behind a locked door, or in the forest's shadow, which remains untold.

Freud's original explanation of this was that the hidden chamber contained real memories of precocious sexuality (Masson, 1984). Subsequently, Freud universalized his theory, making the secret chamber – the unconscious – contain sexual longing and other 'instincts' which Freud attributed to our animal nature. Jung filled the chamber with the shadow – all of those human characteristics which a person wants to deny in themselves (Jung, 1968). The existentialists did not have a place for an unconscious, but Heidegger did consider that a person who does not speak about death and their fear of death falls into mere 'idle chatter'. Klein and her followers include the death instinct as one of those in Freud's chamber. Lacan takes the chamber to be 'the Real': everything about the world which cannot be understood, for which there is no name, and whose effects are therefore unexpected and terrifying.

Fraser's book about myth, *The Golden Bough*, sketches an ur-myth of creation throughout the Mediterranean basin in which it is the earth itself which is the chamber. Every spring, a young man is chosen, an Adonis, who is crowned amid a licentious ceremonial. His crowning coincides with the germination of the corn and the young man is killed, in fact or symbolically, at the time of its harvest. His blood passes into the earth, out of sight, and is reincarnated in the spring. In a comparable ceremony still conducted in Santa Fe, a larger-than-life puppet is burned along with a tape-recording of howls of torment. People write down their troubles and shames and pin them to the puppet to be burnt along with it.

Every one of these formulations contains the following common elements:

- The more clearly a person knows themselves, the more clearly they realize that the knowledge is circumscribed: there is always something more.
- It is most dark just outside the light: there is something particularly fearful about what we do not know about ourselves.
- The strongest light leaves the greatest darkness: the more definite and uncompromising our narrative about ourselves, the more the untold threatens to overthrow it.
- Darkness brings rest and desire: if we stick too closely to a conservative account of ourselves, we become depleted and stale, and we lose our zest for life.
- Darkness brings terror and is the realm of ghosts: what is unspoken threatens to overwhelm us. If we do give the key to someone else, and they enter our darkness, we are forced to confront it too. We are scared that it may destroy us.
- Darkness demands sacrifice, but makes renewal possible.

Readers who have been sympathetic to my attempts to provide an evidence basis for psychotherapeutic practice in earlier sections of this book may be impatient at this point. The formulation above seems poetic rather than scientific, loose rather than precise. Surely things could have been formulated more clearly?

My defence is that psychotherapists have taken the boundaries of their craft to the edge of art, not of science. The psychotherapeutic endeavour, particularly that which deals with human happiness, cannot be pinned down to a procedure. The language describing it has to be suggestive rather than declarative. Working with people who are unhappy because they have become depleted of a desire for life, or who find relationships meaningless, is not scientific work. It is work shared with artists and the religious, not with scientists, because it involves reintegrating into everyday life both the 'highest' eschatological vision, and the 'lowest' scatological feelings.

There can be no prescription of how to work with clients who are finding words for previously unspoken desires or tragedies. The therapist has to draw on their own creativity. Inspiring teachers can help. I would recommend Aichorn (1935), Deurzen (1998) and Winnicott (1949). Many other experienced therapists will have different recommendations.

Two principles do, in my view, inform those therapists who are able to inspire. One is a value: integrity. Rawls (1971) writes that this is the value which can keep us going 'in times of social doubt and loss of faith in long established values' (1971, p. 519), which is often how therapist and client experience their journey into the unknown. He defines integrity as 'truthfulness and sincerity, lucidity and commitment, or, as some say, authenticity' (1971, p. 519). Van Deurzen, particularly, has written about the challenges of authenticity for the psychotherapist (Deurzen, 1997).

The other principle is the therapist's palate. Therapists must be able to accept what their clients tell them without disgust and without shame. Note that this is not to say that no thing should disgust therapists, or that therapists think that no-one should ever be ashamed. Society could not go on if these emotions were not systematically employed in socialization. Nor does it mean that therapists should de-sensitize themselves. Sometimes disgust or shame is an appropriate reaction to a person's intentions. What it seems to me that inspirational therapists are able to do is to look unflinchingly at what has happened in a person's life or inner experience without distancing themself. Fairbairn has formulated this most clearly for me.

He describes the situation when a person's feelings towards someone else are either met with coldness or indifference – a shaming experience – or are rejected as disgusting. If the person can simply detach themselves from the other, then they can also detach themselves from the shame or the disgust. But if the other person is a mother, a lover or a therapist, it might not be so easy to simply put them aside. In this situation the feelings become inhibited by anxiety, but they do not get discharged. They draw a person back: as Fairbairn says, the ego splits and a part of the ego is set up anti-libidinally, against these feelings.

Some of the potential consequences have been discussed elsewhere in this book. A person can 'detoxify' the feelings through a perversion. A person can narrate themselves and their life in such a way as to conceal unpalatable feelings, beliefs or experiences. They may do this knowingly, as a form of deception; in a kind of wishful way, as a form of self-deception; or because they have no words to put to these unpalatable actions, an expression of dissociation. If this process goes further, then a person's commitment to a single, coherent narrative about themself is given up, and there can be multiple narratives. The narrator's belief in these can range from no belief at all – the different accounts are just means of duping others – to complete belief. A person who genuinely believes in two or more different stories about themself is faced with a problem of coherence. One way that people may resolve this is to give up the assumption that there is one person (meaning one narrator), one self or one personality. Having a unique social identity means a person is one person, but does not mean that they experience themself as an individual. One person may experience themself as a community of narrators, personalities, selves or 'I's.

This situation, termed by psychiatrists 'dissociative identity disorder', allows one narrator, one 'persona' to use Jung's term, to tell a story which excludes the shameful or disgusting elements, and it falls to the other narrator, or narrators, to tell what has been excluded. This is the situation described by Le Guin in Omelas. All but one of the citizens tell a story of a graceful life lived in celebration and happiness. Only one – a child – tells a story of fear, deprivation and imprisonment. They are connected because they all live in the same city, and because each knows about the other. But they behave like separate people.

We might all embrace the Omelas solution, and all develop our alters, were it not for shame, that quintessentially social emotion. The laughter of the citizens of Omelas rings false because each and every one of them is tainted by the shame of the child in the locked room. Shame is contagious. There is no healthy escape except by facing it.

I am often struck by the inescapability of honesty. If anything is an unconscious motive, honesty is. In one experiment, volunteers were asked to tell a group of psychiatrists why they should be given home leave from hospital. They were allowed to lie. Many volunteers could control their voice and face so that there were no indications that they were lying. Some could control their arms and shoulders. None could control his or her feet. When the volunteers lied, their feet became restless. It was as if the person could intend to lie, and could manage those parts of the body which were most easily controlled voluntarily, but their involuntary movements told the truth.

A person who is preoccupied with not telling a secret proverbially finds themself remarking on exactly those subjects which would normally lead up to disclosure. Shame and secrets are contrary to our nature as human beings. I believe that each of us can only be happy if we are true to our nature. This does not mean that we can be happy if we behave like animals, for that is not human nature. Nor does it mean that we do what we want, because we may want to do things more as a means of concealing shame or self-disgust than as an expression of joy.

The self of the client, and to a lesser degree the therapist, is narrated in long-term therapy. If the client's anxiety about what is unspoken can be assuaged, then the client may be able to extend this self-narrative to include what Fairbairn calls 'the libidinal object'. The client may be able to speak about desiring a kind of relationship which has otherwise seemed shameful or disgusting, what Ezriel (1950) called 'the calamitous relationship'. But this can only happen if the therapist is not disgusted and does not shame the client by failing to respond to the importance and intensity of the client's feelings.

Long-term therapy requires not just technical skill, but self-knowledge and the right instincts. It's such a tall order that all therapists fall short sometimes. How this might be retrieved is discussed in the next chapter.

The short story about long-term therapy

I am this person, and you are that person because we each have our own body, and because we have an identity attributed to us by Government, banks, neighbours, family members and others. My body includes dispositions to act in certain ways, ways that can be evoked by the emotional meanings that the world has for me.

I am also this person because of the story I tell about myself. This story describes how, as a character, I have developed and changed. It has a plot which is the way in which I have aimed my life towards certain goals, or values, and how I have tried to put myself back on track when circumstance has put obstacles in my way. My story is more or less happy depending on how well I have been able to realize these goals.

If I am not happy, I might turn to a psychotherapist who will first hear my story, and then help me to remake it. I will learn to narrate myself in a new way – one which, if it is successful, will allow me to pursue my values more effectively and to develop my character more fully. Since almost everyone values close personal relationships more highly than any other aspect of life, I will want this new story to shape my character to be one which is attractive or satisfying to other people. I will almost always find that I did not have a very good story previously about what makes a person attractive or satisfying.

How I tell the story is also important. It may be more or less coherent. Only coherent stories will demonstrate that I have been able to achieve what I set out to do. So happy stories are coherent ones. But I may have a coherent story about being ruined, and seeking vengeance. Coherent stories are coherent because one thing follows coherently from another. There is a consistent sense of agency. I might attribute this agency to myself – I am particularly likely to do this in a western, autonomy-orientated culture – or I might attribute it to some other benevolent presence in my life – destiny, say.

However, it may not be possible for me to narrate myself consistently. There may be events which do not square with the happy ending that I want. There may be conflict between myself and other people about what life should be about. These issues are potentially resoluble if, that is, my account of myself is reasonably coherent with that of other people and if it remains coherent over time.

The particular therapeutic challenges of longer-term therapy come about when the 'me' that a person talks about is very different to the 'I' that others experience. I may not feel that I have a definite identity. To put it another way, I may feel that I do not know where 'me' ends, and 'you' begins, i.e. I may have a lack of boundaries. This may lead me to be paradoxically sensitive to any boundary violation. Longer-term treatment may therefore have to concentrate on this issue, and on related issues of powerlessness and threat.

I may know myself, but believe that my values or my feelings are not acceptable to others, who would be ashamed or disgusted by me. I may deal with this by expressing myself very little, or very ambivalently. This will make it difficult for me to have satisfactory close relationships with others. Group psychotherapy may be effective if I want to relate to the other members of the group with sufficient intensity to overcome this inhibition.

However, I may have a strong expectation that members of the group, the therapist, people I meet, even people that love me, will be moved to disgust or shame if they should ever really see me as I see myself. My narrative about myself will be a roman- à-clef, and I will try to mislead or defeat anyone who seems to be getting hold of the clue to what it really means. I will resist them, and I will expect them to be to me as I am to myself, that is, deeply disappointed.

There may be some things about myself which I cannot tell, even though these are not disappointing but deeply exciting. If they came out, they would shame me, but if I touch them in secret, in the dark as it were, they fill me with energy and power. They may be linked to sexuality and to violence. They are the Kali to my Shiva. They have a kinship with addictions and perversions. They may even be perversions or addictions. They are an indication that I could be more than I am, but they are also horrific. They draw me in, and I know that they could entrap me. I cannot be truly happy with another person whilst I harbour such secrets, but I could not be truly happy if I cut myself off from them.

Coming to terms with them, integrating them into myself, may be a prerequisite for happiness and for long-term fulfilment in intimate relationships. It is certainly a requirement for being a competent long-term therapist.

11

Crises, and how to surmount them

Feeling stuck with your client? The client has threatened suicide? Do you dread the next session? Has the client become over-familiar, or unreasonably hostile? Do you feel that it's time to end the treatment, but you can't bring yourself to do it? If so, read on . . .

Psychotherapies progress in different ways. Some seem to be quite straightforward. Others seem to be a series of crises. The most common pattern in longer-term therapy is for there to be a series of sessions in which the discussion between client and therapist seems to be a fairly predictable working out of themes raised in an earlier session. Then there may be a crisis that, if it is surmounted successfully, throws up new themes for working through over the next few sessions.

Some of the crises to be considered in this chapter are shown in Table 11.1.

General principles of managing crises

It would not be possible to write this chapter without some outcome criterion. If a person kills himself, people sometimes say, 'He's better off dead'. If a person remains miserable or confused or frustrated, there will always be someone who says that that person is more realistic about how life really is, than if he or she had been happy or goal-directed or fulfilled. If any outcome is as good as another, there can be no criterion of what constitutes competent psychotherapy. Indeed, there seems precious little value in undertaking psychotherapy at all. I shall assume, therefore, that client and therapist will have agreed on an outcome or outcomes at the start of treatment, and will also have an implicit understanding of how to estimate progress towards that outcome. I shall use words like 'improve' or 'go well' to mean that progress is being made. This usage does not imply that the desired outcome is always fewer symptoms, a better income or a richer sex life, only that the agreed outcomes are being achieved.

It sometimes happens that therapists do not want their clients to do well, and clients sometimes want to stay the same, too. The reasons are usually practical. Clients may not want to lose benefits, or they may have their aims

Table 11.1. A selection of crises

Crisis	Symptom
Failure to progress	Feeling stuck
Boundary violations	Coming late
	Missing sessions
Relationship outside the treatment	
Transference	Disparagement
	Idealization
Psychiatric disorder	Suicidal
	Mania
	Intoxication
Ending	

set on obtaining a good settlement in a marital or occupational dispute. However, duplicity is very rare in my experience. Even when people stand to gain financially in settlements, malingering is the exception rather than the rule in general psychiatry (Deb et al., 1999) and there is no reason to suppose that psychotherapy clients are any more duplicitous.

It is very tempting, when a client does not improve, to think that the client does not want to get better. It is therefore important to remember that this is one of the most unlikely explanations for the crisis. Some therapists argue that clients might want to get better consciously, but unconsciously they want to remain the same. This claim can easily be taken to justify any kind of outcome: if the client gets better, it's the therapist's success, but if the client remains the same or gets worse, it's the client's unconscious that's at fault.

Attributing things to the unconscious is a kind of short hand, like attributing something to destiny. It needs considerable unpacking if we are to take it more seriously. In this book, I have deliberately avoided reifying the unconscious, believing that people may be unconscious of having conflicting intentions, but that does not mean that their conscious has one intention and that their unconscious has another. But, the reader may say, the previous chapter was all about this kind of conflict. Is it not therefore legitimate to explain poor outcome by attributing it to the client's conflicting intentions, even if it cannot be attributed to the client's unconscious?

Yvonne had been severely anxious for many years. It seemed as if her problem was that she was anxious when she ate in front of people, and anxious when she had to speak to strangers in public. She avoided many social occasions as a

result of fear that she would have to do either of these things. After the first two sessions, it was agreed that Yvonne would adopt a modified behavioural approach. At the next session, Yvonne had not kept a diary, as she agreed that she would. She was, however, not willing to talk about this, because she wanted to talk about her relationship with her husband. He worked away for most of the week, and she felt frustrated by his lack of involvement with child care. In the next few weeks Yvonne talked about her worries about her family, a miscarriage, and her mother's secrecy.

Yvonne's therapist, who was a registrar in training, left and reported to his supervisor that he thought that Yvonne was unwilling to give up her anxiety. Certainly she was no better. The supervisor interviewed Yvonne, who confirmed that she was, if anything, more anxious than she had been and was now taking antidepressants. The supervisor offered her a further period of short-term treatment. The first contract was to work on anxiety management. The next was an assertiveness programme. Neither seemed to be of benefit.

Yvonne was in conflict in the sessions about what she wanted from the therapy. She would often say that she didn't know, or that she was in two minds. Sometimes she would tell herself that she just needed to make an effort; at other times she told herself that it was best to make the most of her security at home. Having never really had a home before, Yvonne had poured her energy into creating an ideal environment for her family. Her young daughter had all the toys that could be imagined, and Yvonne liked nothing better than to see her happily absorbed in playing with them.

It would be plausible to argue that Yvonne, who had been a career woman, needed her anxiety to justify to herself and her husband spending so much time at home. She was ambivalent about it, but arguably it was this that held her back from doing something more effective about her anxiety.

Let's say this is true. Is it therefore the case that Yvonne has been offered the right treatment – cognitive-behavioural therapy being the treatment of choice for many people with panic disorder – to which she had failed to respond? Or is it true to say that Yvonne's preoccupying concern was not her anxiety, although it was that which led to her referral, but her ambivalence about becoming more independent? In the latter case, the lack of progress that Yvonne made was not due to her unconscious conflict, but the inappropriate focus of the treatment on anxiety, when the real problem lay in Yvonne's lack of confidence in herself.

Like so many things in psychotherapy, there is no right answer. However, the second explanation, that the focus needs to be changed, seems to be the most facilitative one (Whitaker & Lieberman, 1964), i.e. the one that opens up more therapeutic options.

Personally, I prefer explanations which attribute treatment difficulties to the shortcomings of the treatment or the therapist, to those which atttribute them to the shortcomings of the client. They may be more uncomfortable, but they are more consistent with my values, one of which is 'when in difficulties, try harder', and to me they have a more palatable emotional flavour.

In practice, many crises that arise in psychotherapy can usefully be re-cast as problems in the focus of the therapy (Budman & Gurman, 1983). In fact, three useful principles might also apply in the event of a crisis arising:

(1) Attribute everything that happens to the effects of the therapy unless proven otherwise.
(2) Re-consider the focus of the treatment.
(3) Review the therapeutic relationship.

Attribute everything that happens to the effects of the therapy unless proven otherwise

Communicative therapy (Langs, 1992) is based on the premise that anything that the client brings into therapy is really a comment on the client's feelings about the therapist. This seems extreme, and may have the effect of preventing the client talking about anything other than his or her feelings about the therapist. However, there is an important kernel of truth in it. It is worth considering whether unexpected events or turns in the conversation are actually responses to what is happening in the therapy.

Anya's parents were both family practitioners. Anya, although having been an excellent student, had a breakdown on leaving school and did not go to medical school, as predicted. She did complete a degree in philosophy but this was considered by most of her family to be a kind of superior time-wasting. Anya could not get a job afterwards and, at the time of coming into therapy, was working as a care-assistant.

For quite a few weeks she talked non-stop about her mother to her therapist, herself a female doctor. Despite Anya's preoccupation with her mother, and the increasingly frequent phone calls to her mother that had been taking place, she seemed more and more bitter about the therapy. It wasn't getting anywhere, she would say. The therapist did not understand what really bugged her, and so on, and so forth. After one particular bitter telephone conversation, Anya told her mother that she didn't ever want to speak to her again.

The therapist reported to her supervisor that in the session following the phone call, Anya had gone and sat in her seat, and refused to move despite the therapist's reminder that it was where she, the therapist, normally sat. It was a swivel chair, and the therapist said, rather irritatedly, that she had tried throughout the session to get Anya to concentrate on her feelings for her mother, but all Anya had done was swing round on the chair looking childishly smug. The supervisor asked about the seating arrangements in the room. The therapist explained that she had to use an office in the outclient department and that there was only an office chair by the desk for the psychiatrist, and a stackable chair for the client. Without really thinking about it, the therapist had occupied the chair which was hers by occupational right, the rather higher and more comfortable swivel chair, and she had expected Anya to be in the client's chair.

The supervisor asked if it would be possible for two of the same type of chair to be provided for the therapy sessions, and the therapist said that she would find out. It was possible, and after that both therapist and client used the same type of chair. Some 6 months later Anya told the therapist that she had made such progress that she felt ready to do something with her education at last, and she was going to train as a child psychotherapist.

What the therapist had unwittingly done was to assume that she, the therapist, was entitled to a superior kind of chair and that Anya should have the lower, cheaper, client's chair. It is possible to see, in retrospect, that Anya felt intense frustration at this. It was clearly reminiscent of her family experience when her parents had juggled her and a handful of siblings with the same dexterity and kindly dispassion as they had juggled their practice. Anya's increasingly open frustration with her mother paralleled her frustration with the therapist, who seemed as blind to her assumption of superiority as her mother had been.

Re-consider the focus of the treatment

When one finds oneself as a therapist becoming increasingly angry that the client is not concentrating on what matters in the therapy, and particularly when one starts to think of trying to get the client to do something, it is worth re-considering the focus of the treatment. This is especially important in short-term therapy, where keeping to a focus is the most important predictor of outcome.

However, this does not mean necessarily sticking to a focus which was agreed at the beginning of treatment or sticking to a focus that is theoretically determined. Therapists who do this have worse results (Castonguay et al., 1996). It means continuing to focus on the client's preoccupying concern. This may change as earlier therapy uncovers or clarifies deeper concerns. This might be because the focus shifts from symptoms, to personal predicaments, to relationship problems, as in the case of Yvonne (it is less often the case that the focus shifts in reverse order). But it may also happen that the preoccupying concern becomes more circumscribed, requiring that the treatment also become more tightly focussed.

Bert was a law student. He was referred for panic attacks. He said that the problem was more one of unfocussed anxiety, than panic. He hated homosexuals, and whenever he saw two men walking hand in hand he would experience a wave of disgust, and would then feel anxious for days.

Shortly after the assessment interview, Bert went to Amsterdam. He said that he had gone to test out his sexuality. He allowed himself to be picked up by a man in a bar, and had oral sex. The following day, he went to a (female) prostitute. He said that he could perform with the woman, and did not feel anything for the man. So he had concluded that he was not gay. But when he got anxious, it was the man he thought about, and not the prostitute.

The therapist decided that he should leave a space for Bert to work on his sexual identity. He had a shrewd idea that Bert was going to discover that he was gay, after all.

Bert's initial homophobia was explicable to some degree on the basis of his parents' reported homophobia. But, it quickly became apparent that Bert was struggling against his own homosexual desires and that the focus of treatment was not homophobia at all. Bert was anxious about how his friends, and particularly his family, would take it if they discovered that he had 'come out'.

Review the therapeutic relationship

It is a curious fact that a client complaining about their relationship with the therapist is less cause for alarm than a client complaining about their problem. Normally in a therapy that is going well, both the client and the therapist are content to work with the problem of the moment. Unless there is some specific procedure for reviewing progress like a homework diary, the presenting problem may be almost forgotten. When clients talk about their symptoms, it is because they are searching round for some way of relating to the therapist rather like when people in parties talk about the weather. It is assumed that the weather will always be of interest to the English, and that symptoms will always be of interest to a health professional.

Clients who express their anger, or disappointment, with the therapist are sufficiently trustful of the therapist to know that there will be no retaliation. Usually this indicates that there is, at bottom, a good therapeutic alliance. There are, as always, exceptions.

Constant anger at the therapist, particular of a dismissive or contemptuous kind, usually indicates trouble.

Sam was interviewed during the process of selecting members for a new group. Sam was a stocky young man with a bull neck. He looked like a man in training to be a country squire. It was no surprise that he was studying estate management. It *was* a surprise to discover that he was the survivor of a serious road traffic accident that had led to brain damage. His memory was poor, and his intelligence, although average, was substantially below what it had been, and below that of the other members of his family. He joined the new group being convened by a trainee at the beginning of training, and immediately took against the conductor. Every remark that Sam made was disparaging, often humorously, of the conductor's abilities, his intelligence, his understanding. Sam left after a few weeks.

The conductor failed Sam. Sam identified the conductor as someone he might have been had he not had his accident. It was a kind of malignant mirroring because Sam looked at the conductor and saw reflected back the Sam that might have been, had he not had his accident. He could only deal with this by trying to reduce the conductor and make him less of a threat. But this was no good to the other group members who, right at the start of the group, needed to feel confident in the conductor. The conductor had not predicted this, and did not know how to deal with it.

Flattery or compliments do not usually indicate a good therapeutic relationship, especially if the therapist is not someone who is normally treated in this way. They are more likely to indicate that the client feels insecure, but has come to the conclusion that the therapist is open to this kind of cajolery.

Other signs that there are problems in the therapeutic relationship are if the therapist feels bored or tired during the therapy, or if he or she finds him- or herself relying more and more on technique, particularly if that involves interpretations.

Relationship problems arise between client and therapist, as noted previously in this book, when the client's and the therapist's values diverge. They also occur when the emotional flavour of the treatment becomes unpalatable.

Self-monitoring

It is sometimes possible, after a session when things did not seem to go well, to reflect back and see what went wrong. It is easier to see this when there has been a clash of values, than when the flavour of the treatment has changed as far as the client is concerned.

Therapists can make this self-monitoring more efficient if they spend some time reflecting on the session, especially if they are writing extended notes about the session. It is sometimes easier to be critical of written material than when one is speaking to oneself. Writing up cases for presentation at academic meetings, or for publication, also enhances critical self-reflection.

The General Medical Council has recently introduced new guidelines about the publication of confidential material (http://www.gmc-uk.org/n_hance/good/secret.htm). These are similar to those used by many journal editors up to now. Simply omitting identifying details is no longer considered an adequate protection of client confidentiality.

It is good practice for clients to read the intended text of the publication, at least the part of it that contains an account of their case, and to give their consent, in writing, to its publication. However, this may not be feasible in the case of clients who have been seen for assessment and not been taken on for treatment, clients who have dropped out of treatment, or the clients of supervisees. It is worth distinguishing case histories which are used as evidence, for example a single case study of the efficacy of a psychotherapy intervention, and case histories used as illustration. It is unethical to disguise the former by altering details of the case, or by amalgamating several cases, as this will introduce bias into the evidence. Full consent will be required. In the latter case, I believe that it may be permissible to use 'fictionalized' case material as long as there has been an explicit waiver clarifying that none of the cases described corresponds to a real person. This has been the approach taken in this book.

When a practitioner expects to use case illustrations in teaching or in publications, it may be good practice to notify service users that this may happen (Appendix I).

Recordings

Recording sessions make it possible to review what has happened more systematically. Video-recordings are more intrusive than audio-tapes or minidisk recordings and provide little added value, except for providing verisimilitude in teaching.

Recordings should only be made with the client's express consent, and the client should have the opportunity to renew or withdraw this consent at the end of the recording. Detailed recommendations for consent, storage and destruction of the recording are given in a handbook published by the General Medical Council (http://www.gmc-uk.org/n_hance/good/aud_vid.htm).

Many psychotherapists are reluctant to consider recordings because they believe that having a machine 'listening in' is almost like having another person in the room. This may be less of a problem when the treatment is conducted with more than one person, for example in group or family therapy. Indeed, family therapists have welcomed technological innovations, and often use video-links as a means to provide immediate supervision by a practitioner in another room who has, like the third umpire at a cricket match, the luxury of watching the action without having to participate in it.

Being recorded does alter behaviour. People are less likely to forget themselves, and more likely to present themselves. It increases the sense of distance that a person has from what they say or do. This may be readily compatible with short-term therapy, for example in symptomatic treatment when a person is talking about symptoms that they feel are ego-alien. However, it may act as an impediment in longer-term individual therapy when it is essential that both the client and the therapist are personally involved.

A further, practical drawback of recordings is that they are as long as the actual session. Reviewing the whole of a session effectively doubles the time that the practitioner gives to the session. Watching selected bits of the recording is not the answer. Selection may only maintain the therapist's blind spots.

Supervision

Discussing the case with someone else is an even better opportunity for self-monitoring. That could be a colleague, but it is better if it is a suitably qualified practitioner. Supervision can itself engender some of the relationship issues that therapy engenders. It is therefore important that the supervisor does not have a personal relationship with the supervisee, and probably that the supervisor has had training in supervision as well as in being a qualified therapist.

All counsellors and psychotherapists consider that regular supervision is essential during training. All counsellors and many psychotherapists consider that it is essential for any practitioner. Any mental health professional would consider it advisable, if there has been a crisis in a session, whether psychotherapy or not, to discuss it with a suitably qualified colleague.

Audit

If a therapist uses a questionnaire, as discussed in Chapter 4, and especially if that incorporates some standardized measures, it is possible to ask clients to complete these measures on discharge. If the clinic operates a policy of a 3-month reassessment, as mine has, then the measures can be readministered then, too.

In principle, it is therefore possible to obtain quantitative information about client outcome, and also about untoward effects if these are covered by the questionnaire. This enables individual practitioners to review their success rates with particular clients or particular problems, and to compare these rates with other practitioners. It is also possible to compare rates of untoward events.

Audit like this, which rivals many research projects in its complexity, appeals to clinic administrators. Companies even exist who will provide standardized measures, analyse them and present the practitioner with a comparison between his client's scores and those of a pooled population with the same diagnosis at the same stage of treatment.

In practice, most therapists and many clients find it unpalatable to be continually asked to complete forms. Many therapists find that this level of control over their activities undermines the autonomy and creativity that they value.

In fact, the most useful audit information can be obtained much more simply. As soon as audit is introduced into a department, it becomes apparent that many more clients leave therapy unilaterally, by dropping out, than anyone expected. This proportion can be reduced by training therapists in brief therapy techniques (Pekarik, 1994).

There is often a very high proportion of 'no shows' for assessment interviews, too, especially if there is a long waiting list. There may be other untoward events, such as clients being started on antidepressants, clients being referred to psychiatrists, or the use of emergency services, which will be identified by a simple audit.

Individual therapists can learn much about their own practice by considering in detail why an untoward event happened, and how, if at all, it relates to therapy. This process is augmented if the therapist has a trustworthy supervisor who will be willing to help the therapist in this enquiry without blaming or criticizing the therapist. Services can also compare rates. For example, a service which provides an early assessment interview, but then has a long waiting list for treatment, might compare its no show rates for the first treatment appointment with a service which has a long waiting list for assessment, but then provides a quick treatment appointment.

Audit also provides insights into other factors which influence treatment and treatment decisions. For example, in one unpublished study of the Coventry psychotherapy service, it was found that clients with alcohol problems, as estimated by a score of 3 or more on the 'CAGE' questions (trying to Cut back on drinking, being Annoyed at criticisms about drinking, feeling Guilty about drinking, and using alcohol as an Eye opener) (Bush et al., 1987), were much more likely to be seen for treatment by the consultant than by a trainee.

Manuals

Manuals, and more recently guidelines, are increasingly making the transition from research into everyday clinical practice. Their role in psychotherapy is limited at the moment. Too slavish an adherence to them may indicate treatment failure. However, simple guidelines may help in showing up 'special clients' who have developed an unusual, and possibly untherapeutic, relationship with the therapist. The classic paper by Main (1957) includes many examples.

Personal therapy

All of us have blind spots. We each of us see only a part of our world. This is not a problem for a psychotherapist, but refusing to widen one's vision is. If a psychotherapist cannot bear to see what is there because it is too disgusting or too shameful, or if a psychotherapist cannot bear to hear about something because it is too evil, or obscene, then there is a problem.

Blind spots may not even be so stark. Clients in long-term therapy may have periods when they seem to lose the plot, or become childish, or petulant. Clients in long-term therapy, particularly when it is analytically orientated, may become minutely preoccupied by the psychotherapist, trying to get some clue about whether or not the psychotherapist cares for them, or approves of them. These reactions are normal. They are exhibited by perfectly normal people in other intense, one-sided relationships. But they can seem very strange reactions, and an inexperienced psychotherapist can be quite intolerant of them.

Quite often, psychotherapists, particularly those who intend to undertake long-term therapy, are required to have a period of personal therapy. It is unlikely that this will remove all of the therapist's blind spots, although it may remove some, but it does have the inestimable advantage of teaching the neophyte therapist how very differently therapy seems if you are the client, and not the therapist.

Abuse of power

Possibly one of the most important aspects of being a client is the discovery of the power invested in the role of 'therapist'. Therapists who do not have this experience run the risk of under-estimating their potential for dominating their clients. Psychotherapists, despite any reputation to the contrary, are not lacking in authoritarianism, although they may be more devious than their professional colleagues in expressing it. Bullying of clients by psychotherapists, and bullying supervisees or junior staff, is a real danger. Although having personal therapy will not prevent this, it can make practitioners more alert to this danger, and more ready to scrutinize their own conduct carefully.

Some specific crises considered

Being stuck

Indications of being stuck in therapy are itemized in the Rutgers scale (Messner, Tishby & Spillman, 1992) (see Table 11.2). This is clearly influenced by psycho-analytic theory. Other theoretical approaches might give a different emphasis, or add different items. It is important to remember that being stuck is not a consequence of client failure, but failure of the therapy. How to tackle this is covered in the previous section, on general considerations.

Table 11.2. The Rutgers Psychotherapy Process and Stagnation Scale

Item	Good progress	Being stuck in therapy
Description or exploration of significant material	Yes	No
Development of insight	Yes	No
Emotional experiencing of feelings in the session	Yes	No (Avoidance or covering over by defences would indicate being stuck.)
Emergence of new behaviours, or new ways of interacting, in the session	Yes	No (Enactment of the client's pathology without change would indicate being stuck.)
Direct expression of feelings, thoughts, fantasies and fears about the therapist or the therapy	Yes	No
Straightforward, immediate, and direct communications by the client	Yes	Hesitation, confusion or contradiction in the client's speech would indicate being stuck.
Collaboration with the therapist and the therapeutic task	Yes	No
Focussing on the self in relating feelings, reactions, ideas and events	Yes	Repetitive or excessive dwelling on some aspect of the client–therapist relationship or the therapy without exploration would indicate being stuck.

From Messner, Tishby & Spillman, (1992).

Falling in love with your client, and other kinds of acting out

Developing a wish to see the client outside of the therapy means much the same when the therapist has this wish as when the client does. The therapist has discovered, and fallen into, a feeling of loneliness or emotional isolation which has become too distressing to contain. Acting on this feeling destroys the possibility of reflecting on it, and destroys the possibility of therapy. This kind of action is often termed 'acting out' to bring out this destructive connotation. Every ethical code proscribes having a sexual relationship with a client, but surveys estimate that as many as 10% of therapists may do so. It is inevitable when two adults meet that there may be sexual attraction, and, less frequently, that they may fall in love.

It would be naive to suppose that therapists never fall in love with their clients, or clients with them, and inhuman to penalize therapist or client for this. Many ethical codes recognize this by specifying a cooling-off period between the end of the therapeutic relationship and the first non-professional meeting. If a therapist falls in love with his or her client, the first duty is to ensure that the client's welfare is safeguarded. This will normally mean that the therapeutic relationship is appropriately terminated, which might be by arranging for an alternative therapist to see the client. Following that, there should be no contact between the client and the therapist for a sufficient period for any new relationship developing between them not to be attributable to the effects of the therapy. The therapist finding themself in this situation should certainly seek advice from a supervisor or another experienced colleague.

It is impossible for either the therapist or the client to know, if they act on their wish to meet outside the therapeutic situation, who is meeting. Is it the therapist, or is it an idealized figure of the therapist that the client is meeting? Does the therapist meet the client, or an idealized figure of a suffering victim that the therapist can save? It is difficult to imagine anything humanly good coming out of such a false situation.

Some therapists argue, when they admit to breaking therapeutic boundaries, that they do it for special reasons or to help their clients in special ways. However, it is often the case that therapists who break boundaries have had supervisors who have done so as well. Anecdote suggests that therapists who sleep with their clients are likely to have themselves been the targets of sexual activity by their trainers or supervisors. This would suggest that, as for other abusers, the experience of abuse can sometimes lead to a suspension of commonly held values and their replacement by special pleading.

Falling in love with a client is not itself unethical if a practitioner does something about it before any acting out has taken place. The first step is to discuss the matter with an experienced colleague.

Making demands on the therapist

Are you married? Do you have children? Can I have your home number? Do you have a supervisor? Have you seen anyone like me before? Have you treated anyone like me before? Do you like me? You would say that, wouldn't you? If I tell you something, will you promise not to write it down? Sometimes I might not feel like coming, is it OK if I miss those sessions? These and other questions are examples of questions which therapists may find intrusive. They are asking for information which lies outside the boundary of therapy as far as many therapists are concerned. But they seem innocuous.

Whether one answers a question in psychotherapy depends on whether or not it will continue to be possible to answer similar questions. If the therapist is not willing to answer the question, 'What is your wife's name?' or 'Where do you live?', it is unwise to answer the question, 'Are you married?'.

It is important to keep different kinds of awkward questions separate. Asking 'Do you have a supervisor?' is relevant to therapy, even if it might offend a trainee who feels sensitive about his or her lack of experience. It is quite a different question from 'Are you married?' and needs different consideration.

Questions are a means of imposing a particular kind of relationship on someone. They have a flavour for many people of school, or tribunals, where they are put on the spot. A question imposes the values of the questioner on the person being questioned. 'When did you stop beating your wife?', the often quoted leading question of a famous prosecuting barrister, is offensive because it defines familial violence as 'wife-beating' without allowing the respondent to give his own evaluation of why he has been violent to his wife.

It is advisable for psychotherapists to avoid using questions for this reason. An alternative is to make simple declarative statements. Instead of saying, 'When did you stop beating your wife?', one could say, 'You have told me that violence used to erupt between you and your wife, but you haven't told me whether that is still happening'.

Clients may use questioning as a way of trying to even the score with a therapist who uses many questions. When you are being asked lots of questions, ask yourself if you have asked a lot yourself. If so, try to modify them into statements. And also explain to the client why there is such an asymmetry in your relationship. Explain that therapists ask questions not because they think of themselves as superior, but because people come to them when they are in trouble and the therapist has to find out what the trouble is. When the therapist has a problem and goes for help to someone else, they too have to ask lots of questions.

Some cultures are more opposed to questioning than others. In the West, we expect that authorities that we consult will question us a lot. In Nigeria, as has been mentioned elsewhere in this book, questions are thought to betray ignorance. That is, however, also true in the West. Neophyte trainees, or therapists in the presence of someone they consider to be of higher status, are often unwilling to make statements in case the other person disagrees with them. Many a trainee, when called upon at a case conference to comment, has felt impelled to ask for further information, instead of saying what they think. If this happens in therapy, it is worth the therapist considering carefully what might be undermining the client's confidence.

If the therapist chooses to answer a client's question, he or she should feel entitled to ask one in return. It's usually the same one, a variant of 'Why did you ask that?'. Sometimes it is advisable for the therapist to tell the client that he or she will only answer the question if he or she can ask one of their own.

Questioning may be a way of relieving anxiety. Asking the client, 'Why did you ask that?' may disclose a specific anxiety which the therapist has not expected.

Paul had applied to join a group, but was originally told that it was full. Then he received a letter offering him a place after all. Paul was told before the start of the group by another member that there was a rumour going around that one of the people originally accepted for the group had died.

Paul seemed distressed as soon as the group started. He asked the group conductor whether the rumour was true. The conductor was unsure whether to answer this question. It seemed to break one of the boundaries of the group, that which protected the identity of the member who had withdrawn. But it was clear that this was no idle question on Paul's part. So the conductor said, 'I will answer your question if you will tell us after I do so why it is important to you to know'. The conductor then explained that Robert had been accepted for the group, but had then developed a serious illness and had withdrawn. He had not died.

Paul explained that he had been born 12 months after his mother had had a stillbirth. That sister had been called Pauline, and Paul had felt for many years that not only was he a substitute for Pauline, but that his mother often thought that he was a poor substitute. Paul had become terrified that the same situation would be repeated in the group, and that the conductor might think to himself, 'If only it was Robert and not Paul who had joined the group'.

Some people with restricted interpersonal strategies use questioning as a way of establishing control. It is surprisingly effective if the questioner is sufficiently shameless. To deal with this tendency, the therapist needs to be clear which type of questions he or she is prepared to answer. It may be necessary to explain, if the client genuinely does not know, which questions are acceptable and which are not. But it will also be important to reflect on why the client should feel so lacking in control, and whether the arrangements for the therapy are making this worse, in which case these should be changed if possible.

Being asked for reports

A special sort of demand is when the therapist is asked for a report, for example in connection with a court appearance or a compensation claim. It is always easier to deal with this if the possibility has been discussed beforehand. Therapists assessing clients who are involved in litigation or facing a criminal charge should enquire about the possibility of a report before the treatment contract is established. If there is an explicit agreement that the therapist will provide a report when the time comes, it is possible to combine both roles. However, there may be difficulty if the therapist cannot provide an exculpation and if that is what the client has come to expect.

It is probably better, under most circumstances, to separate the role of therapist from the role of report writer, or medical examiner.

Threats to the therapist

Therapists are rarely physically threatened by their clients, but it may happen. Risk assessment is part of the clinical assessment of every person seen nowadays in a mental health setting. High-risk factors include a history of threatening or aggressive behaviour to previous therapists, being required to see the therapist (e.g. by a court order), a history of aggression or violence in other settings, intoxication whilst attending the therapy, carrying a weapon, and angry thoughts about the therapist. There should also be an assessment of the protective factors. Therapists working in solo offices are more vulnerable.

When there is question about risk, this should be discussed with an experienced colleague, such as a supervisor. Therapists who feel under threat are unlikely to be able to carry out good treatment, and there is little point in insisting that a therapist sees a client unless the therapist is comfortable about doing so.

Intoxication

Intoxication is one of the factors affecting the risk assessment. Clients who regularly attend therapy sessions whilst intoxicated are unlikely to benefit. Any gains that may be made during the therapy are likely to be state-dependent. This should not be a reason for withholding treatment from the client, but only for choosing practical counselling aimed at abstinence or controlled use (see Chapter 8) rather than psychotherapy or therapeutic counselling.

Breakdown

It is always alarming if the mental health of a psychotherapy client seems to be deteriorating. It is easy to panic. Indeed, the commonest reason for deterioration is that the client is becoming so anxious that he or she feels overwhelmed. When a person speaks of a breakdown, he or she often means a severe episode of anxiety.

If the client is having a breakdown, then this will be his or her preoccupying concern. The focus of the psychotherapy should therefore be redirected to this concern, and an appropriate approach adopted. This may be one of the symptomatic approaches considered in Chapter 5, but it is more likely to be an approach that is not psychotherapeutic at all. What clients need most during a breakdown is practical, relevant help, and the psychotherapist is more likely to be needed as an advocate and advisor, than as a psychotherapist.

It is very difficult for psychotherapists to make medical or psychiatric assessments of clients who are established in therapy. One of the first priorities if a psychotherapy client breaks down may therefore be to ensure that the client gets an appropriate and independent assessment. Psychotherapists have to remember that they have a more stringent duty of confidentiality to their clients than many other health professionals. However, the contract between clients and their therapists in the health service will not normally preclude contact being made with another professional with the client's agreement. One of the most important tasks of the psychotherapist may therefore be to assist their client to gain entry into the mental health services.

As in other crisis situations, it is always a good idea to make careful notes, and to discuss any decisions that seem uncertain with colleagues, such as a supervisor.

Therapy breakdown

It sometimes happens, despite a therapist's best efforts at dealing with earlier crises and at ensuring that the pre-conditions for therapy are as good as possible, that the boundaries around the treatment become so insecure that therapy no longer seems possible. Perhaps the client starts coming so late that there is no useful time in which to work, or the client attends so irregularly that there ceases to be a connection between the sessions.

Sometimes clients will attribute the difficulties to practical problems with work or with child care. If these are likely to be long-lasting, the therapist should continue to suggest a moratorium on the therapy, giving the client the opportunity to return and re-start treatment once the practical problems are removed. If the practical problems are a front to the client's personal reluctance to continue in therapy, this proposal will usually result in the client disclosing their antipathy to the treatment.

The therapist should consider carefully whether there is anything about the therapeutic set-up that could be causing the client's antipathy. This is a good moment to discuss matters with a colleague or supervisor.

It is important to remember that it is not the therapist's responsibility to cure the client, but the client's responsibility to do everything that they can to achieve their goals. Therapists should not feel guilt if the client terminates treatment prematurely. In fact, it is much better to agree on termination than to plug along until the client withdraws unilaterally. The therapist should not blame the client, either. Psychotherapy can be no more effective than any other healing art. There are many conditions in medicine which are incurable. Doctors simply do not know enough. There are also many psychological conditions about which therapists simply do not know enough to resolve them. Note how important it is for the therapist to have examined, preferably with a colleague, whether there is anything more that could be done. It is important that when the therapist says to the client, 'We have done all we can, but there is no more that the two of us could do', that is not a mere trope, but a carefully considered conclusion. Clients should not leave therapy thinking that they have failed.

When there has been a breakdown of the therapy, the therapist should be careful not to place barriers in front of the client which may prevent the client from re-considering and seeking psychotherapy in the future, either from the same or from another therapist. Sometimes it is just the human chemistry that goes wrong, and another therapist can succeed with a client that a previous therapist has considered intractably personality-disordered.

Saying goodbye

Endings may be no problem. After all, although many of us might regret the ending of an exciting holiday or a spell of working abroad, we often also look forward to going home and putting our newly created energy into use.

Many short-term therapists include provisions about ending from the first session of treatment. For example, in considering homework, the therapist might say, 'I wonder if this will be something that you will be able to continue after our sessions finish'. It is common for the therapist to remind clients of the session number in other short-term approaches, and to ask the client if he or she is satisfied that the therapy will provide the desired outcome by the time that the planned sessions have come to an end.

Freddy had panic attacks. He had agreed to have four sessions of cognitively orientated treatment and it was the start of the third session. Freddy had proved to be an apt pupil of breathing control, and relaxation. He had had a modified panic attack after his first treatment session, but had been able to tell himself that his chest pain was due to over-breathing, and not cardiac insufficiency. This had successfully moderated his panicky feelings. 'They were bad', said Freddy, 'but not so bad that I couldn't get above them'.

The therapist asked Freddy if he had got enough confidence now to manage a future panic attack after the end of the next session, which was the one that they had agreed would be the final review before a likely ending. Freddy got very irritated. 'I don't know why you keep going on about it', he said, 'It just makes me anxious. I suppose it gives you a comfortable feeling of indispensability'.

The therapist noted the feelings that Freddy had attributed to her, and assumed that they had something to do with Freddy's way of relating to people. He seemed to be a rather insecure person who felt better when they had someone else dependent on them. However, she did not want to pursue this psychodynamic focus. So she asked him what upset him about talking about the ending. Freddy admitted, that whilst he now felt that he could manage his panic disorder when the therapist was on hand to be able to help him, if he couldn't, the idea that he would have no-one to turn to if he stopped being able to 'get above them' was frightening. Again, the therapist felt that Freddy's lack of confidence in himself could be linked to past experiences which might have been explored if that had been the therapeutic focus. However, she again turned her face against them, and said instead, 'You do not think that there is anything that you can do that would make you more confident?'

The rest of the session was spent answering this question. At the end of it, Freddy agreed that he could do several things. He could remember that he had overcome his panic disorder on several occasions now, on his own. He could imagine what the therapist would say. And the therapist said that she would be willing to give Freddy an appointment in 3 months' time if he still wanted that next week.

Endings may not need to be abrupt. After all, this is not the way that people normally break off relationships. Clients can be offered 3- or 6-month reviews, which have the further advantage that they usually provide the therapist with feedback about the durability of therapeutic gains. Therapy can be gradually spaced out, going from once weekly to once a fortnight or once a month, and then once every 3 or 6 months.

Therapists sometimes believe that it is valuable to face ending and separation anxiety 'head on', and that procedures which do not do this are untherapeutic. They may be sometimes. If it is the client who demands them of the therapist, and if they are used simply as devices to get as much of the therapist's attentions as possible, they are. But if the whole of the previous treatment has been carried out in an open and collaborative spirit, it is very unlikely that this coercive element will enter in just at the point of ending.

Ending therapy may mean that the client has to deal with a number of losses. Clients may experience themselves as losing any of the following: the security of a person to whom one is attached, social support, social comparison, access to other health services, invalid status, social contact, and hope. It is easy, however, for therapists to minimize the costs of therapy to the client, and to forget the many other supports and opportunities that everyone has. It is also easy to forget that clients are not so dissimilar to therapists. When faced with difficulty, they have intelligence, life experience and other resources at their disposal to overcome them.

Ending does carry with it a strong emotional flavour for many people who have experienced bereavements or forced separations. Even temporary absence, such as at holiday time, may evoke these flavours. Both therapist and client are most likely to be able to change the meaning if they can anticipate and rehearse the ending. What matters is that the ending should not be seen as an attack on the client's peace of mind. The worst kind of attack is for the client to feel that they have proved too shameful or too disgusting for the therapist to continue to work with them.

Two emotions counteract this flavour: gratitude that the therapy has achieved its goal, and pride in one's achievement. These emotions appertain to the therapy, and are strongest when both client and therapist feel them. The right moment to end is when there is nothing more that needs to be said – when both therapist and client can look back at their hard work and feel both a sense of having accomplished something, and a recognition of how much the other person has contributed to that accomplishment.

Appendix: confidential record

When you come to the service, you will have the opportunity to discuss your difficulties with us. However, we have found that it helps us to have some preliminary information which we ask you to provide by filling in this form. It would be a help to us – and will mean more time for you to talk about your immediate problems with the therapist – if you could send it back to us when you confirm your appointment. If this is not possible, please bring it with you when you come to see the doctor.

Confidentiality

Anything you write to us, or that is written about you by us, will be kept completely confidential and will normally only be seen by the staff directly involved with the University Clinic. However, you may want to note the following.

Should you convince a member of staff that you intend to cause serious harm to another person, the member of staff may be legally required to disclose your intention to the relevant authorities if you are unwilling to do so yourself. This will never be done without your knowledge.

Members of staff in the clinic do undertake research. Occasionally this may mean that a member of the clinic staff wishes to include you in a research project. If so, you will be given information about the project and asked for your written consent. If you refuse, it will not affect your treatment in any way.

Some members of staff or trainees receive supervision. This means that they will discuss your case with a qualified colleague, who will be bound by the same requirements of confidentiality that bind all other staff members.

Members of staff do sometimes wish to use what clients and supervisees have told them in lectures and publications. This is essential as this is a research and teaching department. A member of staff wishing to use information about you in this way must first obtain your consent except if that information is so disguised that no-one, including anyone who knows you well, could recognize you.

Some information will be stored on a computer database which has been registered under the Database Protection Act. This, too, will be confidential. Information from the database may be used for research to improve the service that we offer. If this happens, we will ensure that you can never be identified in any report or publication. Please note that if you decided not to complete the questionnaire, it will not affect our willingness to try to help you, or the type of help that you are offered. You have the right to inspect your entry or to read notes made about you in the clinic. If you wish to do so, please contact the Clinic Administrator.

First name: . . . . Last name: . . . .
Title: (Prof, Dr, Mr, Mrs, Ms, etc.) . . . .
Address:
    Street: . . . .
    District: . . . .
    Town: . . . . Postcode: . . . .
NHS no: . . . . Medical record no: . . . .
Date of birth: . . . . Age: . . . .
Home phone no: . . . . Can we phone you at home? (Y/N): . . . . .
Work phone no: . . . . Can we phone you at work? (Y/N): . . . . .

Your general practitioner is:
Name: . . . .
Address: . . . .
. . . .
Postcode . . . . Phone no: . . . .
Consultant: . . . .

The following information is needed to ensure that our service is being used by people from all walks of life. Whatever your answer, it will not alter your chances of getting the treatment that you need.

Are you male or female? . . . .

Do you consider yourself as white, black-Caribbean, black-African, Indian, Pakistani, Bangladeshi, Chinese, other? (please state) . . . .

What language do you use at home? . . . .

Do you have a religious affiliation? . . . .

If so, what is it? . . . .

Have you *ever* been married or lived with a partner for longer than a year? . . . .

Are you *currently*: single/married/remarried/separated/divorced/widowed? . . . .

Please would you give details of who is living at home with you at the moment, and their relationship to you, indicating which are children: . . . .

Are you in paid employment? . . . .

Please describe your work: . . . .

If you are living with a partner, is he/she in paid employment? . . . .

Please describe his/her work: . . . .

What would you like us to know about your problems before we see you? . . . .

Can you say why you are seeking help now? . . . .

Is there anyone you would like to be involved in your treatment? . . . .

If so, please tell us who: . . . .

Please indicate how disabling you feel your main problem is by putting a cross on the line at the appropriate point:

| | | | | | | | | | | | | | |

I am totally disabled   I have no
by my psychological   problems
problems

and also how distressing you feel your main problems is:

| | | | | | | | | | | | | | |

I am extremely distressed   I have no
by my psychological   problems
problems

Are you a teetotaller? . . . .

If not, please answer the following questions:

Have you ever felt you should cut down on your drinking?   Y/N

Have people ever annoyed you by criticizing your drinking?   Y/N
Have you ever felt guilty or bad about your drinking?   Y/N
Have you ever had a drink first thing in the morning to steady
your nerves or to get rid of a hangover?   Y/N

Family background

Please give details of *all* your brothers and sisters, including half-brothers/
-sisters and step-brothers/-sisters. Please start with the oldest and include
yourself in the list.

Relationship to you	First name	Age now or at death	If dead, your age at death and cause	Marital status	Occupation
[FATHER]					
[MOTHER]					

Were you brought up with your father? . . . . If so, please answer questions
(i) to (v) about him.

(i) His age when you were born: . . . .

(ii) Was he at home: *all* of your life, *most* of your life, *some* of your life, *none*
of your life? . . . .

(iii) His physical health
in the past: . . . .
now: . . . .

(iv) His mental health
      in the past: ....
      now: ....

(v) Would you say you have been close to him
      in the past: ....
      now: ....

Were you brought up with your mother? ....
If so, please answer questions (i) to (v) about her. If not, were you brought up with any other woman? ....
Was her relationship to you a stepmother, grandmother, friend, foster-mother, paid carer? (please ring answer)

Please answer questions (i) to (v) about her:

(i) Her age when you were born: ....

(ii) Was she at home: *all* of your life, *most* of your life, *some* of your life, *none* of your life? ....

(iii) Her physical health
      in the past: ....
      now: ....

(iv) Her mental health
      in the past: ....
      now: ....

(v) Would you say you have been close to her
      in the past: ....
      now: ....

If you were brought up by people other than those you have just told us about, please give details: ....
....
....

Which of the brothers/sisters you have mentioned were you brought up with?
....
....
....

If anyone in your family has had problems with their mental health (nerves), please could you tell us about them: ....
....
....

Could you tell us something about your growing up and your family during

your childhood years? . . . .
. . . .
. . . .

Please tell us about anything that sticks in your mind, including separations, deaths, times away from home, or changes you experienced: . . . .
. . . .
. . . .

Would you consider your childhood years as happy? . . . .
. . . .
. . . .

Were you ill as a child? . . . .

Were you nervous as a child? . . . .

Education

Please give a brief summary of your education, including part-time or evening classes, and periods of professional training.

From	To	Kind of school or institute	Subjects or activities preferred	Standard reached or exams taken

What age did you finish full-time education? . . . .

What aspects of your school days did you like? . . . .
. . . .

What problems (if any) did you have at school? . . . .
. . . .

Overall, did you enjoy school? . . . .

Current lifestyle

Are you in a relationship at the moment? . . . .

If so, are you married/living with your partner? . . . .

Have you ever had children? . . . .

If so, give their age, sex and occupation:

. . . .

. . . .

Please tell us about any particular worries that you have concerning:

Work . . . .

Money . . . .

Housing . . . .

Health . . . .

Partner . . . .

Children . . . .

Have you had any severe stresses, sudden shocks or traumas recently? Please give details: . . . .

. . . .

. . . .

. . . .

. . . .

Health

Have you had any serious illnesses or accidents in your life? . . . .

. . . .

. . . .

. . . .

Have you had previous psychiatric treatment? . . . .

Please give details, including dates and places of any in-client treatment: . .

. . . .

. . . .

. . . .

Have you ever been prescribed tablets for nervous problems? . . . .

If so, please give details: . . . .
. . . .
. . . .
. . . .

Have you had previous psychotherapy/counselling? . . . .

If so, who gave it and what effect did it have? . . . .
. . . .
. . . .
. . . .

Have you participated in self-help groups? . . . .

If so, which groups and what effect did they have? . . . .
. . . .
. . . .
. . . .

Have you ever been recommended self-help literature? . . . .

If so, what was it and what effect did it have? . . . .
. . . .
. . . .
. . . .

Please give details of any medication you are on: . . . .
. . . .
. . . .
. . . .

Have you used drugs not prescribed by a doctor? . . . .
    in the past: . . . .
    now: . . . .

Have you in the past drunk too much? . . . .

Have you ever got into difficulties through gambling? . . . .
. . . .

Have you ever deliberately harmed yourself as a punishment, or in an attempt
to kill yourself? . . . .
. . . .

Do you smoke? . . . .

Please give details of any problems you have had with your weight, including
over-eating, severe loss of weight, dieting, etc. . . . .

. . . .
. . . .
. . . .

Do you consider yourself to be physically disabled in any way? . . . .
. . . .

Do you consider that you have ever been physically or sexually abused? . . .
. . . .
. . . .
. . . .

Do you have any close friends at the moment? . . . .

Have you ever had problems with the police or the courts? . . . .
. . . .

Please write here if there is anything else you would like to tell us before your appointment:

Finally, how did you feel about filling in this questionnaire?

THANK YOU

Professor Digby Tantam
Dilemma Consultancy in Human Relations

© Professor Digby Tantam

References

Addis, M.E. & Jacobson, N.S. (1996). Reasons for depression and the process and outcome of cognitive-behavioral psychotherapies. *Journal of Consulting and Clinical Psychology*, **64**, 1417–24.

Agazarian, Y. & Peters, R. (1983). *The Visible and the Invisible Group*. London: Routledge.

Aichorn, A. (1935). *Wayward Youth*. New York: Viking Press.

Allsop, S., Saunders, B. & Phillips, M. (2000). The process of relapse in severely dependent male problem drinkers. *Addiction*, **95** (1), 95–106.

Amsterdam, B. (1968). *Mirror Behavior in Children under Two Years of Age*. University of North Carolina.

Andrews, B. (1995). Bodily shame as a mediator between abusive experiences and depression. *Journal of Abnormal Psychology*, **104**, 277–85.

Anonymous (1999). *Liddell–Scott–Jones Lexicon of Classical Greek*. Tufts University.

Argyle, M. (1997). Is happiness a cause of health? *Psychology and Health*, **12** (6), 769–81.

Asher, R. (1972). *Talking Sense*. London: Pitman Medical Publishing Co.

Averill, J. (1980). A constructivist view of emotion. In *Theories of Emotion*, ed. R.K. Plutchik, H. Kellerman, Vol. 1, Emotion: theory, research, and experience, pp. 1–20. New York: Academic Press.

Baesler, E.J. (1995). Construction and test of an empirical measure for narrative coherence and fidelity. *Communication Reports*, **8**, 97–101.

Balint, M. (1957). *The Doctor, His Patient and the Illness*, p. International, NY, International Universities Press, xii, 355 pp.

Balint, M., Ornstein, P. & Balint, E. (1972). *Focal Psychotherapy. An Example of Applied Psychoanalysis*. London: Tavistock Press.

Bancroft, J. (1989). *Human Sexuality and its Problems*. Edinburgh: Churchill Livingstone.

Bannister, D. (1970). Science through the looking glass. In *Perspectives in Personal Construct Theory*, ed. D. Bannister. New York: Academic Press.

Bannister, D. & Fransella, F. (1986). *Inquiring Man*, 3rd edn. London: Croom Helm.

Barrett, K. (1998). A functionalist perspective to the development of emotions. In *What Develops in Emotional Development?* ed. M. Mascolo, S. Griffin, pp. 109–34. New York: Plenum.

Barthes, R. (1973). *Mythologies*. London: Paladin.

Bartholomew, K. (1997). Adult attachment processes: individual and couple perspectives. *British Journal of Medical Psychology*, **70** (3), 249–63; discussion 281–90.

Beauchamp, T. & Childress, J. (1979). *Principles of Biomedical Ethics,* Vol. 3. New York: Oxford, University Press.

Beck, A., Rush, A., Shaw, B., et al. (1979). *Cognitive Therapy of Depression.* Chichester: Wiley.

Bergsma, J. & Mook, B. (1998). Ethical considerations in psychotherapeutic systems. *Theoretical Medicine and Bioethics,* **19** (4), 371–81.

Berke, J. & Hyman, S. (2000). Addiction, dopamine, and the molecular mechanisms of memory. *Neuron,* **25,** 515–32.

Bilu, Y. & Witztum, E. (1993). Working with Jewish ultra-orthodox patients: guidelines for a culturally sensitive therapy. *Culture, Medicine and Psychiatry,* **17** (2), 197–233.

Bion, W. (1988). A theory of thinking. In *Melanie Klein Today: Developments in Theory and Practice, Vol. 1: Mainly theory,* ed. E. Spillius, pp. 178–86. London: Routledge.

Blanz, B., Schmidt, M.H., Esser, G., et al. (1990). The importance of early and current risk factors for the development of psychiatric disorders in childhood and adolescence. In *The Public Health Impact of Mental Disorder,* ed. D. Goldberg, D. Tantam, pp. 145–53. Toronto: Hogrefe and Huber.

Bond, T. (1993). *Standards and Ethics for Counselling in Action* (Counselling in Action), London: Sage.

Bouwer, C. & Stein, D.J. (1997). Association of panic disorder with a history of traumatic suffocation. *American Journal of Psychiatry,* **154** (11), 1566–70.

Bradley, F. (1944). *Essays on Truth and Reality.* Oxford: Oxford University Press.

Brandist, C. (1997). The Bakhtin circle. In http://www.utm.edu/research/iep/b/bakhtin.htm: *The Internet Encyclopaedia of Philosophy.*

Brandon, S., Boakes, J., Glaser, D., et al. (1998). Recovered memories of childhood sexual abuse. Implications for clinical practice. *British Journal of Psychiatry,* **172,** 296–307.

Breuer, J. & Freud, S. (1950). *Studies in Hysteria,* transl. A. Brill. Boston: Beacon Press.

Brewin, C.R., Andrews, B., Rose, S., et al. (1999). Acute stress disorder and posttraumatic stress disorder in victims of violent crime [see comments]. *American Journal of Psychiatry,* **156** (3), 360–6.

Brown, B., Nolan, P., Crawford, P., et al. (1996). Interaction, language and the narrative turn in psychotherapy and psychiatry. *Social Science and Medicine,* **43** (11), 1569–78.

Broyard, A. (1990). Good books about being sick. *New York Times Book Review,* April 1st, pp. 28–9.

Budman, S. & Gurman, A. (1983). The practice of brief psychotherapy. *Professional Psychology: Research and Practice,* **14,** 277–92.

Bugental, J. (1976). *The Search for Existential Identity.* San Francisco: Jossey-Bass.

Bush, B., Shaw, S., Cleary, P., et al. (1987). Screening for alcohol abuse using the CAGE questionnaire. *American Journal of Medicine,* **82** (2), 231–5.

Campbell, W.K., Sedikides, C. & Bosson, J. (1994). Romantic involvement, self-discrepancy and psychological well-being: a preliminary investigation. *Personal Relationships,* **1,** 399–404.

Carr, A.C., Ghosh, A. & Marks, I.M. (1988). Computer-supervised exposure treatment for phobias. *Canadian Journal of Psychiatry (Revue Canadienne de Psychiatrie),* **33,** 112–17.

Carr, E.G., Yarbrough, S.C. & Langdon, N.A. (1997). Effects of idiosyncratic stimulus variables on functional analysis outcomes. *Journal of Applied Behavior Analysis*, **30** (4), 673–86.

Carver, C.S. & Scheier, M.F. (1999). Themes and issues in the self-regulation of behavior. In *Perspectives on Behavioral Self-regulation*, ed. R.S.J. Wyer, Vol. 12. Mahwah, NJ: Lawrence Erlbaum.

Castonguay, L.G., Goldfried, M.R., Wiser, S., et al. (1996). Predicting the effect of cognitive therapy for depression: a study of unique and common factors. *Journal of Consulting and Clinical Psychology*, **64** (3), 497–504.

Catalan, J., Gath, D., Anastasiades, P., et al. (1991). Evaluation of a brief psychological treatment for emotional disorders in primary care. *Psychological Medicine*, **21**, 1013–18.

Chessick, R.D. (1990). Hermeneutics for psychotherapists. *American Journal of Psychotherapy*, **44** (2), 256–73.

Childress, A.R., Mozley, P.D., McElgin, W., et al. (1999). Limbic activation during cue-induced cocaine craving. *American Journal of Psychiatry*, **156** (1), 11–18.

Clark, J.J., Leukefeld, C. & Godlaski, T. (1999). Case management and behavioral contracting – components of rural substance abuse treatment. *Journal of Substance Abuse Treatment*, **17**, 293–304.

Clum, G.A., Clum, G.A. & Surls, R. (1993). A meta-analysis of treatments for panic disorder. *Journal of Consulting and Clinical Psychology*, **61** (2), 317–26.

Conan Doyle, A. (1981). *The Complete Sherlock Holmes*, London: Penguin Books.

Coursey, R.D., Keller, A.B. & Farrell, E.W. (1995). Individual psychotherapy and persons with serious mental illness: the clients' perspective. *Schizophrenia Bulletin*, **21** (2), 283–301.

Crisp, A.H., Norton, K., Gowers, S., et al. (1991). A controlled study of the effect of therapies aimed at adolescent and family psychopathology in anorexia nervosa. *British Journal of Psychiatry*, **159**, 325–33.

Crits-Christoph, P., Siqueland, L., Blaine, J., et al. (1999). Psychosocial treatments for cocaine dependence: National Institute on Drug Abuse Collaborative Cocaine Treatment Study [see comments]. *Archives of General Psychiatry*, **56** (6), 493–502.

Crowe, M. & Ridley, J. (1990). *Therapy with Couples*. Oxford: Blackwell Scientific Publications.

Davanloo, H. (1978). Continuum of psychotherapeutic possibilities and basic psychotherapeutic techniques. Basic principles and techniques in short-term dynamic psychotherapy, ed. H. Davanloo, pp. 74–81. New York: Spectrum.

Davanloo, H. (1980). *Short-term Psychotherapy*. New York: Jason Aronson.

Deb, S., Lyons, I., Koutzoukis, C., et al. (1999). Rate of psychiatric illness 1 year after traumatic brain injury. *American Journal of Psychiatry*, **156** (3), 374–8.

DeBerry, S. & Baskin, D. (1989). Termination criteria in psychotherapy: a comparison of private and public practice. *American Journal of Psychotherapy*, **43**, 43–53.

Demitrack, M.A., Putnam, F.W., Rubinow, D.R., et al. (1993). Relation of dissociative phenomena to levels of cerebrospinal fluid monoamine metabolites and beta-endorphin in patients with eating disorders: a pilot study. *Psychiatry Research*, **49** (1), 1–10.

Derlega, V.J., Hendrick, S.S., Winstead, B.A., et al. (1992). Psychotherapy as a personal relationship: a social psychological perspective. *Psychotherapy*, **29**, 331–5.

Docherty, J.P., Marder, S.R., Van Kammen, D.P., et al. (1977). Psychotherapy and pharmacotherapy: conceptual lenses. *American Journal of Psychiatry*, **134**, 529–33.

Dsubanko Obermayr, K. & Baumann, U. (1998). Informed consent in psychotherapy: demands and reality. *Psychotherapy Research*, **8**, 231–47.

Dunnegan, S.W. (1997). Violence, trauma and substance abuse. *Journal of Psychoactive Drugs*, **29**, 345–51.

Dutton, D.G., van Ginkel, C. & Starzomski, A. (1995). The role of shame and guilt in the intergenerational transmission of abusiveness. US: Springer Publishing Co.

Egan, G. (1990). *The Skilled Helper*. New York: Brooks Cole.

Elkin, I., Parloff, M.B., Hadley, S.W., et al. (1985). NIMH Treatment of Depression Collaborative Research Program. Background and research plan. *Archives of General Psychiatry*, **42** (3), 305–16.

Ellenberger, H. (1970). *The Discovery of the Unconscious: The History and Evolution of Dynamic Psychiatry*. New York: Basic Books.

Ellinwood, E. & Kilbey, M. (1975). Amphetamine stereotypy: the influence of environmental factors and prepotent behavioural patterns on its topography and development. *Biological Psychiatry*, **10**, 3–16.

Erickson, M. (1993). Rethinking Oedipus: an evolutionary perspective of incest avoidance. *American Journal of Psychiatry*, **150**, 411–16.

Erikson, E. (1963). *Childhood and Society*. Vol. 2. New York: W.W. Norton.

Erwin, E. (1996). *A Final Accounting: Philosophical and Empirical Issues in Freudian Psychology*. Cambridge, MA: MIT Press.

Evans, R. (1975). *Carl Rogers. The Man and his Ideas*. New York: E.P. Dutton.

Evans, J. & Over, D. (1997). Are people rational? Yes, no and sometimes. *The Psychologist: Bulletin of the British Psychological Society*, **10**, 403–6.

Ezriel, H. (1950). Psychoanalytic approach to group treatment. *British Journal of Medical Psychology*, **23**, 59–74.

Fairbairn, W.R.D. (1946). Object-relationships and dynamic structure. *International Journal of Psycho-Analysis*, **27**, 30–7.

Fallowfield, L.J., Hall, A., Maguire, G.P., et al. (1990). Psychological outcomes of different treatment policies in women with early breast cancer outside a clinical trial [see comments]. *British Medical Journal*, **301** (6752), 575–80.

Fisher, W. (1987). *Human Communication as Narration: Toward a Philosophy of Reason, Value, and Action*. Columbia, South Carolina: University of South Carolina Press.

Foon, A.E. (1986). Locus of control and clients' expectations of psychotherapeutic outcome. *British Journal of Clinical Psychology*, **25**, 161–71.

Foreman, D.M. (1990). The ethical use of paradoxical interventions in psychotherapy. *Journal of Medical Ethics*, **16** (4), 200–5.

Foucault, M. (1973). *Madness and Civilization: A History of Insanity in the Age of Reason*. New York: Vintage Books.

Foulkes, S.H. (1979). *Therapeutic Group Analysis*. London: George Allen and Unwin.

Foulkes, S.J. (1975). *Group-Analytic Psychotherapy: Methods and Principles*. London: Gordon and Breach.

Fowles, D. (1992). Motivational approach to anxiety disorders. In *Anxiety: Recent Developments in Cognitive, Psychophysiological and Health Research*, ed. D.G. Forgays, p. 282. Washington: Hemisphere Publishing Corporation.

Fox, K.J. (1999). Changing violent minds: discursive correction and resistance in the cognitive treatment of violent offenders in prison. University of California: University of California Press.

Frank, J. (1965). Therapist empathy, genuineness and warmth in treatment. *Journal of Consulting and Clinical Psychology*, **30**, 395–90.

Frank, J.D. (1984). Therapeutic components of psychotherapy. *Journal of Nervous and Mental Disease*, **159**, 325–42.

Frank, J. D. (1993). *The views of a Psychotherapist*. Bern: Huber.

Freeston, M.H., Ladouceur, R., Thibodeau, N., et al. (1991). *Cognitive Intrusions in a Non-clinical Population: I. Response Style, Subjective Experience, and Appraisal*, England: Elsevier Science Ltd.

Freud, S. (1910). Five lectures on psycho-analysis. *American Journal of Psychology*, **21**, 181–218.

Freud, S. (1919). Lines of advance in psycho-analytic therapy. In *Standard Edition*, ed. J. Strachey, Vol. 17, p. 159. London: Hogarth Press.

Freud, S. (1940). An outline of psycho-analysis. *International Journal of Psycho-Analysis*, **21**, 27–82.

Freud, S. (1954). *The Origins of Psycho-analysis*. New York: Basic Books.

Freud, S. (1955). *Totem and Taboo*. London: Hogarth Press, 161 pp.

Freud, S. (1965). *The Interpretation of Dreams*. New York: Avon Books.

Fried, D., Crits-Christoph, P. & Luborsky, L. (1992). The first empirical demonstration of transference in psychotherapy. *Journal of Nervous and Mental Disease*, **180** (5), 326–31.

Frijda, N. (1986). *The Emotions*. Cambridge: Cambridge University Press.

Frijda, N. (1988). The laws of emotion. *American Psychologist*, **43**, 349–58.

Frijda, N., Mesquita, B., Sonnemans, J., et al. (1991). The duration of affective phenomena or emotions, sentiments and passions. In *International Review of Studies on Emotion*, ed. K. Strongman, Vol. 1, pp. 187–225. Chichester: Wiley.

Gillon, R. (1994). Medical ethics: four principles plus attention to scope. *British Medical Journal*, **309**, 184–8.

Glover, J. (1988). *I: The Philosophy of Personal Identity*. London: Allen Lane.

Goffman, E. (1956). Embarrassment and social organization. *American Journal of Sociology*, **62**, 264–75.

Goffman, E. (1969). On face work. In *Where the Action Is*, ed. E. Goffman, pp. 1–36. London: Allen Lane.

Goffman, E. (2001). *The Presentation of Self in Everyday Life*, ed. A. Branaman, pp. 175–82. Malden, MA: Blackwell Publishers.

Goldstein, K. (1939). *The Organism: A Holistic Approach Derived from Pathological Data in Man*. New York: American Book Co.

Goldstein, I., Lue, T.F., Padma-Nathan, H., et al. (1998). Oral sildenafil in the treatment of erectile dysfunction. Sildenafil Study Group [see comments] *New England Journal of Medicine*, **338** (20), 1397–404. [published erratum appears in N Engl J Med 1998 Jul 2;339(1):59].

Gottman, J.M. (1999). *The Marriage Clinic: A Scientifically Based Marital Therapy*. New York: W.W. Norton.

Gottschalk, L. (1990). The psychotherapies in the context of new developments in the neurosciences and biological psychiatry. *American Journal of Psychotherapy*, **44**, 321–39.

Gowers, S., Norton, K., Halek, C., et al. (1994). Outcome of outpatient psychotherapy in a random allocation treatment study of anorexia nervosa. *International Journal of Eating Disorders*, **15**, 165–77.

Greenberg, M. & Littlewood, R. (1995). Post-adoption incest and phenotypic matching: experience, personal meanings and biosocial implications. *British Journal of Medical Psychology*, **68** (1), 29–44.

Greenberg, J.R. & Mitchell, S.A. (1983). *Object Relations in Psychoanalytic Theory*. Cambridge, MA: Harvard University Press.

Grunbaum, A. (1986). Précis of 'the foundations of psychoanalysis: a philosophical critique'. *Behavioral and Brain Sciences*, **9**, 217–28.

Haberlandt, K. & Bingham, G. (1978). Verbs contribute to the coherence of brief narratives: reading related and unrelated sentence triples. *Journal of Verbal Learning and Verbal Behavior*, **17**, 419–25.

Haley, J. (1963). *Strategies of Psychotherapy*. New York: Grune and Stratton.

Harman, G. (1999). *Moral Philosophy Meets Social Psychology: Virtue Ethics and the Fundamental Attribution Error*: http://www.cogsci.princeton.edu/~ghh/Virtue.html.

Harre, R. (1979). *Social Being*. Oxford: Blackwell.

Harre, R. (1983). *Personal Being. A Theory for Individual Psychology*. Oxford: Blackwell.

Harre, R. & Gillett, G. (1994). *Discursive Mind*. Thousand Oaks: Sage.

Hartman, L.M. (1983). Effects of sex and marital therapy on sexual interaction and marital happiness. *Journal of Sex and Marital Therapy*, **9**, 137–51.

Hawton, K., Catalan, J. & Fagg, J. (1992). Sex therapy for erectile dysfunction: characteristics of couples, treatment outcome, and prognostic factors. *Archives of Sexual Behavior*, **21** (2), 161–75.

Heber, A.S., Fleisher, W.P., Ross, C.A., et al. (1989). Dissociation in alternative healers and traditional therapists: a comparative study. *American Journal of Psychotherapy*, **43** (4), 562–74.

Heidegger, H. (1927). *Being and Time*. London: Harper and Row.

Heider, F. (1963). *The Psychology of Interpersonal Relations*. New York: Wiley.

Herz, R.S. (1997). Emotion experienced during encoding enhances odor retrieval cue effectiveness. *American Journal of Psychology*, **110** (4), 489–505.

Hicks, T. (1996–2000). Seven steps for effective problem-solving in the workplace http://www.conflict-resolution.net/articles/index.cfm edn.

Hobbs, M., Mayou, R., Harrison, B., et al. (1996). A randomised controlled trial of psychological debriefing for victims of road traffic accidents. *British Medical Journal*, **313** (7070 UR - http://bmj.com/cgi/content/full/313/7070/1438), pp. 1438–9.

Hobson, R. (1985). *Forms of Feeling. The Heart of Psychotherapy*. London: Tavistock Press.

Hollon, S. & Beck, A. (1994). Cognitive and cognitive behavioral therapies. In *Handbook of Psychotherapy and Behavior Change*, ed. A. Bergin, S. Garfield, pp. 428–66. New York: Wiley.

Holmes, J. & Lindley, R. (1995). *The Values of Psychotherapy*, revised edn. London: Karnac Books.

Hout, M.v.d., Merckelbach, H. & Pool, K. (1996). Dissociation, reality monitoring, trauma, and thought suppression. *Behavioural and Cognitive Psychotherapy*, **24**, 97–108.

Howard, G.S. (1991). Culture tales. A narrative approach to thinking, cross-cultural psychology, and psychotherapy. (review) *American Psychologist*, **46** (3), 187–97.

Howard, K., Kopta, S., Krause, M., et al. (1986). The dose–effect relationship in psychotherapy. *American Psychologist*, **41**, 159–64.

Hume, D. (1748). *An Enquiry Concerning Human Understanding and Concerning the Principles of Morals*. Oxford: Oxford University Press.

Hunter, R. & Macalpine, I. (1982). *Three Hundred Years of Psychiatry, 1535–1860*. New York: Carlisle Publications.

Ikeda, M., Mori, E., Hirono, N., et al. (1998). Amnestic people with Alzheimer's disease who remembered the Kobe earthquake [see comments]. *British Journal of Psychiatry*, **172**, 425–8.

Inskipp, F. (1986). *Counselling: The Trainer's Handbook*. Cambridge: National Extension College.

Isherwood, C. (2000). *Lost Years: A Memoir 1945–51*. London: Chatto and Windus.

Jaffe, A.J., Rounsaville, B., Chang, G., et al. (1996). Naltrexone, relapse prevention, and supportive therapy with alcoholics: an analysis of patient treatment matching. *Journal of Consulting and Clinical Psychology*, **64** (5), 1044–53.

Janoff-Bulman, R. (1992). *Shattered Assumptions: Towards a New Psychology of Trauma*: New York: The Free Press, 256 pp.

Jaspers, K. (1951). *The Way to Wisdom*, New Haven: Yale University Press.

Jung, C. (1968). *Collected Works*. London: Routledge.

Kagan, J. (1982). The emergence of self. *Journal of Child Psychology and Psychiatry*, **23**, 363–81.

Kagan, J. (1994). *Galen's Prophecy*. London: Free Association Books.

Kaufman, G. (1996). *The Psychology of Shame: Theory and Treatment of Shame-based Syndromes*, 2nd edn. New York: Springer Publishing.

Kelly, G. (1953). *A Theory of Personality*, 1963 edn. New York: W.W. Norton.

Kelly, T.A. & Strupp, H.H. (1992). Patient and therapist values in psychotherapy: perceived changes, assimilation, similarity, and outcome. *Journal of Consulting and Clinical Psychology*, **60** (1), 34–40.

Kernberg, O.F. (1984). *Severe Personality Disorders*. New Haven: Yale University Press.

Kierkegaard, S. (1960 (1844)). *The Concept of Anxiety*, transl. Thomte. Princeton, NJ: Princeton University Press.

Kierkegaard, S. (1967). *Journals and Papers*. Bloomington, IN: Indiana University Press.

Klein, M. (1946). Notes on some schizoid mechanisms. In *Developments in Psycho-Analysis*, ed. M.H. Klein, P. Heimann, S. Isaacs, J. Riviere, pp. 292–320. London: Hogarth Press.

Klein, M. (1948). On the theory of anxiety and guilt. *International Journal of Psycho-Analysis*, **29**, 25–42.

Klerman, G., Weissman, M., Rounsaville, B., et al. (1984). *Interpersonal Psychotherapy of Depression*. New York: Basic Books.

Kohut, H. & Wolf, E. (1978). The disorders of self and their treatment: an outline. *International Journal of Psycho-Analysis*, **59**, 413–25.

Kolk, B.v.d., Pelcovitz, D., Roth, S., et al. (1996). Dissociation, somatization, and affect dysregulation: the complexity of adaptation of trauma. *American Journal of Psychiatry*, **153** (7), 83–93.

Kopp, M., Litavszky, Z. & Temesvari, A. (1997). The role of dissociation between cardiorespiratory and metabolic responses in angina-like chest pain panic patients. *Behavioural and Cognitive Psychotherapy*, **24**, 215–46.

Kopta, S.M., Howard, K.I., Lowry, J.L., et al. (1994). Patterns of symptomatic recovery in psychotherapy. *Journal of Consulting and Clinical Psychology*, **62**, 1009–16.

Kowalski, R. (1993). *Discovering Yourself. Breaking Walls Building Bridges.* London: Routledge.

Kwee, M.G.T. & Ellis, A. (1997). Can multimodal and rational emotive behavior therapy be reconciled? *Journal of Rational, Emotive and Cognitive Behavior Therapy*, **15**, 95–132.

Lacan, J. (1977). *The Four Fundamental Concepts of Psychoanalysis.* London: Hogarth Press.

Laing, R.D. (1960). *The Divided Self.* London: Tavistock Publications.

Laing, R.D. & Esterson, A. (1964). *Sanity, Madness, and the Family: I. Families of Schizophrenics.* London: Tavistock Press.

Langs, R. (1992). *A Clinical Workbook for Psychotherapists.* London: Karnac Books.

Laplanche, J. & Pontalis, J.-B. (1973). *The Language of Psycho-Analysis.* London: Hogarth Press.

Last, C.G., Thase, M.E., Hersen, M., et al. (1985). Patterns of attrition for psychosocial and pharmacologic treatments of depression. *Journal of Clinical Psychiatry*, **46** (9), 361–6.

Lazare, A., Eisenthal, S. & Wasserman, L. (1975). The customer approach to patienthood: attending to patient requests in a walk-in clinic. *Archives of General Psychiatry*, **32**, 553–8.

Le Guin, U. (1976). *The Wind's Twelve Quarters.* p. 258. Toronto: Bantam Books.

Le Guin, U. (1992). *The Earthsea Quartet.* London: Puffin Books.

Lerner, A., Sigal, M., Bacalu, A., et al. (1992). Short term versus long term psychotherapy in opioid dependence: a pilot study. *Israel Journal of Psychiatry and Related Sciences*, **29** (2), 114–19.

Leshner, A.I. (1999). Science is revolutionizing our view of addiction – and what to do about it. (editorial) *American Journal of Psychiatry*, **156** (1), 1–3.

Leslie, A. (1987). Pretense and representation: the origins of 'theory of mind'. *Psychological Review*, **94**, 412–26.

Levi-Strauss, C. (1983 (1963)). *Structural Anthropology*, transl. M. Layton. Chicago: University of Chicago Press.

Lewis, H.B. (1975). *Shame and Guilt in Neurosis.* Madison, CT: International Universities Press.

Lifton, R. (1989). *Thought Reform and the Psychology of Totalism. A Study of 'Brainwashing' in China.* Chapel Hill, NC: University of North Carolina Press.

Loftus, E. (1997). Creating false memories. *Scientific American*, **277** (3), 70–5.

Lorenz, K. (1966). *On Aggression.* New York: Harcourt, Brace, Jovanovich.

Loudon, I. (1984). The diseases called chlorosis. *Psychological Medicine*, **14** (1), 27–36.

Luborsky, L. (1984). *Principles of Psychoanalytic Psychotherapy. A Manual for Supportive-Expressive Treatment.* New York: Basic Books.

Luborsky, L. & Crits-Christoph, P. (1998). *Understanding Transference: The Core Conflictual Relationship Theme Method*, 2nd edn. Washington, DC: American Psychological Association.

Maas, L.C., Lukas, S.E., Kaufman, M.J., et al. (1998). Functional magnetic resonance imaging of human brain activation during cue-induced cocaine craving. *American Journal of Psychiatry*, **155** (1), 124–6.

Macalpine, I. (1950). The development of the transference. *Psychoanalytic Quarterly*, **19**, 4.

Macdonald, J. (1999). The experience of shame and the emotional isolation of psychotherapy patients. PhD, University of Warwick.

Macdonald, J. & Morley, I. (2001). Shame and non-disclosure: a study of the emotional isolation of people referred for psychotherapy. *British Journal of Medical Psychology*, **74**, 1–22.

Mace, C. (1995). When are questionnaires helpful? In *The Art and Science of Assessment in Psychotherapy*, ed. C. Mace, pp. 203–15. London: Routledge.

Main, T.F. (1957). The ailment. *British Journal of Medical Psychology*, **30**, 129–45.

Main, M. (1996). Introduction to the special section on attachment and psychopathology: 2. Overview of the field of attachment [review] [50 refs]. *Journal of Consulting and Clinical Psychology*, **64** (2), 237–43.

Malan, D. (1979). *Individual Psychotherapy and the Science of Psychodynamics*. Oxford: Butterworth-Heinemann.

Mansell, W. (2000). Conscious appraisal and the modification of automatic processes in anxiety. *Behavioural and Cognitive Psychotherapy*, **28**, 99–120.

Marinoff, L. & Kapklein, C. (1999). *Plato, not Prozac*. New York: Harper Collins.

Marvel, M.K., Doherty, W.J. & Weiner, E. (1998). Medical interviewing by exemplary family physicians. *Journal of Family Practice*, **47** (5), 343–8.

Masson, J.M. (1984). *The Assault on Truth: Freud's Suppression of the Seduction Theory*. New York: Knopf.

McCallum, M. & Piper, W.E. (1990). A controlled study of effectiveness and patient suitability for short-term group psychotherapy. *International Journal of Group Psychotherapy*, **40**, 431–52.

McCubbin, J.A., Wilson, J.F., Bruehl, S., et al. (1996). Relaxation training and opioid inhibition of blood pressure response to stress. *Journal of Consulting and Clinical Psychology*, **64**, 593–601.

McLellan, A.T., Alterman, A.I., Metzger, D.S., et al. (1994). Similarity of outcome predictors across opiate, cocaine, and alcohol treatments: role of treatment services. *Journal of Consulting and Clinical Psychology*, **62**, 1141–58.

Mele, A. (1997). Real self-deception. *Behavioral and Brain Sciences*, **20**, 91–136.

Menninger, K. (1958). *Theory of psychoanalytic technique*. New York: Basic Books.

Messer, S.B. & Meinster, M.O. (1980). Interaction effects of internal vs. external locus of control and directive vs. nondirective therapy: fact or fiction? *Journal of Clinical Psychology*, **36**, 283–8.

Messner, S., Tishby, O. & Spillman, A. (1992). Taking context seriously in psychotherapy research: relating therapist interventions to patient progress in brief psychodynamic psychotherapy. *Journal of Consulting and Clinical Psychology*, **60**, 678–88.

Midgeley, M. (1979). *Beast and Man: The Roots of Human Nature*. London: Methuen.

Miller, W. (1983). Motivational interviewing with problem drinkers. *Behavioural Psychotherapy*, **11**, 147–62.

Miller, W. (1994). Motivational interviewing III. The ethics of motivational interviewing. *Behavioural and Cognitive Psychotherapy*, **22**, 111–24.

Molière (1670). *Le Bourgeois Gentilhomme.* New York: French and European Publications.

Molnos, A. (1998). A psychotherapist's harvest. A to Z of clinical practice and theoretical issues with special reference to brief forms of psychoanalytically based treatment. http://fox.klte.hu/~keresofi/psychotherapy/index.shtml.

Muller, J. (1996). *Beyond the Psychoanalytic Dyad. Developmental Semiotics in Freud, Peirce and Lacan.* New York and London: Routledge.

Musil, R. (1980). *The Man Without Qualities.* New York: Perigee Books.

Mynors-Wallis, L., Davies, I., Gray, A., et al. (1997). A randomised controlled trial and cost analysis of problem-solving treatment for emotional disorders given by community nurses in primary care. *British Journal of Psychiatry*, **170**, 113–19.

Neki, J. (1976). An examination of the cultural relativism of dependence as a dynamic of social and therapeutic relationships. II Therapeutic. *British Journal of Medical Psychology*, **49**, 11–22.

Newman, M.G., Consoli, A.J. & Taylor, C.B. (1999). A palmtop computer program for the treatment of generalized anxiety disorder. *Behavior Modification*, **23** (4), 597–619.

Nietzsche, F. (1977). *A Nietzsche Reader*, selected and translated by R.J. Hollingdale. Harmondsworth, Middlesex: Penguin.

Nisbett, R.E. & Ross, L. (1980). *Human Inference: Strategies and Shortcomings of Social Judgment.* Englewood-Cliffs: Prentice-Hall.

North, A., Hargreaves, D. & McKendrick, J. (1997). In-store music affects product choice. *Nature*, **390**, **132**.

Novalis, P., Rojcewicz, S. & Peele, R. (1993). *Clinical Manual of Supportive Psychotherapy.* Washington, DC: American Psychiatric Press.

Oatley, K. (1990). Freud's cognitive psychology of intention: the case of Dora. *Mind and Language*, **5**, 69–86.

Oatley, K. (1992). *Best Laid Schemes. The Psychology of Emotions.* Cambridge: Cambridge University Press.

Oatley, K., Jenkins, J. & Stein, N. (eds). (1998). *Human Emotions: A Reader.* Oxford: Blackwell.

O'Connor, L.E. & Weiss, J. (1993). Individual psychotherapy for addicted clients: an application of control mastery theory. (review) *Journal of Psychoactive Drugs*, **25** (4), 283–91.

Orwell, G. (1991a). *A Collection of Essays.* New York: Harcourt Brace.

Orwell, G. (1991b (1946)). Politics and the English language. In *Collection of Essays.* New York: Harcourt Brace.

Panksepp, J. (1999). The periconscious substrates of consciousness: affective states and the evolutionary origins of the self. In *Models of the Self*, ed. S. Gallagher, J. Shear, pp. 113–30. Thorverton, England: Imprint Academic.

Panksepp, J., Knutson, B. & Pruitt, D.L. (1998). Toward a neuroscience of emotion: the epigenetic foundations of emotional development. In *Models of the Self*, ed. S. Gallagher, J. Shear. Thorverton, England: Imprint Academic.

Parsons, T., Bales, R.F. & Shils, E. (1951). *Working Papers in the Theory of Action.* Cambridge, MA: Harvard University Press.

Pearson, J.L., Cowan, P.A., Cowan, C.P., et al. (1993). Adult attachment and adult child – older parent relationships. *American Journal of Orthopsychiatry*, **63** (4), 606–13.

Pekarik, G. (1994). Effects of brief therapy training on practicing psychotherapists and their clients. *Community Mental Health Journal*, **30** (2), 135–44.

Pelc, I., Verbanck, P., Le Bon, O., et al. (1997). Efficacy and safety of acamprosate in the treatment of detoxified alcohol-dependent patients. A 90-day placebo-controlled dose-finding study. *British Journal of Psychiatry*, **171**, 73–7.

Perczel-Forintos, D. & Hackmann, A. (1999). Transformation of meaning and its effects on cognitive behavioural treatment of an injection phobia. *Behavioural and Cognitive Psychotherapy*, **27**, 369–76.

Peterson, C. & Biggs, M. (1998). Stitches and casts: emotionality and narrative coherence. *Narrative Inquiry*, **8**, 51–76.

Piper, W.E., Azim, H.F., McCallum, M., et al. (1990). Patient suitability and outcome in short-term individual psychotherapy. *Journal of Consulting and Clinical Psychology*, **58**, 475–81.

Piper, W.E., Azim, H.F.A., Joyce, A.S., et al. (1991). Transference interpretations, therapeutic alliance, and outcome in short-term individual psychotherapy. *Archives of General Psychiatry*, **48**, 946–53.

Popper, K. (1963). *Conjectures and Refutations.* London: Routledge, and Kegan Paul.

Price, D.M. (1999). Relapse prevention and risk reduction: results of client identification of high risk situations. *Sexual Addiction and Compulsivity*, **6** (3), 221–52.

Prochaska, J. & DiClimente, C. (1982). Transtheoretical therapy: towards a more integrative model of change. *Psychotherapy: Theory, Research, and Practice*, **19**, 276–88.

Prochaska, J.O. & Velicer, W.F. (1997). The transtheoretical model of health behavior change. *American Journal of Health Promotion*, **12** (1), 38–48.

Project MATCH, research, et al. (1998). Matching patients with alcohol disorders to treatments: clinical implications from Project MATCH. *Journal of Mental Health*, **7**, 589–602.

Propp, V. (1968 (1927)). *Morphology of the Folktale*, transl. Laurence Scott, revised, 2nd edn. Austin: University of Texas Press.

Putnam, D.E. & Maheu, M.M. (2000). Online sexual addiction and compulsivity: Integrating web resources and behavioral telehealth in treatment. *Sexual Addiction and Compulsivity*, **7** (1–2), 91–112.

Rawls, J. (1971). *A Theory of Justice.* Cambridge, MA: Harvard University Press.

Reis, H.R. & Franks, P. (1994). The role of intimacy and social support in health outcomes: two processes or one? *Personal Relationships*, **1**, 185–97.

Ricks, C. (1976). *Keats and Embarrassment.* Oxford: Oxford University Press.

Rodgers, R.J. & Cole, J.C. (1993). Influence of social isolation, gender, strain, and prior novelty on plus-maze behaviour in mice. *Physiology and Behavior*, **54** (4), 729–36.

Rogers, C. (1974). In retrospect: forty-six years. *American Psychologist*, **2**, 115–23.

Rogers, A. & Pilgrim, D. (1997). The contribution of lay knowledge to the understanding and promotion of health. *Journal of Mental Health*, **6**, 23–35.

Rollnick, S. & Miller, W. (1995). What is motivational interviewing? *Behavioural and Cognitive Psychotherapy*, **23**, 325–34.

Ross, C.A. (1989). *Multiple Personality Disorder*. New York: Wiley.

Roth, A. & Fonagy, P. (1996). What works for whom? A critical review of psycho-therapy research. New York: Guilford Press.

Ruesch, J. & Bateson, G. (1951). *Communication: The Social Matrix of Psychiatry*. New York: W.W. Norton.

Rutter, M. (1980). The long-term effects of early experience. *Developmental Medicine and Child Neurology*, **22**, 800–15.

Sartre, J.P. (1971). *Sketch for a Theory of the Emotion*. London: Methuen.

Schafer, R. (1976). *A New Language for Psycho-Analysis*. New Haven, CT: Yale University Press.

Scheff, T. (1990). *Microsociology: Discourse, Emotion, and Social Structure*. Chicago: University of Chicago Press.

Scheff, T.J. (1994). *Bloody Revenge: Emotions, Nationalism, and War*, pp. CO, US-162. Boulder, CO: Westview Press.

Scheff, T. (1997). *Emotions, The Social Bond, and Human Reality*. Cambridge: Cambridge University Press.

Searle, J. (1983). *Intentionality*. Cambridge: Cambridge University Press.

Shalev, A.Y., Peri, T., Canetti, L., et al. (1996). Predictors of PTSD in injured trauma survivors: a prospective study. In *American Journal of Psychiatry*, **153**, 219–25.

Shapiro, D.A. (1981). Comparative credibility of treatment rationales: three tests of expectancy theory. *British Journal of Clinical Psychology*, **20**, 111–22.

Sharon, N. & Schwartzman, O. (1998). Professional and traditional collaboration in the mediation of family conflicts: the case of Ethiopian immigrants in Israel. *Mediation Quarterly*, **16**, 3–13.

Shiffman, S., Paty, J.A., Gnys, M., et al. (1996). First lapses to smoking: within-subjects analysis of real-time reports. *Journal of Consulting and Clinical Psychology*, **64** (2), 366–79.

Shoham-Salomon, V., Avner, R. & Neeman, R. (1989). You're changed if you do and changed if you don't: mechanisms underlying paradoxical interventions. *Journal of Consulting and Clinical Psychology*, **57**, 590–8.

Skevington, S.M., Mac Arthur, P. & Somerset, M. (1997). Developing items for the WHOQOL: an investigation of contemporary beliefs about quality of life related to health in Britain. *British Journal of Health Psychology*, **2** (1), 55–72.

Sluzki, C.E. (1992). Transformations: a blueprint for narrative changes in therapy. *Family Process*, **31** (3), 217–30.

Smoller, J.W., McLean, R.Y., Otto, M.W., et al. (1998). How do clinicians respond to patients who miss appointments? **59** (6), 330–40.

Smyth, J.M. (1998). Written emotional expression: effect sizes, outcome types, and moderating variables. *Journal of Consulting and Clinical Psychology*, **66** (1), 174–84.

Sophocles (1982). *The Theban Plays*, transl. R. Fagles with introductions and annotations by B. Knox. London: Allen Lane.

Speck, R. & Attneave, C. (1973). *Family Networks*. New York: Pantheon.

Spenceley, A. & Jerrom, B. (1997). Intrusive traumatic childhood memories in depression: a comparison between depressed, recovered and never depressed women. *Behavioural and Cognitive Psychotherapy*, **25**, 309–18.

Spinhoven, P., Vanderlinden, J., ter Kuile, M.M., et al. (1993). Assessment of hypnotic processes and responsiveness in a clinical context. *International Journal of Clinical and Experimental Hypnosis*, **41** (3), 210–24.

Stiles, W. (1999). Signs and voices in psychotherapy. *Psychotherapy Research*, **9**, 1–21.

Stiles, W., Shapiro, D. & Elliott, R. (1986). Are all psychotherapies equivalent? *American Psychologist*, **41**, 165–80.

Stiles, W., Morrison, L., Haw, S., et al. (1991). Longitudinal study of assimilation in exploratory psychotherapy. *Psychotherapy*, **28**, 196–206.

Stoller, R. (1970). Pornography and perversity. *Archives of General Psychiatry*, **22**, 490–99.

Strupp, H. & Binder, J. (1984). *Psychotherapy in a New Key*. New York: Basic Books.

Sullivan, H.S. (1953). *The Interpersonal Theory of Psychiatry*. New York: W.W. Norton.

Szapocznik, J., Kurtines, W., Santisteban, D.A., et al. (1990). Interplay of advances between theory, research, and application in treatment interventions aimed at behavior problem children and adolescents. *Journal of Consulting and Clinical Psychology*, **58** (6), 696–703.

Szasz, T.S. (1960). *The Myth of Mental Illness*.

Szasz, T. (1988). *The Ethics of Psychoanalysis*. New York: Syracuse University Press.

Szmukler, G. & Tantam, D. (1984). Anorexia nervosa: starvation dependence. *British Journal of Medical Psychology*, **57**, 300–310.

Talbot, N.L. (1995). Unearthing shame in the supervisory experience. *American Journal of Psychotherapy*, **49** (3), 338–49.

Tallis, F. & Eysenck, M. (1994). Worry: mechanisms and modulating influences. *Behavioural and Cognitive Psychotherapy*, **22**, 37–56.

Tangney, J.P., Burggraf, S.A. & Wagner, P.E. (1995). Shame-proneness, guilt-proneness, and psychological symptoms. In *Self-Conscious Emotions: The Psychology of Shame, Guilt, Embarrassment, and Pride*, ed. J.P. Tangney, pp. 343–67. New York; NY: Guilford Press.

Tangney, J.P., Miller, R.S., Flicker, L., et al. (1996). Are shame, guilt, and embarrassment distinct emotions? US: American Psychological Association.

Tantam, D. (1984). A prophet in the group. *Group Analysis*, **18**, 44–55.

Tantam, D. (1986). Towards a grammar of nonverbal communication. *Semiotica*, **58**, 41–7.

Tantam, D. (1988). Personality disorders. In *Recent Advances in Clinical Psychiatry*, ed. K. Granville-Grossman, pp. 111–34. London: Churchill Livingstone.

Tantam, D. (1991). Shame and groups. *Group Analysis*, **23**, 31–44.

Tantam, D. (1993). Exorcism in Zanzibar: an insight into groups from another culture. *Group Analysis*, **26**, 251–60.

Tantam, D. (1995a). Empathy, persistent aggression, and antisocial personality disorder. *Journal of Forensic Psychiatry*, **6**, 10–18.

Tantam, D. (1995b). Why select? In *The Art and Science of Psychotherapy Assessment*, ed. C. Mace, pp. 1–30. London: Routledge.

Tantam, D. (1995c). Case reports and confidentiality: psychotherapy. *British Journal of Psychiatry*, **166**, 555–8.

Tantam, D. (1996a). Fairbairn. In *150 Years of British Psychiatry*, ed. G. Berrios, H. Freeman, Vol. 2. London: Athlone Press.

Tantam, D. (1996b). Psychotherapy and traditional healing. In *Psychiatry for the Developing World*, ed. D. Tantam, A. Duncan, L. Appleby, pp. 57–72. London: Gaskell Press.

Tantam, D. (ed.) (1998). *Clinical Topics in Psychotherapy*. London: Gaskell Press.

Tantam, D. (1999a). Meaning, cause and interpretation. In *Heart and Soul*, ed. C. Mace. London: Routledge.

Tantam, D. (1999b). One reason for you, and one for me. The case for new evidential criteria for psychotherapy being needed and what those might be. In *Evidence in the Balance*, ed. C. Mace. London: Routledge.

Tantam, D. & Klerman, G. (1979). Patient transfer from one clinician to another and dropping-out of out-patient treatment. *Social Psychiatry*, **14**, 107–13.

Taylor, M. (1999). *Informal conflict resolution: A workplace case study*. http://mediate.com/articles/taylor.cfm.

Teusch, L. & Bohme, H. (1999). Is the exposure principle really crucial in agoraphoia? The influence of client-centered 'nonprescriptive' treatment of agoraphobia. *Psychotherapy Research*, **9**, 115–23.

Tolstoy, L. (1981 (1886)). *The death of Ivan Ilyich*, transl. L. Solatoroff. Toronto: Bantam Books.

Toneatto, T. (1999). A metacognitive analysis of craving: implications for treatment. *Journal of Clinical Psychology*, **55**, 527–37.

Trigg, R. (1988). *Ideas of Human Nature*. Oxford: Blackwell.

Trigg, R. (1999). *Ideas of Human Nature*, 2nd edn. Oxford: Blackwell.

Troop, N.A. & Treasure, J.L. (1997). Setting the scene for eating disorders, II. Childhood helplessness and mastery. *Psychological Medicine*, **27** (3), 531–8.

Tzschentke, T. (1998). Measuring reward with the conditioned place preference paradigm: a comprehensive review of drug effects. *Progress in Neurobiology*, **56**, 613–72.

Volkow, N.D., Wang, G.J., Fowler, J.S., et al. (1999). Association of methylphenidate-induced craving with changes in right striato-orbitofrontal metabolism in cocaine abusers: implications in addiction. *American Journal of Psychiatry*, **156** (1), 19–26.

von Bertalanffy, L. (1974). The unified theory for psychiatry and the behavioral sciences. *Adolescent Psychiatry*, **3**, 43–8.

von Deurzen, E. (1979). *Existential Counselling in Practice*. London: Routledge.

von Deurzen, E. (1997). *Everyday Mysteries. Existential Dimensions of Psychotherapy*. London: Routledge.

von Deurzen, E. (1998). *Passion and Paradox in Psychotherapy and Counselling*. Chichester: Wiley.

Waller, G. & Smith, R. (1994). Sexual abuse and psychological disorders: the role of cognitive processes. *Behavioural and Cognitive Psychotherapy*, **22**, 29–34.

Weine, S.M., Kulenovic, A.D., Pavkovic, I., et al. (1998a). Testimony psychotherapy in Bosnian refugees: a pilot study. *American Journal of Psychiatry*, **155** (12), 1720–6.

Weine, S.M., Vojvoda, D., Becker, D.F., et al. (1998b). PTSD symptoms in Bosnian refugees 1 year after resettlement in the United States. *American Journal of Psychiatry*, **155** (4), 562–4.

Whitaker, D.S. (1985). *Using Groups to Help People*. London: Routledge and Kegan Paul.

Whitaker, D.S. & Lieberman, M.A. (1964). Assessing interpersonal behavior in group therapy. *Perceptual and Motor Skills*, **18**, 763–4.

Williams, B. (1972). *Morality*. Cambridge: Cambridge University Press.

Winkel, F. & Koppelaar, L. (1991). Rape victims' style of self-presentation and secondary victimization by the environment: an experiment. *Journal of Interpersonal Violence*, **6**, 29–40.

Winnicott, D. (1949). Hate in the counter-transference. *International Journal of Psycho-Analysis*, **30**, 69–74.

Winnicott, D.W. (1965). *The Maturational Processes and the Facilitating Environment: Studies in the Theory of Emotional Development*. New York: International Universities Press.

Winnicott, D. (1988). *Human Nature*. London: Free Association Books.

Winship, G. (1999). Addiction, death, and the liver in mind: The Prometheus syndrome. *Psychoanalytic Psychotherapy*, **13** (1), 41–9.

Winston, A., Laikin, M., Pollack, J., et al. (1994). Short-term psychotherapy of personality disorders. *American Journal of Psychiatry*, **151** (2), 190–4.

Wittgenstein, L. (1958). *Philosophical Investigations*, transl. G.E. Anscombe, 2nd edn. Oxford: Blackwell.

Yalom, I.D. (1985). *The Theory and Practice of Group Psychotherapy*, 3rd edn. New York: Basic Books.

Index